FAT LOSS HAPPENS ON MONDAY

FAT LOSS HAPPENS ON MONDAY

JOSH HILLIS WITH **DAN JOHN**

FOREWORD BY
VALERIE WATERS

ON TARGET PUBLICATIONS
SANTA CRUZ, CALIFORNIA

FAT LOSS HAPPENS ON MONDAY

Josh Hillis
with Dan John

Foreword by Valerie Waters

Copyright © 2015 Josh Hillis
Introduction and Chapters 2, 3, 5, 11, 12 & 16 © 2015 Daniel Arthur John

Exercise photographer: Adam Emperor Southard
Exercise model: Katie Dawers
Author cover photo: Justin Grant

ISBN-13: 978-1-931046-54-1

All rights reserved. Printed in the United States of America using recycled paper. No part of this book may be reproduced or transmitted in any form whatsoever without written permission from the author or publisher, with the exception of the inclusions of brief quotations in articles or reviews.

On Target Publications
P O Box 1335
Aptos, California 95001 USA
otpbooks.com

Library of Congress Cataloging-in-Publication Data

Hillis, Josh, 1977– author.
  Fat loss happens on Monday / Josh Hillis with Dan John.
    pages cm
  ISBN 978-1-931046-54-1 (pbk.)
  1. Reducing diets--Recipes. 2. Weight loss. 3. Reducing exercises. I. John, Dan, 1957– author. II. Title.
  RM222.2.H485 2014
  613.2'5--dc23

2013046438

CONTENTS

FOREWORD IX

INTRODUCTION XIII

CHAPTER 1: FAT LOSS IS EASIER AND SIMPLER THAN
YOU'VE BEEN TOLD 1

CHAPTER 2: PARK-BENCH WORKOUTS 3

CHAPTER 3: EPISTEMOLOGY: TO THE EVIDENCE,
NO MATTER WHERE IT LEADS 7

ONE CHANGE   15

CHAPTER 4: THE HARD TALK 17

CHAPTER 5: REASONABLENESS 21

CHAPTER 6: THE DAY I BECAME THE BEST FAT-LOSS
TRAINER IN THE WORLD 25

CHAPTER 7: THE ELEVEN HABITS 31

CHAPTER 8: MAKING IT WORK 51

CHAPTER 9: ADVANCED FOOD PROGRAMS 71

CHAPTER 10: HOW TO GAUGE PROGRESS 77

CHAPTER 11: SETTING THE MIND TO THE GOAL 87

CHAPTER 12: A SIMPLE WAY TO LOOK AT THE PROBLEMS WITH THE FITNESS INDUSTRY 93

CHAPTER 13: ONE CHANGE REVIEW 99

PULL YOUR WEIGHT   101

CHAPTER 14: SEASONS OF TRAINING 103

CHAPTER 15: THE EIGHT MOVEMENTS 105

CHAPTER 16: GET OFF MY BACK 109

CHAPTER 17: YOU GOTTA GET REAL 111

CHAPTER 18: THE BASIC BASICS 113

CHAPTER 19: HOW TO MAKE A FAT-LOSS PROGRAM THAT WORKS LONG TERM 115

CHAPTER 20: HOW THE MOVEMENT PROGRESSIONS WORK 121

CHAPTER 21: METABOLIC PHASE WORKOUTS 131

CHAPTER 22: ENDURANCE PHASE WORKOUTS 139

CHAPTER 23: STRENGTH PHASE WORKOUTS 149

CHAPTER 24: THE METABOLIC/ENDURANCE/STRENGTH PHASE . . 157

CHAPTER 25: ANSWERING THE NAGGING QUESTIONS 185

BRING IT!   199

CHAPTER 26: THE *BRING IT!* PROGRAM 201

CHAPTER 27: *BRING IT! REMIX* 219

EXERCISE INSTRUCTIONS   233

CHAPTER 28: THE EXERCISE INSTRUCTIONS 235

CHAPTER 29: SHOPPING PLAN 311

CHAPTER 30: THE ONLY GAME WORTH PLAYING 315

INDEX 316

FOREWORD

IT'S ABOUT BECOMING THE KIND OF PERSON YOU SAY YOU WANT TO BE

Imagine two scenarios.

First, imagine you didn't plan and prepare—

You come home at six o'clock at night. The kids are crying, the dog needs to be fed; you're tired and cranky because you didn't plan your snack, so you ate some candy and drank a diet soda from the vending machine at four o'clock in the afternoon.

Now your blood sugar is crashing. You open the refrigerator, but you didn't go to the market on Sunday and pre-prepare anything—so what do you?

You're trying to decide on the fly—you've got to get dinner on the table for the family; you've got to get the dog fed. You're calling for food delivery. In the meantime, you're stuffing a tortilla in your mouth—not because you love tortillas, but because your blood sugar is crashing and you're desperate to get it back up.

Second, imagine you did prepare—

Imagine you open the fridge. You're hungry and you know it's going to take you 30 minutes to prepare dinner, but there's something you can nibble on that's not going to derail your plan.

You slice up a cucumber and have a little guacamole as you're preparing to put the chicken in the oven. And you can put the chicken in the oven because the chicken is there to be put in the oven.

You shopped the day before. You already marinated the chicken and all you have to do is take it out of the refrigerator and let it rest on the counter for a minute while you chop up the veggies, which have already been washed.

You turn on the oven, and you're eating your cucumber with guacamole while you're happily just catching up with your husband or while the dog sits next to you as you listen to music or chill in silence. Then you pop the chicken in the oven. Maybe you steam some broccoli or cauliflower and maybe make some rice if it's on the plan that day, and then in 30 minutes it all comes together and you feel great.

STRATEGY TRUMPS WILLPOWER

You feel great, and it's because strategy trumps willpower. You know it's not about white knuckling, "Don't eat the tortilla! Don't eat the tortilla! Don't eat the tortilla!"

People are always unsuccessful when they wing it. So instead, you set yourself up to not be so ravenous that you stuff the tortilla in your mouth while you're standing in front of the refrigerator. You prepare so you have other options available.

It's not about deprivation. Mostly you wouldn't really have felt more excited to have the pizza delivery. Not only would the pizza delivery have derailed your fat-loss plan; it wouldn't even have made you happy.

The pizza might have gotten there fast, but it's not something you would have enjoyed more than your simply prepared chicken. And now you feel good about yourself because you've done something you're committed to—staying on your plan. You feel proud of yourself…you were able to get dinner in the oven and have it come out and taste good.

And it doesn't need to be fancy cheffy food. It just needs to be a home-cooked meal. There's something so pleasurable about being able to feed yourself and your loved ones that's so much greater than eating the most delicious fast food. There's something more—you're happier with this food.

And it all comes down to planning and preparation and habits. You don't get that happiness if you didn't go to the market when you planned.

Everyone is busy. Whether you work full time or have kids or both, we're all overcommitted and we're all looking for ways to build a better quality of life through simplifying and taking better care of ourselves. And it really starts at the most basic essence—feeding oneself.

We need to feed ourselves in a way that's nourishing on every level.

- Nourishing in that we get the nutrients we need
- Nourishing in that we like it
- And nourishing in that it feeds our goals and who it is we said we want to be

Clients sometimes say, "I can't be perfect all of the time." But it's not about being perfect, and it's not about a fear-based lifestyle. You can have lots of foods to choose from. It really comes down to having quality food on hand, and then choosing not to eat crap.

RULES AND HABITS ARE FREEDOM

I think of a diet as a series of rules. Josh calls them habits, but it's the same thing. If you have a series of rules or habits in place, the diet never ends. A vegetarian will never have to decide whether to order hamburger or steak. It doesn't come up; a vegetarian won't even look at that part of the menu.

When I go to a restaurant, I don't even look at the pasta and the macaroni and cheeses and the pizzas. It's not like it's me fighting myself and working so hard to not eat it; it's just that I have a rule that says I do better when I don't eat white-flour products.

When we have rules or habits in place, it takes away a struggle. The rules are the freedom.

And essentially, your diet, your plan means having some basic rules or habits in place. The rules are not to make you feel deprived in some way. It's exactly the opposite—these are your ticket to freedom. Once those habits are in place, everything else disappears. You don't ever have to struggle about food again.

We all have our own rules—I don't tell a lie; I don't steal. This is how society operates—rules make everything work. It's not bad to have those rules. We don't think, "Oh my God, I hate that we have to stop at stop signs. I just want to roll through the stop signs." I'm happy we have a rule to stop at stop signs so I know what everyone else is doing. It's the rules that make driving on our busy roads even possible.

We use rules like food prep on Sunday, wash and clean the vegetables as soon as you get home, always have water with you, make the diet the priority. Working out is very important also, but fat loss is determined by what you eat, which is really what *Fat Loss Happens on Monday* is all about.

This lifestyle gets easier as you abide by your rules or habits. And these habits make it easier to become the person you say you want to become. Every habit you have either moves you closer to or farther from becoming that person.

JOSH AND *FAT LOSS HAPPENS ON MONDAY*

Josh and I met in person for the first time at a gathering of fitness professionals in Florida. That night at dinner was like we had known each other forever—Josh just plopped down and we started talking. His enthusiasm and passion for fitness was so clear and we connected immediately.

FOREWORD

Josh really gets that everyone has the same struggles, because food and diet and exercise and bodies and self-esteem—it's all messy stuff. And that's where he and I really connect, that we want to help people. We want to give people freedom from some of these struggles.

It's the clarity of Josh's writing and Josh's deep desire to help people that made me want to be involved in this project. How much he cares comes through in all of his writing.

Josh is awesome, and I love the way he writes. The reason his ideas make a difference for people is because his plan is clear, and it's not fancy wizardry. Josh meets people where they are, and leads them by the hand—"Let's put one foot in front of the other and walk forward, and it's okay to freak out, and we're going to keep going."

Fat Loss Happens on Monday is a book that's going to lovingly hold your feet to the fire. You're asking for results, and you're going to get a realistic and manageable plan, wrapped up in eleven food habits to help you toward your goal. You'll also get great workouts, but the magic of *Fat Loss Happens on Monday* is putting the nutrition habits first. Monday is just a metaphor for first—before you get into your workouts, you'll have already done your food planning, shopping, and preparation.

The path is very clear. And it lets you know you can do it, and here's how. It's caring and it's hopeful. I really believe if you follow the *Fat Loss Happens on Monday* program and implement the habits, you'll get results and you can be your own superstar.

Valerie Waters
Creator of the ValSlide & Red Carpet Ready

DAN

INTRODUCTION

One of the turning points of my life and my career as a coach was flying to Granville, Ohio, to join the John Powell Discus Camp at Denison University. I was at a standstill as a thrower and I decided, wisely, that I needed to return to the beginner's mind. The road to true mastery involves those moments where you empty the cup so there's a chance to refill it. I was 35, and I had a bed check every night by a counselor and a bang at the door when it was time to get up in the morning.

It was camp and I camped.

This still stands as one of the best decisions of my life. I was beaten down, melted, and reforged. Moreover, in the years since, my annual visit to Ohio has become a staple of my life, my family's lives, and a reunion of friends, family and people who should be family.

Not every camp or day at camp has been idyllic. In fact, one story stands out that so shaped the rest of my career and my vision of my impact on these few years on earth that I revisit it every time I think I'm finished with my life's work.

We share our camp cafeteria with a cheerleader group. Honestly, the bulk of them are perfectly fine, but that simple truth doesn't make a very good story. This story is no reflection of the excellent staff who have been nothing but kind and gracious to me and my friends and family.

I think I covered my bases here so far. Now…the rest of the story, as Paul Harvey used to say.

Basically, these are several hundred young girls in matching uniforms, matching hair and face glitter. The young ladies in our camp are throwers, certainly beautiful young women, but built on the large and powerful side. In the lunch line, one of the cheerleaders walked up to one of our girls and asked the high school female thrower—

"Are you guys like a fat camp?"

When I heard about this interaction, I was reminded why most people hate high school. The young woman who was asked if she belonged to a fat camp was an all-state volleyball player and received her education for free because of her athletic talents. Yet, she has self-esteem issues. She is tall, strong and muscular, but she doesn't fit into the mold of the 'miss teeny bikini' model of the glamour magazines.

Did she go to her prom? I don't know, but I would be proud to call her my daughter.

With perfect timing, a huge zit would have emerged on the cheerleader's nose. But that's not what happened. Rather, our young cheerleader with her perfect smile marched off to her perfect life.

I was reminded of my father's favorite curse, besides *Pardon my French, but are you a stoop?*—short for stupid. He would say to someone who was greedy, "I hope you get everything you want."

In my experience, getting everything you want is a quick ticket to unhappiness.

I also didn't know until years later that both of my daughters were standing next to these high school girls. Kelly and Lindsay spent time with me at Discus Camp in Ohio in a Daddy Day Care situation for up to three weeks a year. Lindsay commented on what turned out to be the final bit of irony—the cheerleader's plate was filled with all yellow food: mac and cheese, chicken or chicken-ish nuggets and French fries.

The throwers all had a protein serving with vegetables and a salad.

There's a genetic roulette. Some people are born fast and some are born tall. If you're over seven feet tall and grew up in the United States, you probably played basketball even if you wanted to be a basket maker. I can't teach you to make the Olympic final in the 100 meters, and I can't figure out how to get you over seven feet tall.

I also can't make you the cover girl of a fitness or fashion magazine. We can do wonders today with makeup and Photoshop, but we can only go so far. A five-foot-tall cheerleader with a wasp waist is going to look different than a six-foot volleyball girl.

That is all true and that is all good. And it only takes one statement to knock the pillars out from under this truth: *Are you guys like a fat camp?*

Raising daughters, working with female high school athletes and helping with a large number of women in various training situations has made me realize we need a better vision than we're usually offered when working with women.

That's why I like Josh's work so much. It's reasonable. And it's always gracious.

Gracious is probably not the word you expected. It means a lot of things, but what I see in Josh's work is this: kindness. It's reasonable, yes, but it's also kind. The workouts are doable. The goals are reasonable. The path is clear.

And all of this is done with kindness.

Maybe our cheerleader friend asked this in a spirit of kindness and caring and simply didn't understand decorum as well as she needed to. Perhaps, on the other extreme, she was a cruel, evil, awful person.

Frank Layden, the former Utah Jazz basketball coach, always used this wonderful line: "So, I asked my player if he was stupid or apathetic. He said, 'Coach, I don't know and I don't care.'"

I'm leaving the door open for multiple interpretations of the young lady's intent.

There are other stories, of course, and the readers can probably add dozens, if not hundreds, of other stories, too.

One woman told me she was 'so fat, her husband wouldn't touch her.'

A college girl at Utah State liked to stand near heavier girls in the locker room and lament about being so fat, even though she was quite lean. She told her friends, "I like to see how uncomfortable they get."

It's all true. There's nothing—and I can't repeat this enough—nothing concomitantly more public and more private than our relationships with our bodies. Our desire to lean out here and pump up there drives some of us to the edge of life, while others try anything reasonable or unreasonable. For some, money, energy and pain seem to have no boundaries.

We can do better.

We must do better.

Let's get started with a reasonable approach to fat loss. Let's start with a reasonable way of eating and training. Let's leave a legacy of dignity of the human person and respect for ourselves and others.

We can do this.

JOSH

CHAPTER 1

FAT LOSS IS EASIER AND SIMPLER THAN YOU'VE BEEN TOLD

The way you've been doing your fat-loss workouts and diet has been making it harder and more complicated to lose weight.

But it's not your fault.

Virtually everything you see and hear is setting you up to have a harder time losing fat.

The way we talk about fat loss makes it harder, the kinds of workouts we do are designed to make it harder, and the kinds of diets we're taught to think are cool and trendy are all really hard.

It keeps going this way: We do everything the hard way. And we just keep getting older, and we get more responsibilities. Things keep piling up, and losing stubborn fat and getting the body we want starts to almost seem impossible.

But it's *totally* possible. It's exactly the opposite of what you've been told.

The rules have changed. The big revolution in fat loss from 10 years ago saying we needed big movements, circuits, and interval training created its own set of problems.

Workout intensity is a power tool that's been unbelievably overused. We're going to show you exactly when, and exactly how often it should be used for optimum fat loss.

When you use a smart fat-loss system, you get to have the easiest and fastest fat loss possible. Smart, simple, repeatable fat loss requires a different program, and a different mindset—both of which you're going to discover in this book.

A PLAN FOR MAKING FAT LOSS EASY

Going hard all the time is a recipe for failure, for quitting, getting hurt, and losing motivation, or it can be just as simple as fat loss steadily getting harder.

We know we need to cycle all of this.

The trick is, what do you do during the easy workout phases to get results?

Too many easy workouts mean backsliding on your results, getting fatter, and having a harder time.

Fat Loss Happens on Monday is made up of medium and easy workouts that make fat loss doable in real life.

It sounds radical, but it's actually pretty simple if you know what to do.

At its most basic—

1. **We need to make really small changes in food so they stick long term.**
2. **We need a smart plan for getting stronger.**

Making small changes in food that stick long term comes before the workouts. The biggest reason you don't need to do killer workouts is that for fat-loss results, the workouts are secondary to the food intake.

But number two—most people aren't doing a workout that will provide results over the long term.

Most people are doing a workout that *feels* like it gets results. Really, when you leave the gym drenched in sweat and everything is exhausted and you're sore the next day… doesn't it just feel like that should get results?

Workouts that throttle you are sexy. The best-selling workout in the United States today is a DVD set that's five really hard, 60- to 90-minute workouts each week. It looks cool; it sounds cool. It makes people feel tough.

It's the same thing with in-person workout trends. It's all 'hardcore,' 'elite,' 'bootcamp.' Mostly it's running people around until they're totally throttled. It makes people feel like they're doing a hard workout. Like I said, it's sexy. People buy sexy.

But you know what's sexier than that? *Actually getting results.*

There's a great quote by Tony Blauer: "A really bad idea, embraced by millions of people, is still a really bad idea."

In other words, just because it's cool and trendy right now, doesn't mean it's a good idea.

The truth is going to shock you. The program we're using is radically different, and much easier than what you've been 'sold' it takes to get fat-loss results.

This program doesn't exist because I set out to make an easy workout program. This program exists because I set out to create a program that actually works in the real world.

The best-selling DVD set I was telling you about breaks down like this—

Every four weeks—
20 Hard Workouts

I'm not going to lie to you. If you can fit it into your schedule and do it, it works. It just won't work for very long. At best, you'll crash and burn in about two months.

Fat Loss Happens on Monday works like this—

Every four weeks—
Two Hard Workouts
Six Medium Workouts
Four Easy Workouts

We're talking 60% fewer total workouts. And 90% fewer hard workouts. That's a lot less hard work.

And you can get even better fat-loss results. All it takes is for you to make your food preparation the most important 'workout' of the week. Then your actual in-the-gym workouts just need to get you a little stronger over time, and they need to change at pre-planned, regular intervals.

DAN

CHAPTER 2

PARK-BENCH WORKOUTS

My former boss Archbishop George Niederauer has a wonderful way with words. He is the most well-read person I know, and he has this interesting way of simplifying the most complex things into bite-size pieces for the rest of us. He often speaks about two kinds of prayers, the kind where you ask for something and the kind where you just talk with God. A few years ago, he wrote an article about this concept and gave us a simple image to understand it.

In the Tale of Two Benches, Archbishop Niederauer describes sitting on a bus bench. When one waits for a bus, one is filled with expectations. The G bus should be here at 8:11. If I look up at 8:11 and don't see it, I begin to panic. At 8:13, my day is ruined. We want to get off this bench and get going somewhere else! The bus should be here now. Wait…now!

The park bench, however, is a time to sit and listen and watch. We wait for nothing. The local squirrels that showed up yesterday may or may not be here today. And that is okay. We don't call the city squirrel police if they don't show up when we want them to.

Both of the benches in our example might look exactly the same. You might find the same wood, the same metal, and the same back rests in both of our benches, yet our expectations will be radically different. Niederauer uses this image of the bus bench to describe those times we ask—demand—things from God, and the park bench describes those times we're communing with those things in the universe greater than us.

The approach most athletes take to competition is the bus-bench image.

"On Saturday, the 26th, I will defeat all who show up, break all my personal records, find perfection in all I do, and meet the person of my dreams."

This, my friends, is the G bus of sports preparation and of life. It's a tough model to follow. As I look over my 45 years in organized competition, I can only think of a few times when the G bus showed up on schedule.

For most athletes most of the time, and for most of us for most of our lives, the park-bench model is much more appropriate. When you compete, or simply train, take time to enjoy the view, breathe the air, and don't worry about the squirrels! Whatever comes along during your competition or training should be viewed through the lens of wonder and thanks.

My great joy in competing in Highland Games has a lot to do with the friendships made, the variety of events, and the party atmosphere. Highland Games athletes just don't make fools of themselves complaining about a bad performance. The events make a fool of you!

To get a park-bench mentality, you have to realize that at best, very few competitions are going to be perfect. In addition, when the stars arrange for you to have those perfect competitions, you had better not try to mess things up with a lot of extra energy—you just have to let it go.

The park bench also helps with the 20% of competitions where things go all wrong. If you can keep your wits and feed a squirrel or two, you may just salvage this competition.

By the way, nothing frightens your competition more than a serene smile on your face; they'll think you're up to something!

I fully believe that life is a competition. There's just enough Darwin in me, as well as a master's degree in history, to believe that life is tenuous at best, and your survival, without any hint of irony, reflects on your fitness. Without worrying about hyperbole, I feel this is the 'why' of lifetime fitness. Your survival might depend on your fitness, so why are you slamming your head against a wall to get it?

Train hard, but enjoy the competition. Compete hard, but enjoy your training.

One final key point must be kept in mind at all times: NEVER judge a workout or a competition as good or bad solely on that single day.

I often tell new throwers, "Sorry, you just are not good enough to be disappointed."

Judging one's worth as an athlete over the results of single day is just idiocy…and will lead to long-term failure. Epictetus, the Roman Stoic philosopher, tells us, "We must ever bear in mind that apart from the will there is nothing good or bad, and that we must not try to anticipate or to direct events, but merely to accept them with intelligence."

If that is too complex, I have a favorite story.

A farmer had a horse and a son. One day, the horse died. All the neighbors said, "Oh, how bad."

The farmer said, "We'll see."

The next day, the neighbors got together and bought the farmer a new horse. They all said, "That's a good thing."

The farmer said, "We'll see."

The following day, the horse threw the son while trying to break the horse. The son broke his arm. The neighbors all said, "Oh, how bad."

The farmer said, "We'll see."

The next day, the army came to the town and drafted all the young men, save the son with a broken arm. They all died in the first battle. The neighbors said to the farmer, "Oh, how good it was for your son to have a broken arm."

The farmer said, "We'll see."

What does this all mean? First, let things happen and don't judge them as good or bad. Enjoy the opportunity to train and eat well.

Second, find yourself a community of people who support your goal—and be sure you support your goals, too. Do my ideas work in sports and life? We'll see.

So, what would be an example of a bus-bench workout? To be honest, it's the kind of thing most people want. Call it a program, a cookie-cutter approach, or a training manual, but it's that long page after page after page of 'do this' and 'do that' that most people want.

I have done bus-bench programs that have names like—

- Bigger Arms in Two Weeks
- Two Weeks to a Tighter Tummy
- Six-Week Soviet Squat Program

And the list goes on and on. Generally, bus-bench programs have a built-in time, like two to 12 weeks, and if you follow the directions, you should be changed in that time. If not, the program FAILED. Complain away.

I recommend that everyone should have about two bus-bench programs a year. Clarence Bass, a bodybuilder noted for his lean physique and who is known as Mr. Ripped, continues to schedule an annual photo shoot to insist that he has a focus each year to, well, get on the bus. After age 70, it's still working well for him. Many people use January as a time to refocus, and also the weeks leading up to bikini season. I applaud the effort.

The issue I have with most people is that they turn all 52 weeks of the year into the bus-bench mentality. People on internet forums discuss this all the time, how whatever is the latest and greatest is the right answer. Open one of your deep dark cabinets and look at the miracle pills, goos, and patches that have been touted as the answer to all your problems.

I have survived high carb, low carb, high fat, low fat, high protein, and low protein diets, only to learn that most diets are simply the bus-bench mentality at play. And please listen—this is important: Two weeks on the Atkins Induction diet honestly works miracles for some people.

As I often state, it worked so well, I stopped doing it.

Here's the thing to remember. If you faithfully tried 500 calories a day and an injection of beef plasma every day for a few weeks and you failed to achieve your goals, BLAME the program! If it was a success, refocus for a while, readjust your priorities, but don't celebrate with two-dozen doughnuts. One dozen is plenty.

I can't emphasize this enough: The bus-bench approach to training and diet is RIGHT. It's absolutely right about twice a year. Like the old joke about a broken clock being exactly right twice a day, a focused, disciplined attack on a goal is a great thing to do. Just not all the time!

Every aspect of life and fitness is best served by a healthy mix of bus-bench and park-bench mentality. I'm convinced that the bulk of one's time should be spent doing park-bench work.

In this book, Josh outlines a clear park-bench mentality to training most of the time. For many of us, this is difficult, as we tend to want to engage our bodies and train like an army preparing for battle.

There's a time for those hard workouts. There's a time for those strict diets or ways of eating. It's just not all the time.

DAN

CHAPTER 3

EPISTEMOLOGY: TO THE EVIDENCE, NO MATTER WHERE IT LEADS

How do we find the truth? How do we know what we know? These are questions that don't often pop up in books written by strength coaches, but if we're going to cast off the ropes of mistruths and misunderstandings about health and fitness, we have to answer some tough questions.

Listen, you bought the book; I'm not selling you anything else. I don't have a supplement or an 'act now' or anyone standing behind the curtain. How do we know… what we know?

Epistemology is a great word to use at a party. You simply need to stand there with drink in hand, monocle around the eye, and ask, "You make a fine point, my young friend; what is the epistemology of your evidence?"

This will drive away beautiful women and make all the men roll their eyes. This, in fact, is how I kept myself single for so long. However, there's a great value to the word, and it applies to every field. It's the study of how you know what you know.

I spent my undergraduate years trying to balance my academic life with my athletic career. Fortunately, I had a fine group of mentors who understood the needs of the intercollegiate athlete. Athletics never excused me from class work, but it sure made me stand out when I took philosophy classes. I may have been one of the few philosophy students in history to wear a letter jacket.

But I had excellent professors, and among them was an Indian scholar named Dr. Kulkarni.

Dr. Kulkarni had a way of explaining a 4,000-year-old story that kept us both transfixed and wondering how we would handle it on a test. After a few weeks, the names of all the characters would mysteriously slide into a Sanskrit jumble…the basic storylines seemed to meet at some points, then leap into completely unexpected directions. Studying for this class on Far Eastern philosophy after reviewing the breadth of the Hindu canons seemed daunting to the whole class.

A group of us formed a study group and met in one of the school's library rooms one Tuesday evening. We began when one student burst out with a monologue discussing a central concept Dr. Kulkarni discussed nearly every lecture. The student was fascinated by it and wanted our insights. The concept of Dr. Kulkarni's 'droot' really made him interested in continuing with the follow-up course the next term.

"Droot?"

The other students exchanged glances. This was unsettling—we had never heard Dr. Kulkarni discuss the 'droot.'

"Sure, yes," he told us, "he talks about it every day… the 'droot.'"

"Droot? Droot?"

"Oh, the truth!"

Dr. Kulkarni's accent often made a word or two hard to fathom.

"He is talking about the truth!"

At that moment, the student completely changed his demeanor and explained that he knew the truth from his faith, and that his faith's prophet had explained everything and that was final for him.

In one moment, he went from excited scholar to stiff fundamentalist. For him, the case was closed; the book was finished. He was fascinated by the search for 'droot,' but he had no interest in looking for Dr. Kulkarni's truth.

> *"A man gives a diram to each of four persons. The Persian said he would spend his on an angur, while the Arab said he would spend his on an inab. A Turk said he would spend his on an uzum, and a Greek said he would spend his diram on an istabil. These people began to fight with one another.*
>
> *The angur, the inab, the uzum, and the istabil are all grapes."*
>
> ~Jalal-uddim Runi, Masnavi

How do we know the 'droot' of fitness, health, strength, and conditioning?

I often get challenged about how I know that this or that works. Frankly, most of us in the strength and conditioning field have fallen into saying something akin to 'I don't know.' When people use phrases like the Black Box, to explain the process of how one grows after lifting or loses fat after training, I remind them of what J.R.R. Tolkien, the author of *The Hobbit,* said about the use of the term Celtic.

"Celtic of any sort is…a magic bag, into which anything may be put, and out of which almost anything may come… Anything is possible in the Celtic Twilight."

How do I know how my training systems work? I love falling back on this idea of the Magic Bag of Tolkien. We put anything in and almost anything comes out. I have you sprint and lift and soon you look better. Cheers to you and me.

It's funny to think about this so many years later, but my economics professor once stood at the podium and waved his hands to explain Adam Smith's notion of the invisible hand that drives capitalism. Every field seems to have this moment of hand-waving.

Recently, Chip Conrad of BodyTribe told me how the *South Park* television show used this same hand-waving to explain why the Underpants Gnomes (yes, I just wrote Underpants Gnomes) stole underpants to make a profit.

1. Steal underpants
2. ?
3. Make a profit

How we know programs work or don't work is going to look a lot like the second point in the grand scheme of the Underpants Gnomes. At times, and honestly that should read most of the time, we simply have no idea how it happens. We just know it happens.

Frankly, I think it's good enough to know that lifting makes people stronger and we can move on, but it's fascinating to discuss.

Robb Wolf, author of *The Paleo Solution,* offers a concept that really handles the miracle of how doing this with diet and that with exercise works so well: cascades.

Like a snowball gaining size as it rolls down a hill, certain food choices or mistakes can have a cascading effect on the entire system.

As I learned years ago, there are chemicals that in small doses can do wonders for you. In larger doses, they kill you. Choose wisely.

I know from personal experience that a maximum deadlift can take weeks to recover from the hit of the few seconds of pulling the weight off the ground. High-repetition back squats seem to swell up my whole body and the weight stays on for years. Overtraining breaks me. I know all of this, yet I can't always explain how I know it.

From my years of teaching moral theology, I use a simple system for discussing how we choose values. Values, in my classroom, are simply things we value. I realize this seems redundant, but if you think about it and have the opportunity to discuss it with someone else, it makes more sense.

I recently had a conversation with two young men who were convinced they needed to date women with six-pack abs. It was at that moment I realized we valued different things in life. I'm not judging, just observing.

So, how do we discern our values? Generally, I think there are six ways: authority, deductive logic, sense experience, emotion, intuition, and real science.

Without even thinking about it, most of us effortlessly flow from each of these ways to another. When I came out with my book *Never Let Go*, it occurred to me that I could easily re-sort the collection into the various subheadings of *Authority, Deductive Logic, Sense Experience, Emotion, Intuition, and Real Science*. A training lifetime rubs against each of these methods.

Let's look at them.

Authority is probably my personal favorite for my training. When Dick Notmeyer told me to snatch and clean & jerk three days a week, and to front squat and go overhead two days a week, that plan is exactly what I did. "Dick said so" took away all the thought process. Authority, obviously, is a top-down approach to things.

I truly enjoy this. Some of the best successes of my life are when I trust someone else to plan things for me and I just dive in. Examples of this in my career include—

- Throwing under the guidance of Ralph Maughan at Utah State;
- Playing football at any level;
- Doing Alwyn Cosgrove's *Warp Speed Fat Loss program.*

These were all successful for me. I have my own authority programs, like the *Big 21*, where I hand out a spreadsheet with every lift for every day of the program, *Mass Made Simple*, a six-week bulking program with every lift for every day of the program, and a few others. When my athletes follow these, good things happen because, well, I said so!

The authoritative model can often be the most reasonable. Having your own personal mentor is nice (Yoda, Gandalf, Dumbledore, Merlyn, or Ralph Maughan), as you can just trust the process. When you're told, "Take a day off, you look tired," you might take a day because you're tired. If someone has walked this path before, there's a chance he already knows where the pitfalls, traps, and boogiemen are hiding.

The authoritative model reflects the notion of regression better than most of the other models, too. The best and brightest coaches, from John Wooden to 'name the best coach you know,' will all insist on the fundamentals long after you're convinced you know the fundamentals.

I'm telling you to try planks and get back to the basic movements because I have regenerated my career several times doing planks and the basics. Yes, it's hard to hear that the basics are the key because we all love the new and groovy and exciting and secret, but success is rarely found in the exotic.

Basic and boring wins.

Deductive logic can be maddening to define, but in the most general sense, it's the process of reasoning from general statements. Oddly, it works well most of the time. It can be as simple as what I did to become a discus thrower. When I was about nine, I went to the USA-USSR track meet in Berkeley. When I saw the throwers, I noted that—

All the throwers are big and muscular.
All the throwers are very fast.
All the throwers do these interesting movements called techniques.

To be one of them, it seemed, I should get bigger and faster and learn how to throw correctly!

Josh does a nice job of deductive logic with his fat-loss website, where he often outlines a celebrity's training and diet program. He then points out the consistent use of using food logs and basic training moves.

In college, we had the whole family of syllogisms to use and play with in class (Aristotle is a man. All men are mortal. Aristotle is mortal.) but generally people understand this method without all the fuss.

If we have the basic facts, this is an easy method. The problem in the field of strength and conditioning is that we don't always have all the facts. Muscle magazines often push supplements and training programs showing bodybuilders or fitness models who might never have done the workout or taken the product, but will have taken a lot of products only available from people with sunglasses in back rooms. Fourteen-year-old Billy in Nebraska will literally put his health at risk trying to do the arm day of his hero, Mr. Greater Galaxy.

Recently, I gave a talk to the strength coaches of the professional basketball teams of North America. It turns out one can get paid to play basketball. Who knew? I wonder if they're interested in a middle-aged, six-foot power forward.

The problem with basketball (among other things, trust me) is that for years—almost half a century—the sport ignored strength training. I had a friend who told me he worried that lifting would mess up his shot. He was a back-up center at our high school and, thank God, he didn't let training get in the way of his two-point-a-game average.

Yes, sarcasm is just part of what you get from me.

By ignoring lifting, basketball coaches found themselves in a situation where they now are flooded with commercial and personal enterprises of 'do this' and 'do that,' from machines to large bouncing balls to plastic wraps. They have no shared history about what works and what's pure idiocy.

By ignoring strength training for so long, they struggle with reasonableness. The athletes float off to all kinds of trainers, positive and negative, without any ability to say, "The best have been doing X and I too need to do X."

This is the reason deductive logic is so important in this field. It allows us to experiment, but not go too far off the mark.

Without any foundation, it's very difficult to regress. In other words, without the basics and fundamentals of a traditional strength-training platform, it's difficult to go back when injuries, stagnation, or mere off-season issues arise. As a player ages, it's nice to be able to outline a series of regressive movements that will keep him in the game.

But without the tradition, one can't regress.

Basketball will be an interesting study in deprivation. Without the benefit of a tradition in strength training, the very definition of deprivation, we can now observe the sport and coaches attempting to catch up.

Sense experience, too, can be dangerous. This is anything we learn from our senses: taste, smell, touch, see, and hear. Montaigne, the great French author of the sixteen century, gives us some ideas in his great work *Essays*, which simply means attempts in English. After grading thousands of essays in my teaching career, trust me, *attempts* is a far better idea than anything else one can use.

Honestly, a sentence starts with a capital letter and I stand by that no matter what my students write.

Montaigne's motto was *What do I know?* He felt humans would fail in the quest to find certainty and that we have to experience things. With a smile on my face, I remember his firsthand account of being beaten up in a street fight, as he decided to find out, firsthand, what it would feel like to be hit. It hurts.

I can be honest that my journey in strength and conditioning has been no less than Montaigne's leap into a street fight. I can discuss the pros and cons of many programs as I leaped into them, bloodied my face, and came out the wiser. People have asked me many times if my two-year attempts at Nautilus and CrossFit were bad. No. In fact, both experiences opened up some great questions in my head—and some answers—about the role of strength and conditioning.

We can improve on minimal work, but only for so long. We can also learn a lot about human movement by learning and doing a lot of different things, but it's going to move us away from our goals unless our goal is simply to move a lot.

I think one of the things that makes me a reasonable coach are these attempts. I know what it's like to wake up at night with sore joints and a level of body stiffness that demands some intervention from the medicine cabinet. Sometimes the route to reasonableness demands a lot of detours and email messages.

Once again, to quote Ralph Maughan, it's fairly easy to follow this dictum, 'Be reasonable; do it my way,' but sometimes we just have to taste the blood in our mouths. Then I can turn to you and say, "Don't get punched in the mouth."

Sense experience might be a door into understanding regression and, perhaps, deprivation. Getting into a pick-up basketball game with the best in the field will highlight every weakness you have as a player. The universe will scream to you, "Practice the fundamentals!"

You will also become very aware that your genetic gifts may have been deprived in your ability to dominate a game of pure vertical.

Emotion might not work in this discussion as well as the other concepts, but in discussions of what we value, this shows up a lot. It can be explained as the heart flutter we get when we think we're right about something. Most of us have experienced that odd urge toward another person that simply can't be put into words. Joseph Campbell described this as the 'urge of the organs toward each other.' Sure, it can be love, lust, and amore, but it's also the way many people make decisions about God and country and family. Don't confuse me with the facts.

Whenever I feel like I'm caught up in something, I stop for a moment and review what's going on. This is how fads in strength and conditioning come into play. When we see others marching along this new path, perhaps we have this fear of being left behind so we join in. I honestly believe emotions play a huge role in dietary errors, missteps, and lapses. I have been candid before about tears running down my cheeks while deep in a very strict diet, as my response to food could only be described as emotional.

In schools today, we reward kids with candy for turning in their homework. Chocolate is given to show love several times a year, and cake is what we eat when we celebrate a birthday. By tying food to events, we get an emotional hit. It's sometimes good—Thanksgiving and turkey is a great example—and sometimes it's bad.

If we see food as a reward, food is going to be an issue. If we begin to value cakes, sweets, and treats as part of the qualities we have as a person, it's going to be hard to unpack that later with a good training program.

When one finds that moment of 'yes, this is it,' it often comes after some frustration at trying things logically and linearly. The problem, if one wishes to call it a problem, with the emotional approach to learning is unpacking it for the next generation. Standing in front of a group of young warriors and telling them the approach you're demanding is the best approach because it makes your heart go pitter-pat might be the ticket to a new job.

Regression is difficult with emotions, as anyone who has ever had an enflamed heart that cooled will tell you. Of course, the heart grows fonder when deprived, so the strength coach can only offer so much in the matters of love.

Intuition is simply acquiring knowledge without reason. When Luke is lining up to blast the Death Star, the voice of Obi-wan tells him, "Use the Force, Luke." Like emotion, we can't always justify decisions based on intuition.

In the teaching of kettlebells, we often discuss the *Aha!* moment when a drill lights up a person's face with complete understanding. *That's it!* seems to go beyond any ability to use words to explain the insight. Science is filled with the stories of these *Eureka!* moments where everything suddenly comes together.

Dick Fosbury attacked the high jump bar backward and revolutionized the sport. L. Jay Silvester went to his backyard and let his leg hang out a bit in the discus, threw 20 feet farther, and changed discus throwing forever. Bill Koch, the world champion cross-country skier, saw a skater pass him by on a lake and thought he would try that on cross-country skis. The impact forced the sport into two different divisions to deal with this new method.

Reverse-engineering insights like these is nearly impossible. Sherlock Holmes gives us this great skill in *The Adventure of the Cardboard Box*, where Holmes reads Watson's thoughts by watching his eyes. But for us mere mortals, we sometimes just have to enjoy this illuminating insight and be happy that words don't always tell the whole story. I think in the long run, this method is closely allied with authority. Unpacking that *aha* might take awhile, but it's what makes great coaches better than the rest of us.

When we get to *real science*, things get interesting. Greg Gensel, who has been head track and field coach at Utah State University since 1988, told me, "No program has ever been proved to be more effective than DeLorme's."

I argued that we all know we need to increase load and decrease reps to continue to grow beyond the DeLorme Protocol.

"Right," Greg added, "but no one has proved that this has worked better."

He then explained the issues and problems with setting up a scientific study with enough test subjects, enough follow-up, and enough proof to support what DeLorme and Watkins were able to do with polio victims and WWII soldiers.

Certainly, what we do in the weightroom is right…right?

We see the same issue on the diet and nutrition side of things. We can't even get a roomful of experts to agree on what's a good breakfast, or even if we should eat breakfast. Why? There's research that tells us coffee is good, coffee is bad, breakfast is good, or breakfast is bad. Be sure to eat fruit, but not fructose—the sugar in fruit.

Huh?

Exactly.

We know that lifting weights does wonderful and marvelous things for us, but the devil, according to the real science, is in the details.

In my previous works, I've tried to note that the key to true strength training is twofold.

First, ensure the athlete doesn't have any gaps in any movement—don't miss any basic fundamental movements—and then second, be at some standard at each and every movement. If you're strong in every movement, your issues are not in the weightroom. We might need to assess a lot of things to figure out your problem, but the weightroom can be scratched off that list.

"The truth is like a lion. You don't have to defend it. Let it loose. It will defend itself."

Saint Augustine was talking about something besides fat loss for women, but the point stands well in our discussion.

Figuring out these ways of knowing involves one additional step, and here I have punished my students with one of my famous formulas. Remember, you can't divide by zero, but you can multiply by zero and that's easy: You always end up with zero.

Facts times interpretation equals truth.

> *If your facts are true and your interpretation is true, I think you have a truth.*

> *If your facts are false, but your interpretation is true, I think you don't have a truth.*

> *If your facts are true, but your interpretation is false, I think you don't have a truth.*

> *If both your facts and interpretation are false, I think you don't have a truth.*

Position one is where I try to get to on most things. Say I read something from the 1920s, and it's a concept that stands the test of time. I apply it to my athletes and, like magic, it works today.

Positions two and three are where we find much of the advertising in the fitness world. I remember a guy selling me a bottle of chromium picolinate, telling me that a college study found it (and it's always this phrase) 'better than steroids.' I knew the study. These guys also trained four days a week with a combination of Olympic lifting and powerlifting and gained lean body mass. Most people gain LBM lifting weights…especially, as the study forgot to mention, off-season football players coming in after three months off. People who take time off and then train, increase lean body mass.

I don't care how many drops of magic formula you add, it won't be as important as all the rest. Make sure the facts and the interpretation are true.

Position four is the bottom-feeding mess of some of the fitness industry. I've been sucked into this in my past with any number of things and I can admit being a fool. I'm trying to get over it. Does anyone need my bottles of Horny Goat Weed?

It comes down to this: I am not dumb. Nor do I think the legions of coaches, trainers, researchers, and scientists are dumb either. There are some basic issues: Cutting into a corpse is an interesting way to learn about anatomy. Cutting into a living being is frowned upon by polite society. The living, breathing, growing organism called 'you' is pretty complex.

And, it's amazing, too.

Nassim Taleb gives us this genius of an insight.

> *"If humans fight the last war, nature fights the next one. Your body is more imaginative about the future than you are. Consider how people train in weightlifting: the body overshoots in response to exposures and overprepares (up to the point of biological limit, of course). This is how bodies get stronger."*
>
> ~Nassim Nicholas Taleb,
> *Antifragile: Things That Gain from Disorder*

I don't worry so much about the how it happens. I'm sure Robb Wolf's insights on cascading will be a great model for many things, especially something like hormones in the body. But I literally have no need to know how all of this (hands are flapping) happens. Our bodies have more imagination than my hands flapping.

I'm convinced we get stronger in two steps, but I am more than willing to be wrong.

Step one is why you hired me: Strength is a skill. It can be learned. There are tricks to lifting more weight and they are as simple as learning tension and relaxation, learning to wedge under a load, learning to grease the groove and learning that real strength is something that's a practice, not a single workout. In other words, step one is learning to be strong. It takes a while to learn all the great movements, yet an advanced lifter can become 'instantly' stronger by learning this cue or that tension.

Instantly is a funny idea. As Charles Staley told me years ago, saying 'instantly add an inch to your arm in two weeks' sells much better than the same phrase without 'instantly.' For those of us who have experienced that *aha* moment where we failed doing something several times, then were told a new cue and suddenly succeeded, instantly is as close to the magic bag as anything we will experience in life.

Step two is where the real fun begins. Following Robb's insight, step two might simply be called the hormonal cascade. Now, feel free to drop the hormone part as I am sure it's much more subtle and complex at the same time.

I've seen this several times in my life.

The best example is when I met Dick Notmeyer. I had been training with weights for a long time and I was very strong. As a high school senior, I was stronger than most men I've known in my lifetime. I weighed 162 pounds and I was a bench-pressing machine.

Then I met Dick. Four months later, I weighed 202 pounds. That's 40 pounds in four months, 10 pounds a month, two-and-half pounds a week.

How did that happen?

The math won't work, by the way. There's no way I could have consumed enough calories with the calories in/calories out model when I was training so hard, and still exploding in size.

That's the cascade. In *Mass Made Simple*, I offer a six-week training program with only 14 workouts. Guys who do the program always report back that they made the best progress of their lives.

I also get questions like this: If it's so good, why don't you keep doing it?

And I laugh. Obviously, this person has never done the workouts that have pure strength moves, complexes, and staggeringly high rep squats. You can only do it for six weeks. But if you take it seriously, the body will reward you with a cascade.

When you decide to get stronger to support any other fitness goal, don't worry about the how. Correct strength training will get you on the right path. Master the movements and keep your reps, sets, and loads reasonable and repeatable.

Then, enjoy that wonderful gift when your body responds by cascading the hormones and all the whatevers that will make you bigger, leaner, stronger, faster, and abler.

Don't focus on the how. Focus on the do.

This leads us to one of the most important and overarching principles of life.

It's fine when we don't know how it works…if it works.

ONE CHANGE

JOSH

CHAPTER 4

THE HARD TALK

It's time for us to have the hard talk. Now, I get a little nervous every time I have this talk, because I know it's the most important talk we can have about your body composition. I also get a little nervous because I know that when things aren't going well in terms of your fitness goals, this isn't the talk you want to have. There are some parts of it you're not going to like, but here it is: *It's all about the food.*

If you don't like the way your body looks, the problem is always food. Sometimes it's the *quantity* of food. Sometimes it's the *quality* of food.

But it's always the food.

It's never your genetics. It's never how old you are. It's never that you're a man or a woman. It's never that you aren't doing the newest and craziest workout. It's the food. It's the quantity of food, or it's the quality of food.

Once we get real about this, we can get with the facts: The only game we're playing is the game of trying to figure out how to change the quantity or the quality of food you're eating.

That's the key to make this work in real life.

HOW FOOD REALLY WORKS IN FAT LOSS

When it comes to making food work for fat loss, there are only three variables: quantity, quality, and ratios.

That means quantity of food, quality of food, and the ratio of macronutrients, like proteins, carbohydrates, fat, and alcohol.

When we're dealing with quantity, we'll find a lot of diets based on that. These are any type of diets that use points, blocks, or counting calories. This all boils down to different ways of measuring quantity.

Another way people measure quantity is portion size, like the original *Body for Life* diet where a portion of carbohydrates or a portion of protein is the size of the palm of a hand. This is just another way of measuring quantity.

Right now, it's cool to say quantity doesn't matter or counting calories doesn't work. While this is a slick marketing technique, it's just not the truth.

I'll give you a quick story. I used to do Brazilian jiu jitsu. I often ran into people who were professional fighters. Things really hit home for me when I was hanging out with Marcus, a guy who fought at different weight classes. Marcus was a built dude. He was about 8% bodyfat, which is lean. He was about 8% when he fought at one weight class, and he could fight at a weight class 15 pounds heavier and still be about 8% bodyfat. He was lean in three different weight classes.

I asked him about his diet and how he changed weight classes. The quality of his diet was always the same. He always ate about the same foods. The only difference between one weight class and another was the quantity of food he ate.

Don't believe anyone who tells you quantity doesn't matter. Of course, quantity matters. In fact, I would argue that the only thing that determines your scale weight is the quantity of food you eat.

If you've got a highlighter, highlight this: *Quantity equals scale weight.*

Any way you measure quantity, whether it's calories, points or palm-of-the-hand portion size, that's what's going to determine your scale weight. For our purposes, we're going to use calories. Look, I know calories aren't a perfect measurement, but they're the best measurement we have, and the most effective way to track quantity for fat loss.

A note about quantity: They've done numerous studies proving that the people who have the hardest time losing weight are the same people who have the hardest time judging and journaling accurate quantity. Said another way, if the scale isn't moving, you should literally weigh and measure your food to recalibrate yourself to how much you're eating.

The next issue is quality.

Now, quality works on multiple levels. When people are eating fast food, they don't need to worry about whether their eggs are free-range. They need to worry about eating less fast food.

There are a lot of different diets that look at quality. Usually, they recommend a certain level of quality and that's the level of quality you're told to eat.

You need to move through *levels* of quality. If you're eating Ding Dongs and Ho Hos every day, that's the thing to handle. You don't need to worry about not eating a turkey sandwich because it isn't what a caveman would eat; you just need to stop eating Ding Dongs.

As your levels of quality improve, the quantity is going to become less important. This is the concept behind a lot of diets with the idea that you don't need to worry about quantity. It's one of those things where as the quality improves, you're going to get leaner.

I'm going to simplify things a lot. The reality is, quality equals bodyfat percentage.

Whatever the scale weight, your ratio of muscle to fat—how lean you look, how tight you look, how toned you look—is your bodyfat percentage.

Regardless of what the scale says—

Higher bodyfat percentage means more jiggling.
Lower bodyfat percentage means more lean and tight.

Quality is something I coach incrementally. There are different levels to work through, and you don't have the same concerns at one level that you have at the next.

Impacting the quality of food you're eating is so powerful, people have created diets to focus entirely on that. The quality of food you're eating directly impacts your leanness and your tightness or your ratio of muscle to fat. It's one of those things where whatever your scale weight, your ratio of muscle to fat at that scale weight is going to be impacted by the quality.

It really is this simple: *Food quality equals bodyfat percentage.*

As you look at quantity and quality, these both matter a lot. They just affect different things. If your real issue is scale weight, you have to take a look at the quantity.

If your real issue is you're not as lean and tight and toned as you want, you have to take a look at quality. If your issue is both, you have to take a look at both quantity and quality.

FAT LOSS HAPPENS ON MONDAY RESULTS KEY	
YOUR SCALE WEIGHT	QUANTITY OF FOOD YOU EAT (CALORIES)
YOUR BODY FAT PERCENTAGE	QUALITY OF FOOD AND HOW STRONG YOU ARE

FEELING FULL

The last of the three variables we look at in terms of food is ratios. This is another area where you'll see diets entirely based on ratios of protein, carbohydrates, and fat.

For example, *The Zone Diet* equally balances protein, carbohydrates, and fat. Atkins and ketogenic dieters eat no carbohydrates—just protein and fat. And in the 1980s, it was all about low fat.

These are all ratio diets. Usually, when they work it's actually because altering the ratios or providing some kind of rules generally lowers the quantity of calories.

In terms of ratios of proteins, carbohydrate, and fats I don't give people a specific rule. In fact, when I worked at a large gym, we used to survey people to give them a macronutrient ratio 'type.' We found both 'carb type' and 'fat type' people. Basically, what that came down to was some people feel full with more fat. Believe it or not, some people actually do feel full with more carbohydrates. Some people feel the most full with a balance. There really are 'carb type,' 'fat type' and 'mixed type' people.

Just ask yourself—

Do you stay full and satisfied after a meal that's mostly carbs?
Do you stay full and satisfied after a meal that's mostly fat?
Do you stay full and satisfied after a meal that's mostly balanced?

In terms of protein, almost everyone feels more full with more protein in the diet.

Right now, with protein and fat being all the rage, you might assume that *everyone* feels more full and gets better results with more fat.

I have actually had clients who were 'carb types' and felt more full with a higher carbohydrate diet. We would rock it. I helped guys get down to 10% bodyfat and women down to 18% and 19% bodyfat on fairly high carbohydrate diets, as long as they were eating good-quality carbohydrates. This means they were getting all of their carbohydrates from fruits, vegetables, brown rice, and quinoa. It's totally workable.

I don't type people by survey anymore. Now we just take a look at the food journal. We take a look at when they were hungry and after which meals. It's usually pretty simple. We see things like, *Here I had more carbohydrates and I felt more full*, or *Here I had more carbohydrates and I was starving an hour later.*

Things are usually pretty obvious if you look at your food journal, assuming you keep good notes.

There's also a fourth variable, which is timing. A lot of people get into food timing as something they think they should focus on. But timing really isn't an issue. It's one of those things where people talk about what you need to eat or not eat at night or how you need to split food up into six small meals.

This is not something that's been an issue for my clients, and it's not something we're going to work on. It's one of those things where if we get the quantity and the quality correct, you're set. Most of the timing protocols are unnecessarily complicated.

One of my least favorite concepts is six small meals a day. For most people, this just means every single meal they eat is unsatisfying, whereas if you split that into two meals and two snacks, you'd actually get two meals that feel like meals.

I could dig more into this, but all I want to leave you with is that timing is the least important variable in the equation. You want to focus on quantity, quality and the ratios that help you feel the most full, and that's it.

This is the way to think about it—

- *Quantity equals your scale weight.*
- *Quality equals your leanness and tightness.*
- *Ratios equal feeling full.*

CONTEXT AND MINDSET

What we should talk about next is context; it's a mindset thing. Context is not going to change anything we talked about before. It doesn't change what you do. However, by adding new context to it, it changes the *way you do it*. It might change the intensity you have or the level of commitment you apply.

Here's how this works. My specialty is helping people lose stubborn fat. The biggest mistake you can make in losing stubborn fat is to buy into the idea that fat can be stubborn. In fact, there's no such thing as stubborn fat.

Fat is actually the opposite of stubborn. If you think about it from a physiological perspective, fat needs to be maintained. If you don't constantly feed fat, you'll lose it. Fat is like a stray dog. If you keep feeding it, it will stick around forever. If you stop feeding it, it immediately goes away.

One of the things you have to latch onto is that anything making fat appear to be stubborn is a mistake in terms of quantity, quality, or ratio.

Actually, it's just quantity or quality. There is no stubborn fat.

There's usually an issue with preparation or with the way you're tracking such that you're making an error in quality or quantity. That's why you still have the fat. Once you rectify the issue of getting quality and quantity correct, fat can no longer be maintained and you'll lose it.

This is really the basis for the way I coach everyone. It's in view of that context that I make every recommendation. It may seem like a simple or a small thing. But once you get it, everything becomes very clear.

It really boils down to the fact that the quality of food equals how lean and tight you are, and quantity of food equals scale weight. Anything that's stubborn inside either of these is either too much quantity or too little quality. If you stop maintaining the excess quantity and stop maintaining the lack of quality, you'll lose fat.

Here's another way to look at it.

If you have more fat than you want, you need to look at what you're doing to maintain the fat and stop doing that. That's really all there is to it. It's exactly that simple and easy.

Actually, 'easy' is probably not the right word, but it is that simple and it is that clear. If you really use this as the context for all of these tools and all of the strategies you've heard so far, you'll have a new access to fat loss that you didn't have before.

DAN

CHAPTER 5

REASONABLENESS

Let's just get this out first: I believe that a reasonable way of eating and a reasonable training model trump insanity all the time. What's insanity? This idea that you can eat 500 calories for a few weeks, inject yourself with some monkey plasma, and effortlessly lose fat. Insanity is training yourself to exhaustion for 90 days, taking your picture, and then flopping back to the couch for a few years.

	REASONABLE WORKOUTS	TOUGH TRAINING
REASONABLE EATING	*MOST OF THE TIME* REASONABLE WORKOUTS AND REASONABLE EATING	*PEAKING OR PREP* TOUGH TRAINING AND REASONABLE EATING
STRICT DIETING	*POST-PARTY TIME* STRICT DIETING AND REASONABLE WORKOUTS	*EVERY FOUR YEARS... MAYBE?* STRICT DIET AND TOUGH TRAINING

In my last few workshops, I've gone to the whiteboard and illegibly scribbled in my scrawl that earned Ds in handwriting at St. Veronica's School, asking these questions.

What's a tough workout?

Dozens of hands go up, dozens of answers.

I truly enjoy this part as we swim from totally random training programs to sports (run a marathon!) to a multitude of DVD programs and the like. There are programs that can kill and programs that have from 16–50% injury rates inside of six weeks. Remember, this is a room of fitness pros and we still think we need to kill a person to make progress.

What's a reasonable workout?

A few hands go up, a few shy answers like Even Easier Strength.

I discuss hand-waving again and again in my writings. It's this side-to-side hand-shaking wiggle we do with both hands, followed by our mouths saying, "You know," and our shoulders shrugging.

With 'reasonable,' sadly, we seem to not know. I argue that reasonable workouts cover all the basic human movements in a repeatable repetition scheme and an appropriate load, while providing plenty of time and energy for corrective work in any and all areas.

Reasonable seems repeatable.

What's a tough diet or tough way of eating?

Most hands go up with everything from pure fasting or protein-drink-only diets to sheer lunacy.

I had a girlfriend who had a three-day diet. Day one she ate seven eggs—that was it for the whole day. Day two, she had seven oranges and day three was seven bananas. She would lose seven pounds doing this. That, my friends, is a tough diet. I would probably find a three-day fast easier, as my blood sugar would go crazy on the fruit days and turn me ravenous.

Oh, on day five? She put on nine pounds.

What's a reasonable diet or reasonable way of eating?

Crickets.
Nothing.

Blank, uncomfortable stares. As a classroom teacher for 34 years, my one fear has always been passing gas during a lecture. As the seminar group stares back at me, I have one of two thoughts: Either I farted or we have a problem.

I checked. It wasn't me.

Seriously, some of the biggest names in the fitness industry won't raise their hands and tell me what is a reasonable way of eating in this age of one million diets.

Years ago at the Olympic Training Center, we were told to focus on three things.

> **Protein**
> **Vegetables**
> **Clear Water**

Is there anything stunning there? Later, Robb Wolf summarized the most complex eating program in the world (dozens of books by the same author promising all kinds of things, and the problem is always that you don't do it right) with these three memorable lines—

> **More Protein**
> **More Fiber**
> **More Fish Oil**

Please note: I have stolen both of these concepts and I now claim them as my own. Remember, the first time I say something, I'm quoting someone. The second time I say something, I say, "My good friend, fill in the name, always says…"

The third time I say something, I say, "As I always say…"

This is what I remember from my ethics class on the topic of intellectual property.

As I argued in *Mass Made Simple*, I think we know how to eat.

"Honestly, seriously, you don't know what to do about food? Here is an idea: Eat like an adult. Stop eating fast food, stop eating kid's cereal, knock it off with all the sweets and comfort foods whenever your favorite show is not on when you want it on, ease up on the snacking and—don't act like you don't know this—eat more vegetables and fruits.

"Really, how difficult is this? Stop with the whining. Stop with the excuses. Act like an adult and stop eating like a television commercial. Grow up. Now, let's get back to the point: Eat like an adult!"

My point here is important: To begin the process of training and eating reasonably, I have to raise my voice, shake my fist, and wake up the world. Reasonableness has been so lost in the field of fitness, strength and conditioning that striving to get someone to train more reasonably has become unusual, odd, strange, and contrarian.

In junior college, I studied paralegal research at Skyline College. My days were filled with the great canon of Western Civilization and long classes on business and criminal law. The two fields intertwined nearly every day. After we discussed the ideals of classic Greeks, I would grab my bag, walk down the hall, and hear about the basic legal standard.

To understand the law, you must first and foremost understand reasonable and reasonableness. I have always thought this definition of the reasonable person by Percy Henry Winfield to be, well, *reasonable*.

> *"He has not the courage of Achilles, the wisdom of Ulysses or the strength of Hercules, nor has he the prophetic vision of a clairvoyant. He will not anticipate folly in all its forms but he never puts out of consideration that the teachings of experience shows such negligence and so will guard against negligence of others when experience shows such negligence to be common. He is a reasonable man but not a perfect citizen, nor a 'paragon of circumspection.'"*

That sounds like a lot of people I know.

Reasonableness is not only a pillar in the study of law, but it used to be considered one of the rocks of a person of integrity. Integrity, according to my mom, was being one person all the time no matter what the circumstances. I have been at dinner with Cardinals of the Catholic Church, stars from Broadway, professional athletes, Olympians, and fitness models, yet I strive to follow this simple advice from my mother. Ideally, at my funeral you will all be talking about the same guy in my urn or casket.

Integrity comes from the same root as integer. Like a whole number, integrity asks you to be a whole person. I have found, and this is nothing unusual as billions have done it before me, that being reasonable in your thoughts, actions, beliefs and approach to life allows you to handle the contradictions, disparities and unpleasantries of living in community.

My college coach, Ralph Maughan, had a sign on his desk: *Be reasonable. Do it my way.*

Coach Maughan, who was drafted by the Detroit Lions, made an Olympic team as a hammer thrower, won the nationals in the javelin, and earned three medals at the Battle of the Bulge, maybe had more reasons to be reasonable, frankly.

Coach Maughan, part of the Greatest Generation, had seen and done things that were glorious and tragic, and he understood life well. His way was usually a pretty good idea.

Earl Nightingale tells us in *Lead the Field*, the audiotape series that changed my life, "And, to me, reasonableness is another word for integrity: integrity to truth, to the evidence, no matter where it leads…Are you ready to discover 'through experiment and reflection what course of life will fulfill those powers most completely'? That's being true to yourself; that's integrity; that's reasonableness."

To the evidence, no matter where it leads is the drumbeat of my search for better ways to seek and attain our goals in fitness, health, and sports.

An important caveat: *You probably are not getting ready for the NFL Combine.*

My goal in the eighth grade was to play professional football. The Orange Library had two books that changed my life that year, *The Sword in the Stone* by T. H. White and *7 Days to Sunday* by Eliot Asinof. On Wednesday of the seven days, Asinof talked about an undersized linebacker named Kenny Avery, and his story changed my life. If he could do it, I could do it. Pushups, running, tumbling, the hurdles, the shot put, and the discus became my route to the NFL.

I didn't make it. But I became pretty good at the discus throw.

To prep for football, everything is helpful. I use the concept of Quadrant Two to explain collision sports and collision occupations training systems. The number of qualities needed to play football or to work in special operations is staggering. Moreover, the level you need to be at the minimum in all these qualities is truly stunning. The average high school football player is probably faster, stronger, and better conditioned than anyone you know.

To train QII people, your quiver of training ideas has to be jammed full. Sleds, car pushing, Olympic lifting, wrestling, sprinting, hurdling, stadium steps, and everything else you can think of will help someone prepare for the collision sports.

I use the *Mass Made Simple* program up to twice a year for football players, six weeks of a lot of high-rep squatting, complexes, and upper-body work. Frankly, it can be awful. A high school football player needs to do it perhaps twice a year.

You probably don't. This is the caveat, the warning—the sign that says *No Swimming…Sharks* concerning a reasonable approach to training.

The most popular way to sell programs is to use professional football or special operations (think Navy SEALs) or a rugby player in full pursuit as the image to train most of us. But most of us are not playing pro football. Count the number of professional football players in your immediate circle of friends and family. Few of us will make it to one, and those who do will find this might not be true in 3.2 years.

Most of us need to train very simply, very reasonably. Now having said this, I also work with a lot of football players and people whose jobs involve a lot of collisions. I train them differently for a while, until they get where they need to be. Then, usually around age 27, I train them just like I train anyone else.

The warning is this: Enjoy playing football and watching collision sports. Then, remind yourself of who you are day to day, and train appropriately. That's the truth, and believe me, the truth is a hard thing to find in the fitness industry juggernaut.

JOSH

CHAPTER 6

THE DAY I BECAME THE BEST FAT-LOSS TRAINER IN THE WORLD

Back in 2004, I sucked as a trainer. I thought I was giving my clients great workouts, but they got no fat loss results at all.

At the end of the second month, I went to the 24 Hour Fitness Trainer Certification presented by Apex. Back in those days, it was kind of the wild west at 24 Hour Fitness. I can't imagine they still talk like this, but this is what I heard at the time, and it changed my entire career.

The certification instructor was this older, hard, and buffed dude. He growled, "Look, food journals are important for results. If clients don't keep their food journals, I take them in the group exercise room, make them do military-style calisthenics until they puke, and then I make them clean it up. That's what they're paying you for. After a couple times, they get how important the food journal is."

I went back and told all of my clients they had to keep a food journal. Some actually thought I was joking. All of the clients who started keeping food journals immediately began losing scale weight and inches.

All of those who didn't keep a food journal pretty much stayed the same.

I couldn't believe it was that simple.

This is one of the biggest keys for you to understand—if you want results, you must keep a food journal. If you don't keep a food journal, you have no right to expect results.

Later I would learn two tricks that made keeping a food journal easier.

NOTHING IS BAD, NOTHING IS GOOD

I was helping clients get great results just by letting them know that food journals were the key. About 60% of my clients were keeping food journals, and those 60% were achieving life-changing, amazingly great results.

The other 40% didn't feel bad about not getting results because they knew what to do and they just weren't doing it. But still, that wasn't okay with me. The question became, how could I get that other 40% to keep a food journal?

In 2006 I was a coach for the Landmark Education Self-Expression and Leadership Program in Denver. One of the tools of coaching that program is the idea that it isn't morally bad or wrong to not follow your plan. Some things you do forward your goals, and some things don't. Following your plan will take you toward your goal, and not following it usually won't.

But really, nothing is wrong. You're not a bad person if you don't follow your plan.

Taking that into fat loss—nothing you eat is bad or wrong. Nothing you eat is good or right. There's no morality to food or fat loss.

I don't care if you eat Twinkies or eat at Taco Bell. You aren't a bad person if you eat junk food. You aren't a good person if you eat organic veggies with grass-fed beef.

Eating some things will take you closer to your goals.

Eating other things will take you farther from your goals.

There's nothing else to it. In *Fat Loss Happens on Monday*, no one is going to judge what you write down in your food journal.

WHAT IS RESPONSIBILITY?

If you're judging your food journal, you need to grow up. Beating yourself up is the opposite of taking responsibility.

Taking responsibility with food is looking without emotion at actions that work or don't work for your goals.

I discovered people don't keep food journals because they're afraid of being judged. Of course, the normal human thing to do—even when no one else is judging you—is to beat yourself up.

Judging or beating yourself up doesn't make you hot. Judging and beating yourself up doesn't get you back on track. Judging and beating yourself up is totally irresponsible.

Being **irresponsible** looks like—
Feeling bad you didn't eat the right thing (emotion)

Being **responsible** looks like—
*Going to the store, buying good food,
taking it home, and cooking it (action)*

Being **irresponsible** looks like—
Beating yourself up and judging yourself (emotion)

Being **responsible** looks like—
*Writing down everything you eat, and creating
strategies for what you could do differently
next week (action)*

Responsibility is taking the emotion and the guilt out of the equation, and just dealing with actions.

A funny thing happened: When we took all of the bull out of food being bad or good, people could write down what they actually ate. They could come in with a food journal that said, "Sunday I ate seven chili dogs and drank a six-pack of beer," and know it would be totally okay.

Suddenly, 100% of my clients were keeping a food journal. They'd come in laughing when it was filled with terrible stuff, and they'd come in proud when it was all amazingly good food.

But the important thing is, they wrote it all down.

And once it's all written down, we could take a look at it strategically, without emotion, without the impressions of good or bad or right or wrong. We could look at which actions were working for their goals and which actions weren't.

Then, we'd take one small step, like adding breakfast with protein on Monday morning. And that one action that works for the goal would be the *sole focus of that week*. That would be the game: Breakfast on Monday.

And we'd win that game.

When you win lots of small games like that, you get really lean and hot.

TRANSFORM IDENTITY

Let's take a look at deliberately changing the way you talk to yourself and others about—

1. Your body
2. Food
3. Working out

This is about speaking the way someone who has the body you want would speak.

What would _____ (celebrity or athlete) say right now?

People who are fat and out of shape tell a certain set of stories and use the same set of excuses.

People who are in shape say almost exactly the opposite.

You need to choose to say the things that in-shape people say, and believe the things that in-shape people believe.

This is not positive affirmation.

Business philosopher Jim Rohn used to say: "Positive affirmation without action is the beginning of delusion."

What we're talking about with *Fat Loss Happens on Monday* is changing your actions.

People get stuck because their conversations about nutrition and diet don't match their actions. They may be trying a new workout or a new diet, but they still talk like a fat person.

Let me give you some examples.

Fat Talk: I can never resist when you guys bring baked goods to work.

Fit Talk: You guys are going to have to eat the brownies without me this time. I don't eat brownies on Tuesdays, ha ha. Don't worry, I'll make sure to have something sweet on my free day.

Fat Talk: I hate working out. I do it because I have to.

Fit Talk: I used to hate working out, but I found out it doesn't have to be as bad as I thought. On top of that, I feel really good about getting stronger.

Be aware when your ways of speaking don't support your new actions, and change what needs to be changed.

DON'T JOKE ABOUT BEING THE FAT KID

Make sure you aren't trying to do one thing at the gym, and then later say something to friends that contradicts that.

I had a client who always joked about being the fat kid. He was a really funny guy, and he was always joking around, and always made everyone laugh. But his top go-to joke was about being the fat kid.

I'd have him do some exercise he didn't like or that was hard and he'd say, "Oh sure, pick on the fat kid!"

I kept telling him over and over, "Use that joke while you can, because in a couple months you won't be able to anymore." And I'd tell him, "Dude, with the way you're keeping a food journal and working out, you're going to need some new jokes."

Then I changed it to, "Sorry, dude, you need new jokes. You're too strong to be making jokes about being the fat kid," and, "Sorry, dude, fat kids don't keep food journals; you need a new joke."

My favorite at weigh-ins was, "Sorry, bro, fat kids don't lose 3% of bodyfat every month."

Pretty soon all of his jokes were about his hair loss, "Oh sure, pick on the bald guy!"

He had to change his diet, change his workouts, *and* change his jokes to get the body he wanted.

By our last session, he'd lost 50 pounds, was down to 10% bodyfat, and was doing Spiderman pushups and full pull-ups.

Your actions and your speaking have to match. Both actions and speaking have to be aligned so they're both pointing in the direction of your goal.

Ultimately it comes back around to responsibility. All of the 'Fat Talk' is really just a way to abdicate responsibility for your goals. On the flip side, the 'Fit Talk' is a way to take responsibility for your goals.

PROGRESS, EMOTION, AND WOLVES

I've had a lot of clients cry during our sessions. And I'm totally comfortable with crying. The truth is, if something matters to you, it's going to be inherently emotional. That's the flip-side to the previous chapter about responsibility versus emotions. It's okay to be human. It's okay to feel.

Let's take a look at real life.

Usually the clients who break down in tears in front of me are the clients who have goals that are really important to them, and they are *doing the most work*. Now, because they've done the most work, they've already gotten lots of results. It's just that they aren't seeing results right now.

I'll get a client who's plateaued for two weeks, totally torn up because she has a really important goal—a 10- or 20-year high school reunion, a decade birthday, a wedding, an anniversary. She hasn't lost any weight in two weeks. She's concerned about her progress.

What we can do is bring her back to all the ground she's already taken—

- All of the meals she's changed
- The fact that she is planning and preparing her meals and is keeping a food journal
- And the fact that before these two weeks when she plateaued, she lost a pound every week for eight straight weeks

It still comes back to responsibility—but responsibility works both ways. Sometimes it's about being responsible for all of the actions you're already doing right.

If you've been doing everything right and have been getting results, and then you plateau, you've got to recognize everything you've been doing right. And if you continue to do everything right, the plateau won't last long.

If you hit a plateau that sticks for longer than two weeks, it's time to reassess.

1. *Am I really as on point as I think? Check your journal. Re-plan and prepare.*
2. *Is it time to bring up the quality of my carbs and fat?*
3. *Is it time to take a look at advanced food strategies?*

There's the assessment you always have to make: Am I doing everything right, and have just hit a little plateau? Or is it time to reassess my strategies?

Either way, funny as this sounds, it doesn't reflect on you as a person. Sometimes it's just time to reassess your strategy.

When I have a client who's crying, here is what I do. First, I let her cry, and hear her out. It's normal and human to have feelings. We just aren't going to get crushed by them.

Second, we take stock of what strategies she's using and the results she's gotten. Like the example above, most of the time people lose sight of how much ground they've taken since they started. I always like to go back and remind clients of two things.

1. How much weight or bodyfat percentage or clothes sizes have you lost since you started?
2. How much better at meal planning and executing have you gotten? And with this question, I'll go meal by meal. Every meal they've gotten better at is a victory.

I might ask, "Did you ever have protein at breakfast before we started?"

They'll usually laugh and say, "I never even had breakfast before we've started!"

It's one of those funny things, that as humans we have a tendency to only look at the absolute end goal as being a victory. It's easy to forget we'll never get there without hundreds of little victories we stack on top of each other.

There's a Cherokee parable that goes like this—

An old Cherokee is teaching his grandson about life.
"A fight is going on inside me," he said to the boy.
"It's a terrible fight and it's between two wolves. One is evil—he is anger, envy, sorrow, regret, greed, arrogance,

THE DAY I BECAME THE BEST FAT-LOSS TRAINER IN THE WORLD

self-pity, guilt, resentment, inferiority, lies, false pride, superiority, and ego."

He continued, *"The other is good—he is joy, peace, love, hope, serenity, humility, kindness, benevolence, empathy, generosity, truth, compassion, and faith. The same fight is going on inside you—and inside every other person, too."*

The grandson thought about it for a minute and then asked his grandfather, "Which wolf will win?"

The old Cherokee simply replied, "The one you feed."

And I often think about that while coaching my clients about food and the way they look at their bodies. It's always a process. We change all of these little habits, and we take ground in this weight-loss adventure a pound a time. It all adds up.

But the question is, how are you going to feel about it?

You can look at how far you have to go to get to your eventual goal, and 'feed the wolf' that you're not good enough yet, that fat loss is hard and complicated, and that this will take a long, long time.

Or, you can look at how many food habits you've changed, and the pounds you've lost, and 'feed the wolf' of your success with your body, of how much better you look, that fat loss is simple and mechanical, and that you're making great progress.

NINJA SKILLS FOR FOOD

People who are lean are in the habit of being lean. They've practiced eating lean—like a skill. And they've got a lot of reps of practice in for that skill.

You have the body you have because you've practiced eating a certain way. The more you practice eating a certain way, the better you get at it. Call it habit, skill, practice, or just straight-up brain science.

Brain science is remarkably simple: The brain gets more efficient at things it practices.

Eating like a rock star is a skill. The more you practice it, the better you get. But it's not just any skill—it's a ninja skill. You need to practice it like a kung fu master practices kung fu.

Take one meal at a time, and practice that meal. Practice preparing for it, cooking ahead of time for it, portioning it, and setting aside time to eat it.

The Four Ninja Food Skills to Practice

1. **Shopping Ahead of Time**
2. **Prepping and Cooking Ahead of Time**
3. **Portioning the Meal Ahead of Time**
4. **Scheduling Time for the Meal Ahead of Time**

Each of these skills needs to be practiced. You will record how you do in your simple food journal.

The more often you practice these skills, the better you get at them. You will literally rewire your brain to eat better.

You should practice one meal per week. Like a ninja or a kung fu master—work on one skill to mastery. Practice lots of reps of that meal. Get a rep in for that meal every week.

Master that one meal—for example, breakfast on Monday morning. Spend your main effort that week on shopping for breakfast on Monday, prepping for breakfast on Monday, portioning breakfast on Monday ahead of time, and even scheduling how to wake up early enough to eat breakfast on Monday.

Only after having mastered breakfast on Monday do you move on to breakfast on Tuesday.

YOUR TWO MOST IMPORTANT WORKOUTS

Your two most important 'workouts' each week are—

1. Journal Review, Meal Planning, and Shopping for Food
2. Preparing, Cooking, and Portioning Food

The initial idea was for the workout week to look like the following, with every other 'workout' being food-related.

> MONDAY: Hard Workout
> TUESDAY: Medium Workout
> **WEDNESDAY: Journal Review, Meal Planning, and Shopping**
> **THURSDAY: Preparing, Cooking, and Portioning**
> FRIDAY: Easy Workout
> SATURDAY: Off
> SUNDAY: Off

But that causes too much gear-grinding in most people's heads. Everyone thinks about each week starting with Monday. And that's one of the reasons people put their most important workouts on Monday. The revised workout week takes advantage of that.

> **SUNDAY: Journal Review, Meal Planning, and Shopping**
> **MONDAY: Meal Preparing, Cooking, and Portioning**
> TUESDAY: Hard Workout
> WEDNESDAY: Off
> THURSDAY: Medium Workout
> FRIDAY: Off
> SATURDAY: Easy Workout

*Note: Usually people end up doing a mini food prep again on Wednesday or Friday also.

Your Monday 'workout' is your food preparation. It's your most important workout of the week, *and we're smart enough to put the most important things first.*

Until you make the switch in your head that food preparation is the most important workout of the week, you'll forever be caught in the trap of trying to get your results through workouts. And we know that workouts will never get you there.

Write this down:

Working out and getting stronger is *required*, but it is *not sufficient* for hitting your fat-loss goals.

You already know this. Years of experience have already shown you this.

We just don't want to believe it. The truth is, just going to the gym and working out but getting no results is more comfortable than making changes to how we eat.

And that's why we make small changes…over time.

JOSH

CHAPTER 7

THE ELEVEN HABITS

HABIT 1	PLAN	Plan your meals for the week, either on Sunday or Monday. Grid your free meals ahead of time.
HABIT 2	SHOP	Go shopping for the food on your plan, either on Sunday or Monday.
HABIT 3	COOK	Prepare, cook, and portion the food on your plan on Sunday or Monday.
HABIT 4	JOURNAL	Keep a daily food journal. Review your food journal weekly, either on Sunday or Monday.
HABIT 5	PROTEIN	Make sure you're getting protein at every meal. Shoot for three-quarters of a gram of protein per pound of target bodyweight, per day.
HABIT 6	CALORIES	Review your food journal for total calories consumed. Compare your total calories to your weekly weight change.
HABIT 7	SLOW	Eat slowly. A meal should take at least 15 minutes.
HABIT 8	80%	Stop eating when you're 80% full.
HABIT 9	HEALTHY FAT	Make sure you're getting good fats at most meals. Add good fat to meals you normally feel hungry after and see if that helps you feel full.
HABIT 10	QUALITY CARBS	Check the quality of your carbohydrates. Are you getting most of your carbohydrates from brown rice, quinoa, brown rice pasta, sprouted-grain bread, fruit, and vegetables?
HABIT 11	GRATITUDE	Keep a gratitude journal—every day, write down one thing you like about your body, are proud of about your body, or are grateful for about your body.

BONUS HABIT 12: YOU'RE A SEA-MONKEY!

If there were two more bonus habits, they would be water and sleep. Lack of either one is going to make you extra hungry.

The first extra habit is water intake. Water is this magical elixir that transforms your body! Okay, not really. It's actually the other way around: It's totally essential, and if you don't drink it, you'll be weirdly hungry all the time. People can completely sabotage fat loss just by feeling extra hungry when they're dehydrated.

Remember those dry sea-monkeys you could just add water to? That's you. With water you spring to life! Without it, you're just a crusty, lifeless shrimp in a plastic bag. I'll be honest, I don't really have anywhere for this metaphor to go, but I figured you'd be more likely to remember to drink water if I gave you something silly to think about.

Remember, if you're dehydrated, you're going to be weirdly hungry all the time. You don't want to be hungry all the time, so you don't want to be dehydrated.

It's generally accepted that you can tell if you're dehydrated by your pee. If you don't ever pee, you're dehydrated. If you pee and it's dark yellow, you're dehydrated. If you pee and it's straw-colored or clear, congratulations! You have enough water in you to sustain human life and normal body function.

BONUS HABIT 13: DON'T STARE AT THE SUN!

The second bonus habit is sleep. If you're chronically sleep deprived, you'll feel like you have super-powers when you add more sleep. And if you don't have enough sleep, you'll crave sugar and starch, and you won't want protein or vegetables.

The main problem with lack of sleep is that those who have serious issues with it are usually people who can't do anything about it, like nurses or doctors who work crazy hours, or moms whose kids wake them up all night. In those cases, you really just need to be aware that on nights when you don't get enough sleep, you're going to crave fast food, and you're not going to want the good food you planned. Know that, and get your head ready ahead of time.

On the flip side, if you're sleep deprived because you're staying up watching late-night TV, you get to choose between TV and fat-loss results. Our bodies like to wake us up with the sun and go to bed at night. Unfortunately, screens (TV, phones, computers, e-readers, tablets, pads) are just bright enough and interesting enough to keep us awake way too late. If you want to get more sleep, stop staring at the sun—turn off the screens earlier.

THE ELEVEN HABITS IN REAL LIFE: IT'S MESSY

The mistake I made with the first two versions of the habit section was that it was too…clean. Too simple. Things never actually work like that.

So there are several strategies I use.

The eleven habits are legit. And you could, theoretically, just work on one per week and have everything work out dandy. The only issue is, I've never actually done that. I use a certain sequence of habits with some clients, and another sequence of habits with others. And some people will use one sequence of habits for a while, and then need to switch to another sequence.

That's real life. Things change. You have different needs at different times. You may get great results with one of the sequences at one time, and then later stall and need something a different sequence offers. That's okay. That's what this really looks like.

The commonalities are that in all of them, we only focus on one habit per week. And many of the habits overlap. Here's a glance at our habit strategies.

1. *By the Numbers Strategy (aka the Just Gimme the Results!)*
2. *Planning and Preparing Strategy*
3. *Win One Meal at a Time Strategy*
4. *Fullness Leads to Fat Loss Strategy*
5. *Mindfulness Strategy*
6. *Maintenance (aka the Let's Talk about Something Else Strategy)*

THE *BY THE NUMBERS* STRATEGY, AKA JUST GIMME THE RESULTS!

This strategy is where online food journals really shine, because you can see the numbers so plainly.

This is always our first stop when coaching food. If we can keep it this simple, let's do it. We coach you straight off of the macronutrient content and calories in your online food journal.

It's really this simple: Start with three-quarters of a gram of protein per pound of bodyweight (this is the protein habit). Then get the calories to where you are losing a pound per week (this is the calories habit). Then, as a bonus, we increase healthy fats a little, and reduce carbohydrates a little (this is the macro habit).

Secondary habits we can work on include making sure the quality of the carbs and fats works. Usually it's my experience that if the numbers are right, people aren't doing crazy things with the quality, but just in case, we can check on that.

If you already have the shopping, preparing, cooking, and planning habits down, this is the fastest way to results. This means you're already doing habits one, two, and three, so we start with habit four.

I start everyone with this model, and then see if planning, preparing, and cooking are issues. About 50% of clients can just take the *By the Numbers Strategy* and run with it.

BY THE NUMBERS: FIRST SEQUENCE

HABIT 4	JOURNAL	Keep and review your food journal.
HABIT 5	PROTEIN	Make sure you're getting protein at every meal. Shoot for three-quarters of a gram of protein per pound of target bodyweight, per day.
HABIT 6	CALORIES	Review your food journal for total calories consumed. Compare your total calories to your weekly weight change.

Each strategy has two sequences of habits, including some of The Eleven Habits, and excluding others. Pick the strategy that hits what you need the most, and that strategy will focus you on the sequences of habits that will make the most difference for you right now.

Rotate through the three habits of the first sequence, focusing on one each week.

When you're effective with the habits in the first sequence, move on to the habits in the second sequence.

BY THE NUMBERS: SECOND SEQUENCE

HABIT 9	HEALTHY FAT	Make sure you're getting good fats at most meals. Add good fat to meals you normally feel hungry after and see if that helps you feel full.
HABIT 10	QUALITY CARBS	Check the quality of your carbohydrates. Are you getting most of your carbohydrates from brown rice, quinoa, brown rice pasta, sprouted-grain bread, fruit, and vegetables?

If you can get the protein and the calories right, you can get results. Your journal is your scorecard for your protein and calories, and if it's accurate, your results will always match the numbers in your journal…eventually.

Secondarily, as the quality of your fat and carbohydrates improves, it'll supercharge the results you're getting from getting the calories and protein right.

Look, we know that the master key is this—

FAT LOSS HAPPENS ON MONDAY RESULTS KEY

YOUR SCALE WEIGHT	Quantity of food you eat (calories)
YOUR BODYFAT PERCENTAGE	Quality of food you eat and how strong you are

So the *By the Numbers Strategy* is to track those numbers, and adjust for maximum results. It's the fastest and most direct route to awesome results. And a lot of times, it's just that simple.

But for when it isn't, we have other strategies.

THE PLANNING AND PREPARING STRATEGY

This strategy can exist in an online food journal or paper food journal, but the rubber really meets the road in your day planner or calendar app.

Like the *By the Numbers Strategy*, we're only going to focus on one habit per week. Here we're working with the first three habits, all having to do with planning, shopping, cooking, and then journaling how you did with the planning, shopping, and cooking.

PLANNING AND PREPARING: FIRST SEQUENCE		
HABIT 1	PLAN	Plan your meals for the week, either on Sunday or Monday.
HABIT 2	SHOP	Go shopping according to your plan, either on Sunday or Monday.
HABIT 3	COOK	Prepare, cook, and portion your food every Sunday or Monday.
HABIT 4	JOURNAL	Keep a food journal daily. Review your food journal weekly, either on Sunday or Monday.

Each strategy has two sequences of habits, including some of The Eleven Habits and excluding others. Pick the strategy that hits what you need the most, and that strategy will focus you on the sequences of habits that will make the most difference for you right now.

Rotate through the four habits of the first sequence, focusing on one each week.

When you're effective with the habits in the first sequence, move on to the habits in the second sequence.

PLANNING AND PREPARING: SECOND SEQUENCE		
HABIT 5	PROTEIN	Make sure you're getting protein at every meal. Shoot for three-quarters of a gram of protein per pound of target bodyweight, per day.
HABIT 6	CALORIES	Review your food journal for total calories consumed. Compare your total calories to your weekly weight change.
HABIT 9	HEALTHY FAT	Make sure you're getting good fats at most meals. Add good fat to meals you normally feel hungry after and see if that helps you feel full.
HABIT 10	QUALITY CARBS	Check the quality of your carbohydrates. Are you getting most of your carbohydrates from brown rice, quinoa, brown rice pasta, sprouted-grain bread, fruit, and vegetables?

PLANNING IS USUALLY NUMBER ONE

For a long time I hung my hat on food journaling. I didn't realize until later that the food journal was primarily my tool as a coach to know where to impact the clients' plans. And that's what really made the difference—*the plans*.

Once I began to have clients only come to me for food-journal coaching, it became immediately clear that what most people need is just to plan things ahead of time. That's the number one habit.

A food journal is still supremely important; after all, you're your own coach—and you need your food journal to see what happened. You'll use it to make the next week's plan.

If you think about it like personal finance, it'll make sense. Your budget is your plan, and your checkbook is your food journal.

Most of my food-journal clients do daily plans. Every night they do a quick plan for the next day.

Note: People don't always follow the plan 100%, but they have a plan.

Three things you always need to know—

> **Plan:** *What's the plan for tomorrow?*
> **Action:** *What am I eating today? The plan I made yesterday is happening right now!*
> **Food Journal:** *Did I follow the plan yesterday?*

Jim Rohn once said, to paraphrase, that the plan is the most important thing. If you don't have a plan for today, today is lost. Start planning tomorrow.

The cool part about having a plan is that it's like seeing the future. You can take a look at the obstacles that might come up tomorrow, and handle them ahead of time. Do you need to go to the market? That's a huge stumbling block for a lot of people—they fail on their nutrition every day, not realizing that going to the market and getting quality food is more important than going to the gym.

In Bill Phillip's *Eating For Life Food Journal*, he says most people know all of the obstacles they are going to run into in their meal plans if they just think things through. He had a very simple exercise that's genius. Look at this—

What are the three biggest obstacles I'm going to run into with food?

1. _____
2. _____
3. _____

What are three structures I can put in place to overcome those three obstacles?

1. _____
2. _____
3. _____

The whole idea of a structure is that you put something in the plan or in the physical world to help you overcome the obstacle. For example, if you know your spouse isn't going to want to eat on the plan, that isn't a surprise—you know that ahead of time. A structure you can put in place is to come up with a list of meals that both fit your plan and that your spouse will like. Or figure out how to modify the portions. Or figure out how you can both eat different things and be okay with it. These are all things you can plan ahead of time to make this work.

If you have to eat out often for work, a structure could mean looking at the menu ahead of time and picking what you want before you arrive hungry. Find the best option available on the menu so you can just order that when you get there.

You can see when the problem is shopping…if you have a plan.

If you have social events, you can think those through ahead of time. Priceless!

If you're preparing to eat out, you can plan what you're going to eat. If you're visiting family, you can plan what you're going to say when it comes to food choices. If you're making dinner, you can plan when you're going to make dinner.

And all of these things, seen ahead of time, can be changed. Maybe you just need to make tomorrow night a free meal. If you know that ahead of time, you can make it part of the plan instead of feeling like a failure when you cave.

You have all the power if you have a plan.

THE *WIN ONE MEAL AT A TIME* STRATEGY

Coach one meal at a time (breakfasts/lunches/dinners).

One meal per week—

- Focus on finding recipes for those times
- Work on planning for those times
- Work on preparation for those times

- Works for anyone who says 'I always struggle with XYZ meal'

WIN ONE MEAL AT A TIME: SEQUENCE ONE

HABITS 1–3	BREAKFAST	On Sunday or Monday: Plan, shop, and cook all of your breakfasts for the week.
HABITS 1–3	LUNCH	On Sunday or Monday: Plan, shop, and cook all of your lunches for the week.
HABITS 1–3	DINNER	On Sunday or Monday: Plan, shop, and cook all of your dinners for the week.
HABIT 4	JOURNAL	Keep a food journal daily. Review your food journal weekly, either on Sunday or Monday.

Again, each strategy has two sequences of habits, including some of The Eleven Habits and excluding others. Pick the strategy that hits what you need the most, and that strategy will focus you on the sequences of habits that will make the most difference for you right now.

Rotate through the four habits of the first sequence, focusing on one each week.

When you're effective with the habits in the first sequence, move on to the habits in the second sequence.

WILL CHANGING ONE MEAL REALLY MAKE A DIFFERENCE?

In the beginning it may seem silly to work on breakfasts, or only changing breakfast on Monday. But don't think about it as changing one meal. *Think about how changing breakfast on Monday means changing 52 breakfasts per year.*

This is how we make long-term changes.

One other note—if you get stuck anywhere along the path or if you need to back up, that's fine. It doesn't matter if it takes you one week, six weeks, or 24 weeks to master a daily meal. You've still changed your life forever. No matter how long it takes, every change you make will show up in your body.

This is not nearly as sexy of an idea as 10-minute abs or insane crush-you-to-death workouts. But this is what works in real life: *small changes, with consistency, over time.*

Work on that one meal each week. Each time it comes around, get better at planning for it, shopping for it, and cooking for it. It's about mastery.

Don't move on to mastering breakfast on Saturday if you're still struggling with breakfast on Tuesday. One

WIN ONE MEAL AT A TIME: SEQUENCE TWO

HABITS 5 AND 6	BREAKFAST	Make sure you're getting protein at every breakfast. Compare your calories at breakfast to your weekly weight change.
HABITS 5 AND 6	LUNCH	Make sure you're getting protein at every lunch. Compare your calories at lunch to your weekly weight change.
HABITS 6 AND 6	DINNER	Make sure you're getting protein at every dinner. Compare your calories at dinner to your weekly weight change.
HABITS 9 AND 10	BREAKFAST	Make sure you're getting good fats at breakfast, and check fullness after breakfast. Check the quality of your carbohydrates at breakfast.
HABITS 9 AND 10	LUNCH	Make sure you're getting good fats at lunch, and check fullness after lunch. Check the quality of your carbohydrates at lunch.
HABITS 9 AND 10	DINNER	Make sure you're getting good fats at dinner, and check fullness after dinner. Check the quality of your carbohydrates at dinner.

step at a time…be where you are. It's okay to be new at this—this is probably the first reality-based fat-loss program you've ever done.

If you're on the other side and discover that the first week you end up changing 12 meals—a whole bunch of breakfasts *and* lunches!—that's totally fine, too. In fact, that's awesome. But when you look back at the week to decide whether it was a successful fat-loss week, only look at the meals that were your habit change for the week.

In other words, if the first week you changed a whole bunch of breakfasts and lunches but only needed to work on breakfast, only review breakfast. Did you get at least one breakfast better than when you started? And next week, did you improve at least one lunch from when you started?

That's why I don't care if you change one breakfast the first week or all of the breakfasts. It just needs to be a little better than the last time you planned breakfast—at least one meal better. You could change your whole meal plan in three weeks, or 18 weeks.

THE *FULLNESS LEADS TO FAT LOSS* STRATEGY

With our fullness strategy, you can use a paper or an online food journal. A paper journal can be a great way to take notes about how you felt. An online food journal will give you more precise protein, carbohydrates, and fat percentages.

Many people find that eating slowly is completely game changing. Sometimes in the initial consultation when I ask clients if they eat quickly, they start laughing. This is a red flag.

Past eating speed, it's also a matter of getting the macronutrients right. We're going to hit this with a three-pronged attack.

We're going to play with the ratios. This isn't one of the habits we're focusing on, other than protein intake, so it warrants special mention.

Most people feel more full with a higher percentage of protein.

Some people feel more full with a higher percentage of carbohydrates.

Some people feel more full with a higher percentage of fat.

We look for quality of carbohydrates. It's no surprise that people feel more full after eating an apple than they do after a candy bar. And yet almost no one plans their meals this way. Always ask yourself: *Is this meal going to make me more hungry or more full?*

Healthy fats are important. Fat triggers feelings of fullness, so this one is a no-brainer.

As far as the ratios of macronutrients go, this is easy to fix. Take a look at your food journal and notice which meals you feel full after, and after which meals you feel hungry. Make a special daily note about fullness in your journal, and when you do your weekly review, let this influence your future meal decisions.

Look for a few things in your journal—

Do I feel more full with meals that have more protein?
Do I feel more full with healthy fats?
Do I feel more full when I get lots of vegetables?
Do I feel more full after quality carbohydrates?
Do I feel extra hungry when I don't get protein?
Do I feel extra hungry when I don't get healthy fats?
Do I feel extra hungry after refined carbohydrates?
Do I feel extra hungry after eating sugar?
Do I feel extra hungry after having juice or soda?
Do I feel extra hungry after missing a meal or an afternoon snack?

Ask those questions of your journal, and let your notes be your guide.

FULLNESS LEADS TO FAT LOSS: SEQUENCE ONE		
HABIT 7	SLOW	Eat slowly. A meal should take at least 15 minutes.
HABIT 4	JOURNAL	Keep and review a food journal. Note which meals you feel full for a long time after, and which meals you feel hungry after.
HABIT 5	PROTEIN	Make sure you're getting protein at every meal. Shoot for three-quarters of a gram of protein per pound of target bodyweight, per day.
HABIT 9	HEALTHY FAT	Make sure you're getting good fats at most meals. Add good fat to meals you normally feel hungry after and see if that helps you feel full.
HABIT 10	QUALITY CARBS	Check the quality of your carbohydrates. Are you getting most of your carbohydrates from brown rice, quinoa, brown rice pasta, sprouted-grain bread, fruit, and vegetables?

*Again, each strategy has two sequences of habits, including some of The Eleven Habits and excluding others. Pick the strategy that hits what you need the most, and that strategy will focus you on the sequences of habits that will make the most difference for you right now.

Rotate through the five habits of the first sequence, focusing on one habit each week.

When you're effective with the habits in the first sequence, move on to the habits in the second sequence.

FULLNESS LEADS TO FAT LOSS: SEQUENCE TWO		
HABIT 8	80%	Stop eating when you're 80% full.
HABIT 6	CALORIES	Review your food journal for total calories consumed. Compare your total calories to your weekly weight change.

The first habit of the second sequence is to stop at 80% full. If there's a punchline to this strategy, that's going to be it: *We're going to do everything in our power to have you feel as full as possible, and then we're going to stop before you get totally full.*

Unfortunately, people have confused being 'stuffed' with being full. And so, especially in the beginning, the normal, healthy, proper portions aren't going to get you to 100% full—aka stuffed.

Most of the people who are 'naturally skinny' and 'don't ever have to diet or think about food' are just people who naturally stop at 80% full. We could argue if that's genetics, or that they were never told by their parents to clean their plates, or whatever. Regardless of where the habit came from, *you're going to have to practice stopping at 80% full.*

Think about it as if you're training yourself to eat like someone who's naturally lean.

Most things having to do with hunger are just habits. Start the long-term process of training yourself to make food choices that feel more filling, and then be done at 80% full.

The last habit, of course, is checking to make sure you're eating calories that help you actually get results. Another way you can think about fullness and calories is that usually feeling 100% full means your body will stay the same, and feeling 80% full sets your body up to lose fat.

As always, check your calories against results to verify your success with the strategy.

THE *MINDFULNESS* STRATEGY

First off, with this strategy you'll use a paper food journal, not an online food journal. This is going to have a lot to do with how you feel, and you need room to write. Also, this strategy deliberately doesn't look at the macronutrient numbers, but instead mainly focuses on food quality.

I think everyone should spend some time in this strategy. Some people get amazing results here and are able to use this strategy all the way until they hit their goals. Other people may get some great results here and shift their mindsets, but then may plateau in results and need to switch to one of the other strategies to get to the next level of results.

Feel free to switch between strategies to get what you need, when you need it. It's normal for your needs to change as you progress and change. You won't be the same person a year from now as you are at the start of this journey.

Instead of writing a lot about this strategy, I'm going to instead include an email I wrote to one of my coaching clients, as it gives a lot of life to this strategy. You'll find the letter right below the habit notations below.

MINDFULNESS: SEQUENCE ONE

HABIT 11	GRATITUDE	Keep a gratitude journal—every day write down one thing you like about your body, are proud of about your body, or are grateful about your body.
HABIT 7	SLOW	Eat slowly. A meal should take at least 15 minutes.
HABIT 8	80%	Stop eating when you're 80% full.
HABIT 4	JOURNAL	Keep and review your food journal. Write down how you felt, in terms of energy fullness, after each meal.

Again, each strategy has two sequences of habits, including some of The Eleven Habits and excluding others. Pick the strategy that hits what you need the most, and that strategy will focus you on the sequences of habits that will make the most difference for you right now.

Rotate through the four habits of the first sequence, focusing on one habit each week.

When you're effective with the habits in the first sequence, move on to the habits in the second sequence.

MINDFULNESS: SEQUENCE TWO

HABIT 5	PROTEIN	Make sure you're getting protein at every meal. Shoot for three-quarters of a gram of protein per pound of target bodyweight, per day.
HABIT 9	HEALTHY FAT	Make sure you're getting good fats at most meals. Add good fat to meals you normally feel hungry after and see if that helps you feel full.
HABIT 10	QUALITY CARBS	Check the quality of your carbohydrates. Are you getting most of your carbohydrates from brown rice, quinoa, brown rice pasta, sprouted-grain bread, fruit, and vegetables?

Here is the email I wrote to one of my food-journal coaching client who had a concern about body image, her relationship to food, and health. She was also concerned about how being obsessed with body image might impact her kids, and wondered if she should stop tracking food and instead just focus on health. Notice how it totally maps onto the Mindfulness Strategy.

This is absolutely THE BEST inquiry to be in!

Three things.

- We can totally work on having a better relationship toward food!
- We absolutely can shift the context from weight to health!
- Both of those are a cop-out for not tracking!

Tracking

I like to use money as a metaphor, because everyone can relate to it, and it's easy to count.

Some people are obsessed with money at the cost of everything else in their lives. Obviously that's bad.

Some people never think about money—they don't balance the checkbook; they overspend and rack up debt. For basic financial health, that doesn't work.

Tracking food is all about *context*. When people come to me and say they want to eat healthier, we *absolutely* track their food.

Your food journal is your checkbook register for your food. If you want to pay your bills, you need to know what's in your bank account. It would be crazy to never look at your bank account and just hope for the best.

Relationship to Food

As far as having a relationship to food—here is the fun but hard part: *It's all made up.* We could argue about what's been given to you by the media, your peers, and your family, but what you have now, wherever you got it, it is now your job to either keep feeding it, or to feed it something else.

For the relationship to food I like to use that old Cherokee Indian story I told you on page 28.

It's the same for body image.

Wolf #1: Talking to yourself about *hating* parts of your body, constant *comparison* to others, trying to *dominate* your body, trying to *use* your body as a tool for acceptance.

Wolf #2: *Appreciating* all your body does, *focusing* on your favorite parts of your body, *practicing gratitude* for your body, *cutting off* negative body thoughts that pop up—they never stop popping up, you just stop feeding them—*being proud* of your body, and *being inspired* by what your body can do.

And we can play the same game about food.

Wolf #1: Being *resentful* of eating healthy food, *feeding* negative thoughts of missing out because of not eating crap, *justifying* being *lazy* about healthy food, talking about how *hard* it is to eat healthy, *complaining* about how healthy food isn't what you really want.

Wolf #2: *Appreciating* how healthy food makes you feel, *focusing* on your favorite healthy foods, *practicing gratitude* for getting to eat healthy food, *cutting off* negative food thoughts that pop up—they never stop popping up, you just stop feeding them—*being proud* of eating in a way that fuels a strong healthy body, and *being inspired by* what eating good food does for you.

There's a really great book on cognitive therapy for body image and food called *The Beck Diet Solution*. The short version is this: Mostly we have a bunch of really crappy preprogrammed thoughts and ideas about food and body image, and we need to purposefully cut ourselves off from those and practice new thoughts. And *The Beck Diet Solution* has a bunch of structures for doing that.

Here is what I am going to have you start with—

1. Write your food journal entries in an actual paper journal instead of using an online journal.
2. In your journal, in addition to what you ate, write down how you felt—if eating that way made you feel better or worse in terms of things like energy and fullness. You can also journal any other feelings you had about food each day.
3. For your gratitude practice, each day you'll finish your journal entry with one thing you really love about your body. It can be anything, but really *do the work on this one*. Think of something. It could be the way your hair looks that day, or it could be that you're happy you could do lunges, or you're happy you have eyes to see the day's beautiful sunset. Whatever it is, figure out something to write. Gratitude about your body is going to be one of your most important disciplines.

4. Focus on that word *discipline*. One of the quickest and easiest ways to feeling good about your body is to develop discipline.
   — Discipline about healthy food
   — Discipline about maintaining a strong body through your workouts
   — Discipline about daily gratitude

Focus on your disciplines more than anything else. People actually have healthier feelings and thoughts about their bodies from their *disciplines* than they do from any kind of results.

This is the BEST kind of work you can be doing!

Important note on mental health: Most people have some degree of negative mental chatter about body image, food, and fitness, either from time to time or even a lot of the time. And most people can use the two-wolf metaphor to realize they don't necessarily get to choose the thoughts that pop up (thanks a lot, media!), but they can choose which ones to feed. And through that, you can slowly chip away at disempowering contexts for your body, food, and fitness, and create or feed empowering contexts. But if you get stuck here and feel crushed by body image or your relationship with food, consider checking with a therapist or counselor. I've had clients work with these habits and simultaneously work with a mental health professional, and it's amazingly awesome.

THE MAINTENANCE STRATEGY

Most people really have no idea what to do after they hit their fat-loss goals. Here are two options.

- Find a fitness, strength, endurance, movement, or play goal.
- Put food and workouts on autopilot for a while.

If you're looking for a new goal, there are all kinds of things you can do depending on what's fun for you. You could do anything from focusing on snowboarding to learning to breakdance to whatever you want.

Or you could set a performance goal—increase your strength or endurance. For ideas on strength and endurance goals, see the section about structured refeeds on page 74. You get the picture: Find some other activity-related goal, and work toward that. Put the food priority on the back burner for now.

The other option is to put the food and workouts on autopilot. What!?!? Heresy! Everyone is supposed to make fitness their number one priority forever, right?

Not really. You might have work commitments that ebb and flow; you might have kids who are sometimes in school and sometimes on summer vacation; you might be going to school. There are a million things that ebb and flow in life, and they require more or less time.

It's okay to have your workout and diet priorities flow in seasons. This is natural. Motivation moves in cycles. Your time and energy moves in cycles. It's okay to have times when you get into your workouts and when you pay some attention to your food, but when neither is a major priority.

In that case, the *Pull Your Weight* workouts beginning on page 101 are reasonable workouts to just do two or three times per week, and the maintenance habits are perfect to keep an eye on food without spending a lot of attention on it.

Whichever direction you decide to go, your food habits can look like this—

	MAINTENANCE STRATEGY	
HABIT 5	PROTEIN	Make sure you're getting protein at every meal. Shoot for three-quarters of a gram of protein per pound of target bodyweight, per day.
HABIT 7	SLOW	Eat slowly. Each meal or serving should take at least 15 minutes.
HABIT 8	80%	Stop eating when you're 80% full.
HABIT 11	GRATITUDE	Keep a gratitude journal—every day, write down one thing you like about your body, are proud of about your body, or are grateful about your body.

WHICH STRATEGY IS FOR YOU?	
Start here	BY THE NUMBERS STRATEGY
If planning is a challenge	PLANNING AND PREPARING STRATEGY
If certain meals are challenging	WIN ONE MEAL AT A TIME STRATEGY
If you feel hungry all the time	FULLNESS LEADS TO FAT LOSS STRATEGY
If relationship with food is challenging	MINDFULNESS STRATEGY
After you've hit your fat-loss goals	MAINTENANCE STRATEGY

WHICH STRATEGY SHOULD YOU USE?

Whichever strategy looks the most different from what you're doing right now will probably yield the most striking results.

I'm always looking for what's missing that will take a client's food plan to a higher level. That's what there is to look for—which of these models is going to add what you're missing?

The cool thing about fat loss is that it's so totally clear: You either lose fat—*the diet is working*—or you don't—*it's not working*.

All of these models should work unless you're just repeating things you've already done. In other words, they already worked, but you've achieved all of the results you're going to get out of that model. All of these models work. It's really about which one will work the fastest for YOU.

We started with the most common strategy, and worked our way through the others. You could do the same thing: Start with the first one and see where you struggle.

And if you don't struggle with any of those, just keep rocking the first model until you've lost all the fat you want to lose, and you're lean, hot, strong, sexy, and awesome.

THE POINT OF THIS IS MASTERY

Most people suck at food choices, and at planning, cooking, reviewing, and logging. And that colors all of their results forever.

The idea here is to work on one habit at a time. You'll have a sequence of three or four habits that you'll keep repeating. With each week you repeat a habit, the concept is to take it a step deeper, to get better at it.

> *People drastically underestimate the skill involved in planning.*
> *People drastically underestimate the skill involved in cooking.*
> *People drastically underestimate the skill involved in keeping and reviewing a food journal.*

These are things that are worth putting time into, and to slowly measure your progress.

I have people work on either one habit per week, such as planning, or one group of meals at a time, like breakfast, but I only grade them on *one meal at a time*.

For example, let's say you grid out your meals for a week. Fifteen of your meals sucked, and seven meals were on plan. This week the habit to work on is planning, and because you plan, this week only 14 meals suck and eight meals were on plan. Is this week successful? OF COURSE! This week was a HUGE win!

And then next week when you're working on cooking, hopefully working on cooking takes you from 14 sucky meals and eight on-plan meals, to 13 sucky meals and nine on-plan meals.

Sure, the goal of that cooking habit is to cook all of the meals for the week on Sunday or Monday, but it's a process. I just want you to be better at that habit than you were before. It's easy to see on the grid, and easy to count. And if you count the sucky meals and the on-plan meals, and the on-plan meals go up by at least one, you've taken major ground.

Small moves repeated weekly, actually stick.

FOOD PLAY

The first four habits have to do with food, and changing what you eat.

It should be obvious that eating what you eat gets you the body you have now. And if you want to take your body in a different direction, you need to make different food choices.

Eating at 'the next level' sounds all well and good, except that means you're buying things you haven't bought before and you're cooking things you haven't cooked before. It's going to be new. New can be exciting and fun, or it can be scary and overwhelming.

Let's make it fun. We're going to play games.

HABIT 1	PLAN	Plan your meals for the week, either on Sunday or Monday.
HABIT 2	SHOP	Go shopping according to your plan, either on Sunday or Monday.
HABIT 3	COOK	Prepare, cook, and portion your food every Monday.
HABIT 4	JOURNAL	Keep a food journal daily. Review your food journal weekly, either on Sunday or Monday.

Planning Games

Planning is a fun habit to play with, because it leads to everything else. Here are some planning games you can play.

- Find a new recipe
- Buy a new cookbook
- Ask your fittest friend for a favorite healthy meal
- Search the web for a new vegetable
- Search the web for a new kind of fat
- Search the web for a new carbohydrate
- Search the web for a new fruit
- Search for the healthiest place to eat out in your town
- Search for a cheap healthy place to eat out in your town

Shopping Games

Shopping games are where the rubber meets the road. Buying new stuff can be an adventure—what is this new food? How do I know if it's ripe? How long will it last? Do I even know where to get it?

- Buy a new vegetable
- Buy a new kind of fat
- Buy a new pseudo-grain or sprouted grain
- Buy a new fruit
- Shop someplace new, like a farmer's market, co-op, or health-food store

Shopping games can be really cool. People talk about how they love to travel and see new places. You can have the same kind of exploration fun with food. It's amazing how interesting a new kind of food can be in planning for, shopping for, and preparing. On top of that, at the local farmer's market you can find a lot of that small community feel we often look forward to when traveling.

Here is a list of some foods you can get started exploring that may be new to you.

- Kale—try blending up a little in a protein shake
- Clarified butter—try cooking with it
- Coconut oil—try cooking with it
- Avocado oil—try cooking with it or using it for salad dressing
- Extra-virgin olive oil—try three parts oil to one part balsamic vinegar with salt and pepper instead of your usual salad dressing
- Quinoa—instead of pasta, bread, tortillas, or rice
- Spouted-grain bread—instead of normal bread. It goes in the freezer or refrigerator; put it in the toaster to defrost it
- Sweet potatoes
- Yams
- Frozen fruit—easy, keeps for a long time
- Frozen vegetables—easy, keeps for a long time
- Pre-cut frozen peppers and onions—great for cooking with when feeling lazy
- Jar of minced garlic—lazy awesomeness

Cooking Games

This one takes care of itself. With your new recipes from the preparing games or your new foods from the shopping games, now you get to do something with them!

Give yourself extra time for cooking new things. New recipes might take twice as long…or longer.

This is also a good time to check in on the food you purchased: What's ripe? How do you know if it's ripe? What went bad? How long did it last? Are there things I can do to make it last longer?

Food Journal Review Games

The big game here is usually substitution. Take a look at what doesn't work as well as you'd like it to, and see if you can swap it with something else.

Snacks are a good option for the substitution game. Can you swap out a bad snack for an apple and almonds?

Advanced Food Games

For the people who are already on top of this, but want to stretch themselves, of course there's a new level of games to play.

- Try playing the locavore game: *How much of your produce can you get locally?*
- Try playing the seasonal game: *How much of your produce can you get in-season?*
- Try playing the flavor game: *What's the most amazingly delicious recipe you can come up with?*

Honestly, I don't know if local and in-season food sourcing is going to impact your fat-loss results, but I do know the produce you get is going to taste awesome. People often find they can get fruit and vegetables that taste 10 times better for the same price or sometimes even less.

And, it's totally a fun game to play.

SUCCESS STORY: SHARON SHINER
We found what works for me, and it could be repeated.

When I started working with Josh, there were a couple big changes to my diet. The first was portion control; I had become cavalier about my eating and was overeating, thinking it was okay since I was exercising. For instance, fresh coconut meat is a fine snack, but I ate way too much of it, not paying any attention to fat and carb grams. Once I started eating more protein during the day, also I found the urge to snack after dinner went away.

The second big change Josh suggested was the concept of carb cycling, eating high carb a few days a week and low carb the other days. That was a huge change that turned out to be quite successful for me. I learned I couldn't really manage the high-carb days, and the lower-carb, higher-fat days were better.

The third change was to considerably increase the amount of protein, and on the days I ate less protein than my body needed, I was the most hungry. I'm also convinced that eating the right amount of protein guided me to my strength gains.

Logging the food using Josh's instructions made a huge difference in my success. It was an eye-opening exercise to see how much food I was actually eating versus what I thought I was eating. And as I was trying to hit a certain number of fat, carb, and protein grams each day, I wanted to be spot on. It became a game—how close to the required number of grams could I get? It was good to be able to go back and look at what I had eaten on a particular day when I felt strong or when I felt off to see what I might have done to feel that way.

I started to realize my own strength through this process. I've never doubted my strength, but it's taken some time to get to a point where I started seeing myself as a strong person. I might be petite, but my strength is not!

Josh made it clear that we found what works for me and that it could be repeated. At times I have a real 'all or nothing' attitude, meaning it's either all good or all bad. I started to shift from feeling bad, to seeing something wasn't really bad; it was a hurdle in the cycle and things would turn around.

Realizing my strength has had a huge impact on my life. I've had a tough road with a child who has special needs, as well as some major changes in other parts of my life. Being physically strong has given me the mental strength to handle these situations.

I've also been approached by colleagues for advice, training, and coaching, which to me is the greatest compliment and affirmation of my strength I could ever get.

Trusting in a process and sticking to it can be scary, but if you do it, results will come. Thanks, Josh, for showing me how to accomplish all this.

SUCCESS STORY: AARON PEARSON
Getting Leaner and Stronger at the Same Time

I spent nearly four months trying to gain weight, and then it was time to shed the fat. The idea was simple: Use the winter months to gain both weight and strength. I ate whatever I chose, while following Wendler's 5-3-1 method for strength gains.

Then I contacted Josh to let him in on my plan and asked for his guidance. His method was so simple, it was crazy. Everything starts with a food journal in order to make the appropriate adjustments. I was to start by adjusting the quantity of food until the scale weight began to drop. Eat protein with every meal. Make adjustments to fat and protein based on how my body composition changed. We made carbohydrate and fat adjustments based on energy levels and feelings of constant hunger.

According to Josh the biggest difference between the typical fat-loss client and me was the strength issue. His clients don't usually care about strength gains. Most of them are willing to sacrifice strength in order to achieve fat loss. My goal was slightly different—I wanted to make significant strength gains in the process.

My plan was simple: Follow Josh's fat-loss program while continuing to follow Wendler's 5-3-1 method. I stayed on the same strength program I used to gain weight during my new plan to lose weight. All of this was done without adding cardio or dietary fat-loss supplements. This was nothing more than hard work and clean eating and NO TREADMILL!

By the end of week five, things seemed to be falling into place. If anything I lost weight too fast. I was down to 166 pounds and 12.5% bodyfat. My squat was up to 355 pounds, with a new deadlift max of 455 pounds. I felt better than I had in a long time. I ate less, dropped weight, and was getting stronger than ever. By week six I intentionally slowed my weight loss. I weighed in at 165 pounds, which happened to be my goal weight.

I am far from finished when it comes to getting stronger. The body fat will continue to decrease, but honestly, it's not a priority for me any longer. What's more important is maintaining my current weight while greatly increasing my strength. So far my numbers look like this: My squat went from 315 pounds for a one-rep max to 315 for five reps, and 365 pounds for my one-rep max. My deadlift went from a one-rep max of 435 pounds to 435 for two reps, with a one-rep max of 455.

SUCCESS STORY: PAIGE GAYNOR SCHMIDT
Planning Makes All The Difference

As a teacher, I am consistently planning, teaching, monitoring, and adjusting my lessons. I transferred this same philosophy to fitness and nutrition. When Josh assigned a food log, it helped me create a plan for what I was going to eat that week, while monitoring and reflecting on what went well and where I may have slipped and needed to fix something for the following week. The food log kept me honest.

There were many faculty meetings I sat through with a huge birthday cake next to me; the smell of frosting was intoxicating, but I didn't want to have to log that I ate an unplanned piece of cake. It was also helpful having Josh review my food log each week and discuss what choices were positive, such as eating more protein than carbs, replacing a snack with almonds, or avoiding the tastes of candy and sweets, or talking about where my food choices took a downward turn.

Each week I stepped on the scale, I held my breath and hoped for the best. My hope was that the scale would reflect my hard work in fitness and healthy food choices that week, or the scale would be my ally and help me cover up if I had made a poor judgment in food or missed the gym or a run. It was motivating when I saw the results on the scale, and the pounds were coming off at a consistent rate.

I used two systems throughout my weight-loss journey. The first was the free day as Josh calls it. This was where I ate really well for six days, and on the seventh day, I could let loose a little and enjoy the desserts, drinks, and fast food that were my guilty pleasures. I just put them in a 24-hour period instead of having them trickle into my diet throughout the week. The other method was a 'three free meals a week' plan. This was for the weeks when I knew there would be several functions such as a holiday party, concert, or special event, and I couldn't plan for one free day. The key would be to plan the three free meals in advance so it wouldn't turn into a free week.

I'm still using many of the strategies I learned when I was initially on my weight-loss journey. For example, my husband and I plan what we're going to eat for our meals before I go grocery shopping for the week.

By having my husband onboard with my weight-loss journey, we can encourage each other to make positive decisions and lifestyle changes. We want our son to grow up in a home where food is important, but healthy food choices and exercise are the keys to a healthy, happy lifestyle.

SUCCESS STORY: DANIEL M.
It's about 'better,' not perfect.

I had been eating a lower-carb diet, but what really changed when I began working with Josh was tracking food and logging it. Tracking and logging changes everything, especially if you do it after every meal. You know exactly what you can and can't eat based on the macro and calorie counts. What was cool about working with Josh is that he didn't blink an eye, or try to get me to eat his way. We made small, incremental tweaks to what I was already doing.

What logging is about is awareness. You become aware of what you're eating in a much different way. Once you're aware, you can make better choices.

My workouts were terrible, honestly horrible. The first month my hands were a wreck. The second month I was insanely sick. The third month I thought I could lift the same amount of weight I did when I was 25 pounds heavier. You know what? It didn't really matter. The important thing was I was showing up three to five times a week and putting in the work using a program my body was inefficient at.

If the "goal is to keep the goal the goal," as Dan tells us, you can't worry if you have a crappy workout. Is it working—are you losing fat? Are you losing weight? Are you losing inches? Yes? Then keep going. Drop the weight you're trying to lift if you have to, but keep going.

I was doing a lot of straight-ahead strength work like Pavel's Power to the People program or the 40-Day Program. I hit the same exercises several days a week with low volume. I felt good and got stronger, but it wasn't inefficient enough to drive fat loss.

What I think most people need is better, not perfect. If you're working toward getting better, you will get there. There are going to be compromises, and you just have to decide what you're willing to compromise. If you try to be too hard core, you're going to end up blowing yourself up.

You have to keep yourself sane and reasonable, and keep the focus on doing the most important things consistently, day after day.

SUCCESS STORY: JAMIE PAUL
Mindfulness, Stars, and Freedom from the Perfection Trap

I love tracking the way Josh recommends! I'm getting SO much more out of this process using a physical journal and tracking everything from mindfulness and food habits, to my sleep and my workouts…all on one page. I wish I had started tracking this way sooner.

All I have ever done in the past when trying to lose fat was some kind of tracking based on the rules of the diet. Whether it was counting calories, counting macros, or even counting the number of hours in a daily fast, there was always a way to be better at a diet.

Getting swept up in the various rules of different diets ultimately led to numerous episodes of addictive overeating—the mindless, repetitive, trance-like state of nonstop food-to-mouth activity that often lasted from dinner until bedtime. From there, I engaged in subsequent cycles of guilt, followed by renewed dedications to follow the rules even tighter.

I finally realized this approach was not working for me. Rather than quitting, the first action I took to break out of this cycle was to start writing my food records in a marble composition notebook. I wrote down everything I ate, even when it was 'ugly.'

Stars and exclamation points have been my grading system, except that there's no true scoring system. Every meal or snack in which I ate mindfully and without distraction receives a star. Any awesome thing I do throughout the day gets a big, fat, inked-in exclamation point, whether it's leaving three bites of ice cream behind after I felt like I was satisfied or made a new PR in the gym.

One of the biggest differences for me was spending more focus on the positive habits I was creating around meals, and feeling good about those habits even if the food quality wasn't 100% ideal. I'm a bit of a perfectionist, so focusing on every little victory where I could get it has been a game changer. In addition, I'm trying to shift some of my thinking patterns, so I'll often write extra notes about the day and the choices I made. From my journal, I'm learning what's working and what isn't.

Following food rules was easy enough, but for a long time spending anything over five minutes to eat a meal and to do it without distractions was real work. I soon realized being present in front of food without eating it created quite a bit of anxiety. I still struggle with this a bit, but it feels less excruciating than it did at first.

Another bonus of tracking mindfulness with pen and paper is the amount of time it takes. It's become a therapeutic ritual to spend a few moments of my morning updating the previous day's entry, to reflect on how the day went, and if necessary, to write how my choices made me feel. Not only am I figuring out which choices work and which don't, I get to spend a few minutes in quiet solitude.

JOSH

CHAPTER 8

MAKING IT WORK

FIRST THINGS FIRST

At every step, we put the most important things first.

1. **Shopping, preparation, cooking, and food journal review** are the most important things, so we put them first in the book, first in the habits, and they're the first 'workout' of each week.
2. **Protein** is the most important part of the meal, so we think about protein first when we plan meals. Protein always comes first. Healthy fats come second. Carbohydrates come third.
3. **Getting stronger,** over time, is the most important part of the workout. In our workouts, we put strength first—well ahead of sweat, soreness, cardio, or total workout time.

This whole book could be organized by those three points, in that order.

But the point of this mini-chapter isn't to revisit those three points; it's to highlight *that they're in order*.

Really, until you start working on the food planning, preparation, and cooking, you have no business even going to the gym. Monday, of course, is just a metaphor for first, and so we put the food planning and preparing on Monday.

If you're new to food planning and preparation as a fat-loss goal, that's okay. We've broken it up into small weekly steps.

THE PROTEIN SOLUTION

People always ask me how to add more protein. I'll tell you this: If you're asking how to *add more,* you're already lost.

First: *Why three-quarters of a gram of protein per pound of bodyweight?*

We want optimal performance. We want you to get stronger, so you can get leaner and hotter as you lose weight. If we don't get you stronger and add or keep muscle, you'll get skinny-fat. Skinny-fat is when you look starving; you've lost weight, but you still don't look healthy or fit, and you still feel jiggly. Skinny-fat is when you've lost weight, but it literally makes no difference in how you look.

The reason we say 'fat loss' instead of 'weight loss' is because we want you to look hotter. To look hot, you need to lose fat *and gain or maintain muscle*. For most people, that means losing weight *and* getting stronger. That means we need to strength train *and* get enough protein.

On the following page, there's a table of organization position stands from ADA, ACSM, JISSN and the IOC, and current research on the protein needs of strength-training athletes and dieting athletes from AARR. Three-quarters of a gram of protein falls at the top end recommendation for some and the bottom end recommendation for others—I think it's a reasonable recommendation given the information we have. It has worked for my clients for both maintaining lean mass and promoting fullness, although you should do your own research and experiment with your own body.

At times I've coached up to or over a gram of protein per pound of bodyweight, but it seemed unnecessary. At times I've let people go lower than three-quarters of a gram of protein per pound of bodyweight, and sometimes people lost muscle—they got skinny-fatter. I settled on three-quarters of a gram of protein per pound of bodyweight because it just works for losing fat and for holding on to muscle. I later found it matched the ACSM/ADA/DC and JISSN position papers, which made me happy.

If you're really interested in the most current research on protein and body composition, I recommend a subscription to the *Alan Aragon Research Review*. Alan notes that while academia and the RDA recommend 0.8 grams of protein per kilogram of bodyweight—that's 0.36 grams of protein per pound of bodyweight—the current research doesn't support that. Research shows that getting enough protein to maintain muscle during a fat-loss program starts at around two times the RDA (0.71 grams of protein per pound). Check the *Alan Aragon Research Review* October 2013 and June 2013.

PUBLICATION	PROTEIN/KG	PROTEIN/LB
Position of the American Dietetic Association, Dietitians of Canada, and the American College of Sports Medicine: *Nutrition and Athletic Performance* – 2009	1.2–1.7g for strength training athletes	0.54–0.77g
Journal of the International Society of Sports Nutrition position stand on protein and exercise – 2007	1.4–2.0g	0.63–0.9g
Dietary protein for athletes: from requirements to optimum adaptation—Phillips SM1, Van Loon LJ. *J Sports Sci.* 2011;29 Suppl 1:S29–38. doi: 10.1080/02640414.2011.619204.	1.8–2.0g	0.8–0.9g
Interview with Eric Helms about his latest peer-reviewed publication on protein needs of lean, trained athletes in an energy deficit—*Alan Aragon Research Review* October 2013	2.3–3.1g	1.0–1.4g
Effects of high-protein diets on fat-free mass and muscle protein synthesis following weight loss: a randomized controlled trial, Pasiakos SM1, Cao JJ, Margolis LM, Sauter ER, Whigham LD, McClung JP, Rood JC, Carbone JW, Combs GF Jr, Young AJ., FASEB J. 2013 Sep;27(9):3837–47. doi: 10.1096/fj.13-230227. Epub 2013 Jun 5. via *Alan Aragon Research Review* June 2013	2x RDA, 1.6g	0.8g
Fueling the Vegetarian (Vegan) Athlete. Fuhrman J1, Ferreri DM., *Curr Sports Med Rep.* 2010 Jul–Aug;9(4):233–41. doi: 10.1249/JSR.0b013e3181e93a6f. American College of Sports Medicine	1.6–2.0g for strength training athletes	0.7–0.9g
International Olympic Committee consensus paper on *Nutritional Requirements for Athletes* – 2010	1.2–1.6g	0.5–0.7g
Phys Sportsmed. 2009 Jun;37(2):13–21. doi: 10.3810/psm.2009.06.1705. Protein for exercise and recovery. Kreider RB1, Campbell B.	1.4–2.0g	0.63–0.9g

On top of holding on to muscle while losing fat, shifting the calorie balance a little from carbohydrates and fat to protein really works to help trigger fat loss.

THE TRICK TO GETTING YOUR PROTEIN REQUIREMENT

The biggest trick is not to think about *adding protein*. What you need to do is start thinking *food IS protein*. When planning a meal, start with protein. Carbs and fats are fillers to add after the protein is handled.

If you think of food as carbohydrates, the battle is lost before it starts.

> Remember—**Food = Protein**
> *Carbohydrates and fats are fillers to add after protein is taken care of.*

How it looks in real life—

1. **Choose protein:** fish, chicken, beef, pork, poultry, eggs, or dairy.
2. **Choose seasoning:** Italian, Mexican, Indian, Asian, American, and so on.
3. **Choose a fat:** avocado, olive oil, grapeseed oil, almonds, cashews, and so on.
4. **Choose vegetables:** romaine, broccoli, asparagus, and so on.
5. **Choose a carbohydrate:** quinoa, brown rice, fruit, and so on.

This is the opposite of how most people plan meals. Most people start with a carbohydrate, and they add protein if they have room. And they almost never think about good fats.

If you start with protein, it becomes easy to add more protein if you need to. If you're eating three ounces of salmon, and you aren't getting to your protein goal by the end of the day, make your meal four ounces of salmon. Simple.

In fact, it's really, really, really simple.

While I've given you a starting target for protein in the habits section—three-quarters of a gram of protein per pound of target bodyweight—that's just a starting point. We always want to be aware of bodyfat percentage—ratio of lean, hot, sexy muscle to jiggly fat—instead of scale weight, because scale weight could be either.

Ultimately, the goal is to make you hotter. And hotter is leaner. Sometimes we need a big change on the scale to get lean. Sometimes we don't need any change on the scale. Lean means sexy, tight muscle. And muscle means metabolism. It's in your best interest to hold on to as much muscle as possible—you'll look hotter and you'll have a faster metabolism.

If you're losing scale weight and you lose *strength*, it's a huge indicator you need to add more protein.

The game we're playing is, you want to get stronger while you're losing fat. While I always like to test bodyfat with my personal clients, I realize not everyone reading this will have access to a good way to get tested. A good enough indicator of losing muscle is if you're getting stronger—adding reps, moving up to heavier kettlebells, or doing harder variations of the bodyweight exercises. If you're getting stronger, you're probably doing okay on protein.

Protein is your friend; start every meal with it.

MAKING HEALTHY FAT EASY AND DELICIOUS

By now we all know that healthy fats are good for metabolism and good for feeling full. We also know they're super high calorie, and if we overdo them, we'll overdo our total quantity of food in terms of calories.

The joke I used to always make was: *Low-calorie and low-fat diet = angry and hungry all the time.*

Really, you need to have enough good fats to feel full.

That's the rub.

We need healthy fats to feel full.

We need to always be conscious about not eating too many calories.

Oh wait—They're super delicious.

And that's the best part—good fats are fairly easy to prepare and make your proteins or vegetables taste amazing. Italian dish? No prob, put pesto sauce on your chicken. Mexican dish? Awesome, add guacamole to your chicken! Tastes delicious, is easy to prepare, and is chock-full of good fats that will have you feeling full, with a healthy metabolism.

For salads and veggies, a splash of olive oil and a dash of salt and pepper, maybe a pinch of oregano or a few sprigs of cilantro, and you're good to go. Olive oil is an awesomely healthy fat. If you get bored with olive oil, you can play with flax oil on your salad instead.

LEAN AND SEXY FAST FOOD

A smart play is to always have stuff on hand that's easy and fast. Protein powder for protein shakes is an obvious choice. Fully cooked chicken is awesome, as is good quality deli meat. You can eat it straight when you need protein.

Fruit is really great for that—takes no prep time, just eat it. Almonds are also an already done deal.

Zero prep time is a really good thing, and it makes your life a thousand times easier. And easy is what you want in fat-loss nutrition.

VEGETARIAN CONSIDERATIONS

Here's the thing about being a vegetarian—you have to switch your mindset from 'if it isn't meat it's okay' to the idea of a plant-based diet.

And then, on a plant-based diet you have to always be thinking protein. There are tons of plant-based protein options. **Like everyone, you still need to make protein the foundation of your meals.** Then add good plant-based fats. *And only then* add plant-based carbs.

Plan your meals like this—

1. Plant-based protein
2. Plant-based fat
3. Healthy, unprocessed, plant-based carbs like fruit, brown rice, or quinoa

The American Council on Sports Medicine, after their review of current research, came out with a position paper on protein for vegetarians that could be summarized as follows.

- Vegetarian athletes need the same three-quarters of a gram of protein per pound of bodyweight that omnivorous athletes need for optimal performance.
- It's totally possible to get three-quarters of a gram of protein per pound of bodyweight on a vegetarian diet.

Plan your meals: protein, fat, carbohydrates, in that order. What it really comes down to is that vegetarians play by the same set of rules as omnivores. If you start with carbs as the base, you've already lost.

It's totally possible to get all of your protein from plant-based sources. And if you're a lacto-ovo vegetarian—up for eggs or dairy—it's super easy. And then if you add fish…

The big thing is to check your daily protein intake using an online food journal. You'll find that even though you're getting some protein from quinoa and beans and nuts, you'll probably have to add more protein from a mostly protein source like tofu or tempeh, or even a hemp or pea protein powder. The carbohydrate-based protein such as quinoa isn't enough, nor is a fat-based protein like nuts enough all by itself.

The other thing to watch out for is there's a lot of processed crap food, especially cheap processed soy. This is essentially vegetarian fast food. Don't fall into the trap of thinking that because it isn't meat, you don't have to be concerned with quality.

It all comes back to the same thing—vegetarians have the same rules as omnivores: Quality of food and quantity rule the day.

REVIEWING OUR NEW HABITS

Let's look at what our habits are about.

- The first three habits are all about planning and preparing.
- The fourth habit is the scorecard for your planning and preparation.
- The fifth and sixth habits are about quantity, and the ninth and tenth habits are about quality—so you can re-plan and prepare more effectively.

So really, most of the habits have to do with pregame and postgame. Habits seven and eight are the only two habits that actually impact the game while it's happening.

| HABIT 7 | SLOW | Eat slowly. Each meal or serving should take at least 15 minutes. |
| HABIT 8 | 80% | Stop eating when you're 80% full. |

It's a completely game-changing way to look at food consumption.

EAT SLOWLY AND STOP WHEN YOU'RE 80% FULL

Habits seven and eight are two habits I got straight from John Berardi, creator of Precision Nutrition, in a talk he did at a Perform Better Summit. John is a nutrition-habits genius, so when he said, "Eating slowly might be *the* most important habit you can implement with your clients," I ran home and dropped this into the programs of all of my clients who were struggling with food quantity.

It's been interesting to apply these habits with my food journal coaching clients. It creates an amazing mindfulness about food that we never had access to before. Now I wouldn't know how to coach food without them.

Most people find they eat so fast, they never have time for the body to even get the signal that they're full, which takes at least 15 minutes. You might put a clock on it shooting for 15 minutes, and initially feel like *10* minutes is an eternity to finish a meal. That's a red flag that for you, this may be the most important habit of the entire program.

I think you'll find if you slow down your eating and then stop when you're 80% full, it will change your entire experience of eating. You'll enjoy your food more; you'll feel the right amount of fullness; and you'll get in touch with healthy quantities of food in a way you never had before.

BUMPS IN THE ROAD

When working on weight loss, we all want our scale weight to go straight down, but usually it has some bumps back up. Cut yourself some slack on this one.

It would be great if scale weight and bodyweight just get better, better, better forever. The reality is, it's almost always two steps forward, one step back…two steps forward, one step back.

Don't get discouraged by the one step back.

In my personal training career, I've never had one client whose bodyfat percentage dropped down like a straight line. It's always down and then a little up, down and then a little up. All we care about is that over time, *the trend is down*.

As long as the scale weight or the bodyfat percentage is down every month, we don't care if it's up one week.

Bodyfat percentage and scale weight will go up a little, down a little, and it's fine… so long as it's mostly down.

WHICH IS THE BEST DIET?

Answer: *Any of them.*

Seriously, I've had clients get great results doing *The Zone, The Paleo Solution, The Abs Diet, Apex's Calorie System, Eating Clean, Cheat Your Way Thin, Eating For Life*…the list goes on.

This is why I tell people to collect *diet cookbooks*, not diets. Diets, for the most part, are all the same. And, for the most part, they all work.

I'll tell you right now that you can and actually should buy as many diet books as you can find. I just want you to play this game with each one when you get it: Look at it and ask yourself, 'Is this diet based on quality of food? Is it based on quantity of food, or is it based on ratios?'

What you'll find is that nearly every diet book says almost the same thing. If it's good, it's going to say most of the same things I've told you in this program. It's going to tell you to eat better quality. You need to reduce quantity. You need to alter the ratios in some way, although some diets have their magic ratios. Occasionally, you'll read something about timing. But, there are only these four possible concepts they can cover.

Every time you see a new diet book, ask yourself, 'Is this about quality, quantity, ratios or is it selling timing?' Look at whether the diet is based on whatever its gimmick is or whether it's really a smart, balanced diet based on all three, but is just pointing to one as a gimmick to sell the book. That would actually be ideal.

In reality, *diet is about quality, quantity, and ratios.*

Often you'll find a diet isn't balanced. It's a diet entirely about quality, a diet entirely about quantity or a diet entirely about ratios. That's fine, too, because now you can recognize it. You can think, 'Okay, so the author's thing is all about *that*.'

Often the author is speaking to a certain market or a certain demographic. For that demographic, a certain one of the three may be a little more important. Maybe they've worked with a demographic or a certain type of client and having that perspective worked well for them. That's fine, too, and now you can recognize what they're saying.

Sometimes it will be a quality-based diet. The author is assuming if you increase quality, quantity will shift to a better level by itself. You'll see a lot of diets based entirely on quantity that leave out quality. That's probably not a good idea. It might get you closer to your goal, but it won't get you all the way.

Now that you have this filter, you can get any diet book you want, and the reason I recommend this is because I want you to get the recipes. I want you to collect as many recipes as you can. When starting a diet for health, fitness, fat loss, or to look better, many people start eating totally bland food. They'll have steamed broccoli with no seasoning and a naked chicken breast. Why not add some hot pepper sauce, some tomato sauce, some cilantro, or some onions?

I want you to get in the habit of collecting the recipes connected to these diet books. You'll get easy recipes that are totally delicious, which will make this whole thing work a lot easier.

You can even get the X-Y-Z Diet cookbook where you just get the recipes and they don't tell you anything about the diet. This would be even better—you could just collect recipes.

Magazines like *Cooking Light* have a lot of readers who have gotten great results because they're in the habit of using the rules we've discussed. People know the rules—the three different variables we're playing with—to lose fat, lean up, and get the body they want. They collect recipes that fit those rules. Be on the lookout for recipes for whatever diet you choose, as long as you evaluate it, filter it, figure out the message and the marketing, and decide if you agree with it. Then grab all the great recipes.

People spend way, way too much time trying to find the right diet, when in fact, 90% of the clients I've ever had really needed to work on the habits that would have made *any* of these diets work.

It's kind of like why the movie *The Karate Kid* is so terrible. Don't get me wrong, I love to watch it, but it's *the worst lesson in the world*: You can win it all if you find the magic move.

This is the way that most people treat diets, 'If I can just find that one magic diet.' In reality, it's a lot more like *Rocky*—a training montage that details months of working on all of the required skills. He runs, he hits the heavy bag, he spars, he does mitt work, he jumps rope, he hits the speed bag, he spars some more. This is all on top of a lifetime of training.

And by the end, he's got all of the skills required. No magic move, just lots of heart and lots of skills.

Stop looking for new diets. Instead, go to work on The Eleven Habits.

EVALUATING AN EATING PROGRAM

Now that we've established what matters—*the habits*—we can discuss the three things you should look at when evaluating an eating program. You'll notice that all of the diets mentioned above meet these three criteria, and that's what I mean when I say they're all pretty much the same.

There are three things we need in a good nutrition program.

1. More protein *than the average person eats*
2. Fewer calories *than the average person eats*
3. Better quality of carbohydrates and fat *than the average person eats*

Remember: The average person is fat. According to WebMD, 63.1% of Americans are overweight or obese. You don't want to eat what the average person eats.

Those three things might sound vague, but they aren't. Remember, it all comes down to a simple equation.

FAT LOSS HAPPENS ON MONDAY RESULTS KEY	
YOUR SCALE WEIGHT	Quantity of food you eat (calories)
YOUR BODYFAT PERCENTAGE	Quality of food you eat and how strong you are

You always know where to look. *If the scale weight is too high, you need to eat fewer calories.*

If you aren't as lean as you'd like to be, *first you need better quality of food*, which includes more protein, and better quality carbohydrates and fat.

Then you need to get stronger in your workouts. In this program, that would be lifting kettlebells for more repetitions or using heavier kettlebells, and doing body-weight movements for more repetitions or moving up to harder versions.

It's actually very simple if you let it be…

…and that's what clears out all of the nonsense we hear from media, well-meaning friends and family, and fitness gurus who actually don't know anything about fat loss. We skip the nonsense, and get right to The Eleven Habits—which are really just how we strategically impact your quantity and quality of food.

HOW MANY CALORIES?

This has to be the number one question I get: *How many calories should I target per day?* And I know most people have formulas for this kind of thing, but I don't.

I'm a test-and-adjust kind of trainer. And that's what you're going to do here. *Let your life be your ultimate fat-loss guide.*

All you need to do is keep a food journal for a week. At the end of the week, average your daily calories.

AM I EATING THE RIGHT AMOUNT OF CALORIES?	
IF YOU LOSE MORE THAN THREE POUNDS PER WEEK	You're eating too few calories
IF YOU LOSE ONE TO TWO POUNDS PER WEEK	You're eating the right amount of calories for fat loss
IF YOUR WEIGHT STAYS THE SAME	You're eating maintenance calories
IF YOU GAIN WEIGHT	You're eating too many calories

It's remarkably simple. You're going to use that system every week going forward.

We might as well just start with that.

What I like about this is that it side-steps all the questions about how active your life is, how much muscle mass you have, whether you're a woman or man. Like everything in this program, we start with you, in your life, where you are right now.

If you were at maintenance calories and you want to lose weight, drop your calories by 200 calories per day. Check back in a week and see what happened. If you lost a pound of fat, awesome. Stay at that level of calories until it doesn't work anymore.

When you plateau, you can try dropping the calories again.

It should be noted that there are bottom limits. According to the American College of Sports Medicine, 1,200 calories per day for a woman is the absolute minimum. For men, they say the lower limit is 1,800 calories. The concept is to not go lower, despite what some crazy people will tell you.

If you've been at that bottom limit of calories for any length of time, you should be ready for one of the advanced nutrition strategies we'll talk about at the end of this section. You're probably due for a refeed, and we can see if over the long term we can get you lean at a higher caloric intake.

For everyone else, just start with where you are, and work your way down. Take a hard look at portion sizes, and look to true-up your portion sizes on a regular basis.

> Remember: Quantity isn't everything.
> But it is scale weight.

SYSTEMS, PLANS, AND MORE SYSTEMS

I love systems. I love plans. I'd recommend you *always* have a plan.

The plan usually changes.

A million things could derail a plan. As they say…"the best laid plans of mice and men."

The important thing is to have a plan. If you have to change it—know why you're changing it. For example, if I have a client who gets sick, we may back up a step.

If someone gets bored easily, I may mix up the order of exercises every workout so it feels different. If people get overwhelmed by the second cycle where we train multiple adaptations per week, we'll go back to the first cycle where we train one adaptation per month. The plan can change a little.

If a certain way of building the habits doesn't work, we may take two weeks per habit. Or we may use a completely different system. Sometimes people can move faster, and instead of changing one habit and one meal, we'll change one habit for all of their breakfasts. Or we'll change one habit for all of their lunches.

Or maybe we just work on Monday, and we work on Monday for a whole month.

There are a lot of ways we can approach this. But the principle never changes: *Change only one thing per week*. Know which meal or meals are the ones you plan to *win* at.

PLAN YOUR FREE MEALS AHEAD OF TIME WITH THE GRID

	MON	TUES	WED	THURS	FRI	SAT	SUN
BREAKFAST	X	X	X	X	X	X	X
LUNCH	X	X	X	X	X	X	X
SNACK	X	X	X	X	X	free	X
DINNER	X	X	X	X	free	free	X

The Plan: Mark your free meals at the beginning of the week so you know when they're coming up. This is assuming four meals per day—three meals and one snack—but you could just as easily grid three meals.

Actual: At the end of the week, fill in a new sheet with what actually happened, and add up your score. In the example above, she had 25 on-plan meals and three free meals. Count the boxes marked 'X' for on-plan meals, and the boxes marked 'free' for free meals—that's the goal!

You can also use the grid to plan how to get better each week.

Example #1: Let's say last week you had 15 on-plan meals and 13 free meals. You could use the *Planning and Preparation Strategy* to try and improve that number. If next week you can get to 17 on-plan meals and 11 free meals, you'd have improved by two meals per week! You could keep doing that, working toward eventually getting to just 3 free meals per week.

Example #2: Let's say you look at your grid and see that all of your breakfasts and lunches were on-plan, and all of your dinners were free. You could use the *Win One Meal at a Time Strategy* to work on your dinners.

The Compliance Grid is something John Berardi mentioned in an interview years ago, and it's been an absolutely essential part of how I evaluate clients' food since then.

If you keep your food journal on paper instead of online, you can grid it right on your journal. Just put a red box around all the free meals, then count the number of free versus planned meals for the week.

ABOUT FREE MEALS AND FREE DAYS

Right off the bat—if you get 90% of your meals right, you don't need to worry about the other 10%.

Free *days* seem to work better than free meals for most people, at least in terms of the mental game. I've seen more people able to stick to free days, because there are such clear starting and stopping points. Free meals can sometimes start with three per week, and then turn into five per week. It can get away from you.

But everything is individual. I've had clients get great results with a free day every week, and I've had clients get great results with a few free meals spread out over the week. Know thyself: Usually the clients who do well with free days have trouble with free meals, and the clients who do a few free meals during the week have trouble doing a full free day.

And that's the thing; it's individual.

I've had clients where their first food journals had *27 free meals*. And every week we just worked them down to one less free meal. And they lost 3% bodyfat per month, going from 27 free meals per week to 23 free meals per week, to 19. It amazes me sometimes that it's that simple.

On the flip side, I've had clients who only had one free meal per week, and only after a hard workout. Without skipping too far ahead, this would usually be a client who's due for a structured refeed, which you'll find in the advanced section.

And that's my point. Everyone is different. We use the same physiological principles, but then factor in different backgrounds and motivations and histories and habits.

I can't tell you how many times when people are stalling on fat loss, they've got the idea of 'maybe I should have fewer free meals.' We look at the food journal, and they're having three free meals per week.

Let me tell you, three meals per week is never the problem. Let's take a look at the other 18 meals, and see if there's something we need to tighten up there.

Always, without fail, we find sloppiness in the 90% of the on-plan means. These are the meals to work on. Really, if you get the 90% right, you've earned the right to eat whatever you want on your free meals.

And that's the way to look at your free meals—like you can have whatever you want…whatever you want in terms of *quality*. Have some cookies. Have some pizza. Have whatever you want in terms of quality.

But changing quality isn't a license to binge. You don't need to force-feed yourself a whole bag of chocolate chip cookies because it's your free meal.

1. If at any time you're sick to your stomach, the free day or free meal is over.
2. If you feel stuffed or over full, your free day or free meal is over.

FREE DAYS AND FREE MEALS MAKE IT WORK IN REAL LIFE

The first and most important thing for actually making any of this work in real life is to schedule free meals or free days. If you're not having free meals or free days, you're making things way too hard on yourself, and you're making this much less sustainable.

First, there's the psychological aspect. If you know you can't have something ever again, you're going to go crazy wanting it.

Second, when you know you can have whatever you want once a week, it removes not just the cravings, but also the food-pusher situations. This happens when someone at work offers you a homemade super-deluxe peanut-butter chocolate cupcake. You can say no, knowing you can have chocolate on your free day…in a couple of days.

Next, it gets us out of the totally damaging mindset that certain foods are bad or evil or are going to kill us. You can have whatever you want, in moderation.

Some people actually get to a point where they can flow and manage free meals on the fly. And they can dance between freestyling sometimes, and other times if that freestyling starts showing up negatively on the scale or in the bodyfat percentage, they can start gridding their free meals and planning more rigidly again.

A free day can be used to boost your metabolism when you've been dieting hard. If you've ever dieted really hard and had the experience of feeling your metabolism come to a grinding halt, you know you need a free day. It's one of those things where a free day every week up-regulates the metabolism. It lets your body know you're not dying. It keeps your metabolism from crashing.

Here's what you need for a free day to jumpstart your metabolism.

The day has to be high in carbohydrates.
It has to be high in fat.
It has to last at least six hours.

These are things to keep in mind in terms of keeping the metabolism going.

You will be amazed at how hard you can get away with dieting without your metabolism crashing if you include a free day. You would also be amazed at how little dieting it takes for your metabolism to come crashing down if you don't plan a free day.

Here's the last mistake people make with their free days: They spend their free days plowing through two gallons of ice cream and two bags of chocolate chip cookies, while sitting alone in front of the TV. At the end of *that* free day, they're not very satisfied. You can do this if you want, but it's a wasted opportunity.

My experience in dealing with a lot of clients is that typically people are happiest about their free days when they use them for something social. You could go out to dinner with your significant other, have a nice meal, a bottle of wine and dessert. You could have chicken wings and pizza with friends.

When you use your free day in a social setting, it's like you get something really good for yourself. It's more like the freedom to eat whatever you want versus purposely shoving down all the junk food you can find. It's one of those situations where it's a choice that will make you happier. I strongly urge you to choose your free day when you have the coolest social event of the week.

PREPARATION VERSUS WILLPOWER

You're going to eat what you have access to. You're going to eat the stuff in your home. You're going to eat the stuff you have at work. You're going to eat whatever is there and whatever was prepared in advance.

When you get home from work, when it's time for dinner and if there's nothing good in the kitchen, it's a recipe for disaster. I don't care how much willpower you have, you're going to crash and burn.

You're setting yourself up to fail.

You need to stock the refrigerator in advance of actually needing the food. You're going to need to go shopping twice a week because real food spoils. You're going to need to pop into the store or the farmer's market a couple of times a week and get real food, just enough to last for a few days.

When you prepare food, prepare it in bulk. When you cook something, have all four burners going at the same time. If you can have two burners on your stove preparing protein, and two burners on your stove preparing carbohydrates, you're rocking.

Here's an example.

On the first burner, you could be cooking two pounds of ground buffalo Italian-style with oregano, basil, onions, salt, pepper, and maybe some stewed tomatoes.

On the second burner or maybe on a George Foreman grill, you could be cooking Mexican-style chicken breasts with cumin, salt, black pepper, maybe a splash of red pepper sauce, onions, and bell pepper. You could add fresh cilantro at the end.

On the third burner, you could be cooking brown rice pasta, a type of pasta that's just brown rice and brown rice bran.

On the fourth burner, you could have some quinoa and broccoli.

This would be an example of how to cook all at the same time, maybe three meals with one kind of protein and carbohydrate, and three meals with a different protein and carbohydrate.

Then portion everything in Tupperware so it's pre-packaged into meals.

Put the meals that will last for the next two or three days in the refrigerator. Take everything that's left over and put it in the freezer.

What you've done is set yourself up to win.

You've set yourself up to have your own healthy TV dinners.

Another thing you can do is to always have on hand a pound of good luncheon meat like Boar's Head pepper turkey or whatever is tasty to you. Have a bunch of fruit and some nuts.

Let's say you're in a bind and missed preparing your food. You don't have a ready-made Tupperware of ground buffalo and brown rice. You can always make yourself a snack plate. Snack plates are the best ever. Get some sliced turkey; maybe cut up some strawberries or banana. Throw on 10 almonds. There you'd have protein, carbohydrates, and fat. It's all healthy, handy…perfect. And it took literally two minutes to prepare.

In your refrigerator, keep the world's easiest and fastest fast food.

When your kitchen is set up like this, you're set up to win. You'll get home and it's actually easier to eat good, healthy food that will help you get lean than it is to eat stuff that will make you fat. When you're set up like this, fat loss doesn't take a lot of willpower.

Screw the whole willpower-motivation thing. You don't want to have to use willpower or motivation. Set yourself up to win. Make it easier to win and to eat good food.

We used to call this swimming downstream. You can swim upstream and make it really hard where it will take a lot of willpower. Or you can set yourself up to win, surround yourself with lots of good food, and swim downstream. Make it easy.

Let's take a look at restaurants.

There are magazine articles and books written about what to eat when you go to a restaurant. But I'm going to make it really simple.

- Every restaurant has some kind of salad and chicken.
- Most restaurants will have fish with vegetables.
- Many restaurants have a steak salad.

When you go out to eat, those are your three options. Get one of those and you're done. Don't make eating out any more complicated than that.

PREPARATION AND FOOD PUSHERS

The next thing to talk about is social considerations, and this is huge.

Most people are food-pushers.

Taryn Bagrosky, Ms. Fitness USA 2010, once told me her parents still try to give her all kinds of baked goods, even when she has a show coming up. It's not just you. It's everyone who is surrounded by people trying to feed them things that don't work on the food plan.

Most people just don't get it, and that's okay. They're really trying to be nice and giving.

The same way you need to be physically prepared with the right kinds of foods in your home and at work, you need to be socially prepared. You need to know ahead of time what you're going to eat and what you're going to say.

Something amazing I learned from Anna Messinger: *Don't ever say you can't eat something; say you don't.*

If you say you can't, it sounds weak. *Can't* almost makes it sound like you're being victimized by your food plan, "Oh, I'm sorry, I can't eat pizza; it's not on my plan. What? No, no really I shouldn't. Which plan? Oh, I read this book…"

This sounds like you're not in control, and people are much more likely to question you about why you can't eat things, and sometimes will even push you to justify why you can't.

Saying you don't is stronger, and doesn't require justification.

Saying *I don't* is a declaration about what you stand for, "Oh wow, pizza for the whole office—thanks, that's really thoughtful. I brought lunch; I don't eat pizza during the week. Lucky you guys, more for you."

FOOD JOURNAL AND RE-PLANNING

The food journal is the lynchpin that holds all of this together. If there's only one thing you learn from this discussion, it's that you have to keep a food journal.

I'm going to repeat this: *All of my clients who keep a food journal get results.*

There are different ways to keep a food journal. You can keep a written food journal, or you can keep an online food journal, or keep one on your phone.

If you keep a written food journal, I recommend using a calendar and not an actual journal. The upside of using a calendar to journal your food is that you can't cheat and skip a day. All of the days are already there, so you can't 'forget' a day's logging.

Or if you skip one, at least it'll be clear.

The upside of keeping a written food journal is that it's easy and portable. Nothing is easier than writing food down. Written food journals are great for tracking quality because you can skim it so easily for review.

THE WAY I SCORE A FOOD JOURNAL

First I go through and put stars by all the meals that have protein. Next I circle all the meals that break the carbohydrate and fat rules on the client's level, remembering the different carbohydrate levels, explained below. I'll circle those based on where we are, and then just eyeball it each week.

"Okay, this week was about 80% on point," or, "This week was about 90% on point."

THEORETICAL CARBOHYDRATE LEVELS	
STARTING LEVEL	Cut out sugary desserts, alcohol, and all beverages containing calories.
MID-RANGE LEVEL	Continue to avoid sugary desserts, alcohol, fast food, and all beverages containing calories. Now cut out foods that come from a drive-through, a microwave, or a convenience store. Limit portion size per meal of white flour, white rice, and pasta to the size of the palm of your hand, or to one slice.
STRICTEST LEVEL	Limit carbohydrates to fruit, vegetables, sprouted-grain bread, brown rice, and quinoa.

*Carbohydrate quality levels are a continuum with many shades of gray. These levels were designed as a way to grade the food journal. You would move to more strict levels only as needed to continue to progress.

That's how grading a written food journal works. It's pretty much all grading the quality of food.

Online and phone app food journals are killer. They're great, because not only will they track quality, but they'll also track ratios and quantity for you. It's the best possible option. You get to see your ratios, your quantity, and your quality each day, and you can also track these over time.

I love reviewing the reports and seeing the averages because it helps people see that one off-meal doesn't ruin the whole plan. Nor does one great day set them up for everything they need. It really is the average of what you're doing over time that gives you the body you want. That's super cool.

Where a written food journal ends up being mostly about looking at the quality of your food choices, an online food journal ends up being mostly looking at calories and macronutrient ratios.

These are the details of food journals, but the real money in a food journal is that you actually know what's going on. We humans have this amazing ability to fool ourselves. It's not like you're deliberately lying to yourself. There's just something about the human brain that omits the details it doesn't like, and focuses on what it does.

With all of my clients, we review measurements, scale weight and bodyfat percentage every month. If you're not getting the results you want in terms of the metrics—the actual hard metrics—it's time for us to have that hard talk.

Ninety percent of the time, if you're not getting the results you want, either you're not keeping a food journal, or you're missing something, like forgetting to write something in your journal. This is where the hard talk really becomes the hard talk, because we have to get legitimate.

The other 10% of the time, you've been totally accurate in your food journal, but it hasn't gotten you all of the results you want. We can go through your food journal and see all of the places where things aren't lining up. It's where you're eating food that doesn't work for your current level, or you're eating too much.

If you're eating too much, we adjust. If you need to level-up your food choices, you can go to the next level on food choices.

When we have the journal to dig into, there's no mystery. It's totally clear, because you've tracked it…and we can see it.

I want you to realize if what you're eating doesn't work, you're not a bad person and you're not failing. You're just using strategies that aren't working.

By strategies, I mean the ways you're preparing food, or not preparing it, aren't working. Food preparation—the planning, shopping, and cooking—really is a skill. That's all there is to it. We need to go back through your food journal and look at the times you failed to prepare and plan for the following week, as well as when to add more preparation time.

I have clients who completely stop working out. All we do is spend a one-hour training session planning the food for the next week, talking about the social events and what they'll say when people try to push food on them. We talk about what they do when work spills over into their preparation time, how they take food to work, and how they prepare for dinner.

We get them prepared.

Other clients text or call me after they've gone to the store and bought good food. That was their thing—their big stumbling block was making it to the store often enough.

I really want you to get that. You can look at your food journal and know exactly the life situations that are going to arise that will throw you off. You can look back to see where you've been thrown off, and come up with a strategy to plan around it for the future.

The whole story is in your food journal.

I don't want to beat this to death. But it's important to understand that every strategy you need to put into place is just a matter of preparation.

Everything you need to prepare for can be found in your food journal at the places where things went off-plan. It wasn't a matter of willpower. It wasn't a matter of motivation. It wasn't what your parents taught you about food.

It was the lack of preparation.

Have a session every single week when you use your food journal to get real about what happened. And then make a plan for the following week.

You should get pumped about finding things that went wrong, because that's where you get to attack. You get to make your war plan for the next week. You get to see, plain as day, exactly what you need to do to get the results you want.

The first level of the food journal is writing down what happened. An advanced food journal—a super ultra mega food journal—is to split each page into a planned side and an actual side.

If you're doing an online food journal, which I recommend, you're going to have to do your planning in a separate place. That's totally okay. You can plan in a Word document. You can plan by writing things down. There are even apps just for planning that also automate your grocery list.

It's a little cumbersome to have one app for planning and shopping, and another app for tracking. You may find you gravitate to doing either one or the other, whichever has the bigger impact on eating well during the week.

Let's say you planned to have an omelet for breakfast, a protein shake in the middle of the morning, and a turkey breast with some brown rice at lunch. You can go back and review, 'Okay, I missed having the omelet for breakfast. What happened there? Well, I didn't have any eggs.'

What happened was not a failure of motivation. It was just that you didn't plan and didn't have eggs in the fridge. You discover it really came down to shopping.

Okay, when can you go shopping next week?

When you're dealing with your food journal like this, you get strategic. It changes things—it's no longer an emotional thing. It isn't whether you're a good or bad person. It isn't motivational. It's simply strategy.

You can also look at it this way. Let's say that you have eggs, but you woke up late. You didn't have time to prepare the eggs. That was the issue. If the issue became that you didn't have time to prepare the eggs and you can't get more time in the morning, the only way to solve it is to go to sleep earlier.

"Next week, can I go to sleep 20 minutes earlier so I can wake up 20 minutes earlier and I'll have time to prepare eggs?"

Now, here's where it gets really crazy. You can say, yes or no. You get to decide.

"There's no way I'm going to go to sleep earlier, so that means there's no way I can have eggs in the morning."

That's okay. *You just need to be real about it.*

Instead, maybe you need to get a protein shake you can blend in 10 seconds, or maybe you need to eat lunch meat and fruit in your car while driving to work. These are all different choices you can make while getting strategic. This works if you can look at your plan versus what actually happened—in a totally mechanical way—and think, 'Here's what happened. Here's what worked. Here's what didn't work. What can I do differently next week?'

Look at your food journal, see what happened, and consider strategically. Then plan the next week using the plan. You can get very tight with what works and what doesn't work in your real life.

There's absolutely nothing you can do better, no better spent time for the leanness of your body.

Skip a workout, but don't skip planning.
Skip a workout, but don't skip food preparation.
Skip a workout, but don't skip going to the store.

You'll be so much more effective if you get the food right first.

If there's anything I want you to get out of this material, it's that your food journal time, both writing and planning, are the keys to the kingdom. It's everything you want. Food is the magic to getting the body you want, and your journal will tell you if you're getting the food part right.

Food Journal Session

Now we're going to do a food journal coaching session. I'm going to coach you as if we're sitting looking at your food journal together. I invite you to re-read this coaching session while you're evaluating your food journal for the first couple of weeks until you get the pattern down.

The first part of the food journal coaching session is about measurements, which we discuss on page 78. I want you to rotate through measurements every week. One week you'll measure bodyfat percentage. One week you'll measure scale weight. The next week you're going to measure circumference measurements.

Before you measure whatever it is you're going to measure this week, think about what you wrote in your food journal *last week*. You don't need to open it. I just want you to think about it. I want you to guess whether your measurements are going to get better or worse. Take a second and guess what your measurements will show.

Then measure yourself.

Now that you've measured, take a look at whether the measurements matched up with what you thought they were going to be. Speculate on whether it's an accurate measurement.

Now take a look at the measurement versus what it was three weeks ago. Did it go up? Did it go down? Think about the last three weeks. Does it make sense that it went that way?

The three-week measurement is probably more accurate than a weekly measurement. You should put a little more stock in how it relates to three weeks ago. Then you should look at how it relates to this particular week.

Now, we're going to take a look at your food journal. Go through each day first. On each day, is there protein in every meal? How does the total quantity look? Does it look as though the quantity is set up to lose fat?

How is the quality of the carbohydrates? Does this look like the quality of carbohydrates you would expect in a fat-loss diet? Then look at good fat. Is there enough good fat for you to feel full? Is there so much good fat that it's increasing the quantity—the calories?

After you've taken a look at that for every day this week, note whether you kept a food journal every day of the week or whether you missed a day. If you have an online food journal, set it up so you can look at the average for the week. If you have a written food journal, eyeball it or actually go through and calculate your averages.

Is there enough protein to maintain muscle and feel full? Look at the total quantity for the week—the average quantity for the week. Is the average quantity for the week such that you're losing fat?

Next, look at the average ratios for the week. In looking at the average ratios, does it make sense you felt as full as you could have or do you think you're a little hungrier than you need to be because the ratios are off?

In looking at all of that, go back and review the measurements. Ask yourself whether the measurements are accurate. If you think the measurements are accurate, you get to become strategic.

If you don't think the measurements are accurate, completely disregard them this week. You'll know based on next week's measurements if you're going in the right direction.

For now, make a guess as to whether the measurements are accurate based on what you saw in the journal, or whether they were just off this week. Either way is fine.

Next, we go back through your food journal to see what's missing. Is there anything missing in terms of planning or strategy that you can do better next week? It could be as simple as the fact that you didn't get protein at every meal, so you add protein next week. It could be as complex as a need to prepare for a specific situation next week.

Choose one thing to strategically improve next week *and that's it.*

After writing that one thing down, take a look back through the week to see what you did correctly. Look at the things that really worked. With the systems you set up, how did you win? What was the planning? What was the food journaling? What are the things you did that had you winning?

If you had a terrible week and the only thing you did correctly was keep a food journal, celebrate. The food journal is the baseline for everything. Anything above and beyond that, you should celebrate as well. Find as many things as possible that you did correctly last week.

Regardless of your results, take the case again this week that this entire process is mechanical and strategic. You're not bad if there was something missing and you're not good if there was nothing missing. You aren't even good if you did everything right.

I just want you to take a look at this as the simple machine called fat loss. Be curious about how it all works, what's working for you in your life, what might work better…and play the game. This is a machine you're tinkering with for fun.

You should have one thing to add that was missing last week. You may actually have weeks where there's nothing missing. Most of the time you'll probably have something missing that you can add to the next week. You'll also have something you did correctly last week that you can make a point to repeat next week. You'll now have these two things to take into next week.

With these two things in mind, plan out next week meal by meal. You're going to go through every day next week and plan it meal by meal. If you have a paper food journal, you're going to write on one side of the paper. If you have an online food journal, you can open a Word document with the two windows side-by-side. Meal by meal, plan the next week and set yourself up to win.

Look for things that come up that will be hard and might throw you off. Plan when you need to do your shopping. Plan and schedule when you're going to do your food preparation, when you're going to portion the foods, the times you're going to eat and what you're going to eat.

There you go. You're all set for next week. You're ready to go. You have a plan.

Regardless of what happened last week, last week is over and you have a plan for next week. You may not follow the plan exactly, but you have a plan. You're ahead of 99% of people.

You have strategies. You have one thing you're going to do that's new to the plan. You have one thing that really worked for you last week that you're going to make sure to do again.

You're ready to rock! Off you go!

DO I HAVE TO DO MY FOOD PREPARING ON SUNDAY AND MONDAY?

You can do your food preparation whenever you want. You can do it all Sunday. You can do it all Monday night. If your week starts on an odd day, you can do it all then.

The point is to have it all done before you do your first workout of the week.

In fact, even if you do your cooking for the week on Monday night, you'll still need to have Monday *day* sorted out ahead of time.

I have some advice about that: Eat the exact same breakfast, same lunch, and same dinner every Monday. *Avoid all thinking. Just eat the same thing on Mondays.*

We used to call this reducing friction. Thinking, deciding, new planning, choosing—this is hard. It's friction.

If at the very least your Monday food plan can just repeat every week, you'll start each week on the right foot, without nearly as much effort as if you re-planned every week.

JOSH'S WORLD'S EASIEST MONDAY FOOD PLAN FOR WOMEN

Breakfast

Protein shake blended with—

- Whey Protein—Two scoops in water: 200 calories / 36g protein / 4g fat / 12g carbs
- Banana—One: 121 calories / 1g protein / 0g fat / 31g carbs
- Kale—Two leaves: 34 calories / 2g protein / 0g fat / 34g carbs
- Fish Oil—Five capsules: 45 calories / 0g protein / 5g fat / 0g carbs

Lunch

- Premium Sliced Deli Turkey—Four ounces: 120 calories / 28g protein / 2g fat / 0g carbs
- Apple—One: 72 calories / 0g protein / 0g fat / 20g carbs
- Almond—18 nuts: 192 calories / 7g protein / 17g fat / 7g carbs

Dinner

- Seasoned Ground Turkey—Six ounces: 240 calories / 30g protein / 12g fat / 0g carbs
- Brown Rice Pasta—One-half cup (cooked): 97 calories / 1g protein / 0g fat / 24g carbs
- Tomato and Basil Pasta Sauce—One-half cup: 50 calories / 1g protein / 2g fat / 10g carbs
- Broccoli—One cup: 31 calories / 3g protein / 0g fat / 6g carbs
- Extra Virgin Olive Oil—Two tablespoons: 240 calories / 0g protein / 28g fat / 0g carbs

- Garlic—One teaspoon: 4 calories / 0g protein / 0g fat / 1g carbs

Total: 1,445 calories / 110g protein / 69g fat / 145g carbs

THE HOW AND THE WHY

If you look at those meals, you'll see everything is easy. And easy is good when we're looking for less friction.

We start the day with a protein shake—easy. It's a really easy way to start the day with a pretty awesome amount of protein. And we're blending up some kale into the protein shake—you can't really taste it, and it's a super easy way to get some extra veggies. Bananas are easy…doing great so far. After the protein shake, take your fish oil supplement for the day. Awesome.

At lunch, we go to the market and get four ounces of deli meat. I choose turkey, but it could be chicken or roast beef or whatever you like, and however they season it so it tastes good. Easy. Then add some almonds for a healthy fat, and add an apple. The day is looking amazingly healthy and lean so far.

Dinner is the only meal that requires any actual cooking, but I've made that easy for you, too. Get the ground turkey that's already seasoned. Cook that up, then add tomato sauce. We're using a little bit of brown rice pasta—a half-cup isn't much. It's basically going to be meat sauce 'seasoned' with brown rice pasta.

Then we've got broccoli with two tablespoons of olive oil. In this meal, you're actually getting most of your energy from the healthy fat in the olive oil, instead of from the carbs in the pasta.

I listed broccoli, but it doesn't matter what kind of vegetable you use. Get a ton of it frozen, and keep it in the fridge. If you want to steam it, great. If you want to sauté it with garlic, great. If you're short on time and just boil it with the last couple minutes of the pasta, fine. You can even stir the broccoli and the olive oil into the pasta. That works great!

What I want you to take away from this is that everything was deliberately made as easy as possible.

What if you really wanted to make it easy? You could go get your dinner at Chipotle.

Get the salad, skip the salad dressing and rice and beans, and just get this—

- Romaine lettuce: 10 calories / 1g protein / 0g fat / 2g carbs
- Double portion of chicken: 380 calories / 64g protein / 13g fat / 2g carbs
- Tomato salsa: 20 calories / 1g protein / 0g fat / 4g carbs
- Guacamole, 3.5 ounces: 150 calories / 2g protein / 13g fat / 8g carbs

Meal total:

560 calories / 68g protein / 26g fat / 16g carbs

And that way you wouldn't have to cook at all.

Feel free to adjust portion sizes to the appropriate amounts.

And you can switch out the vegetables, proteins, and carbs—everything changed for your preferences.

The point of this is to start making the whole process easier on yourself. And this is just an example of how you could do that.

Make it easy.

JOSH'S WORLD'S EASIEST MONDAY FOOD PLAN FOR MEN

Breakfast

Protein Shake blended with—

- Whey Protein—Two scoops: 200 calories / 36g protein / 4g fat / 12g carbs
- Banana—Two: 242 calories / 2g protein / 0g fat / 62g carbs

- Kale—Two leaves: 34 calories / 2g protein / 0g fat / 34g carbs
- Fish Oil—Five capsules: 45 calories / 0g protein / 5g fat / 0g carbs

Lunch

- Premium Sliced Deli Turkey—Six ounces: 180 calories / 42g protein / 3g fat / 0g carbs
- Apple—Two: 144 calories / 0g protein / 0g fat / 40g carbs
- Almonds—18 nuts: 192 calories / 7g protein / 17g fat / 7g carbs

Dinner

- Seasoned Ground Turkey—Eight ounces: 320 calories / 40g protein / 16g fat / 0g carbs
- Brown Rice Pasta—One cup (cooked): 193 calories / 1g protein / 0g fat / 14g carbs
- Tomato and Basil Pasta Sauce—One-half cup: 50 calories / 1g protein / 2g fat / 10g carbs
- Broccoli—One cup: 31 calories / 3g protein / 0g fat / 6g carbs
- Extra Virgin Olive Oil—Two tablespoons: 240 calories / 0g protein / 28g fat / 0g carbs
- Garlic

Snack

Finally, you'll get a snack of a protein shake that's just protein powder. It won't taste as good as a jazzed-up shake, but it's super portable. Grab a blender bottle, water, some protein powder, shake it up, and knock it back. Takes 10 seconds. You can do that in the middle of the afternoon if you get hungry. Or you can do it late at night if you normally get the munchies then. Easy!

- Protein Powder: 200 calories / 36g protein / 4g fat / 6g carbs
- Water

Total:
2,053 calories / 172g protein / 77g fat / 225g carbs

CELEBRATE AND BE HAPPY

This is going to sound kind of silly, but it's the thing we do that actually makes the most difference: *We celebrate changing habits.*

It's completely the opposite of what human beings naturally do. Normally people say, "I'm going to be SOOOO happy when I get to my end goal!"

And then they wait until the end to have any feeling of happiness or satisfaction.

It's kind of a bummer, because fat loss is hard enough that if we don't get any kind of reinforcement along the way, we probably won't make it. Changing habits is hard.

In fact, changing habits is the whole deal.

When I have clients who are changing habits but stall on results, I never worry. I know they're doing the right things and they're going to get results. If results stall for a week, it's no big thing; results ramp up the next week.

But if I have a client who's struggling with making a change in habits, it keeps me up nights wondering how we can make a smaller change, or a different change, or add more structure or accountability to make that habit stick.

It's all about the habits.

You should celebrate changing habits like they're birthdays. Seriously, if this is the first time you've had protein at breakfast in 10 years, it's actually a bigger deal than your birthday—it's rarer. In fact, you only have about 30 meals you really get to change, and you'll have a lot more birthdays than that.

That's the first reason you need to celebrate these habit changes—they drive results.

The second reason is something I learned from Mike Wunsch, a trainer at Results Fitness who is a genius about the mental game of training: *There's no reason to wait for happiness.*

Most people aren't actually happy about anything in the fitness journey until they hit the final goal. Depending on your goal, that could be a long way off!

Getting to your goal is built on these little habit changes along the way. Sure, you should be happy about the long-term goal. And you should also be happy about the medium-term goals like, 'I'm down a pound this week!' and then, 'I'm down a pound this week too!' and on and on…

But you might never get there if you don't recognize and be happy about those smaller habit changes—like planning that one breakfast or adding protein to that lunch, or whatever change is planned for that week.

Now we'll take it a couple steps further.

I once heard the best reason to set a goal is to become the kind of person who could achieve it.

Usually what we want out of a goal is to feel good about who we are and how we look, and to be liked and respected. And that's even just a step toward something more, like being more connected to people who matter to us, and to more freely give and receive love. It's an expression of who we are, and who we want to be for ourselves and for the people we care about.

You have more access to being the person you want to be—the person who can achieve your goal—when you *are being that person right now.*

> *And right now that person would celebrate and be happy about the little victories.*

CHAPTER 9

ADVANCED FOOD PROGRAMS

ADVANCED FAT-LOSS FOOD PROGRAMS

People often say there's no difference between beginner and advanced—that *advanced* just means you're better at the basics than beginners are. This is mostly true. Unfortunately, straight lines don't always work with the human body.

In fat loss, the basics of quality, quantity, and macro ratios never change. You have to get those right.

And the basics of getting those right—The Eleven Habits—don't change either.

Advanced is what you do after you've got that all down, and have maxed out your results. Results is a key word here—*you've already gotten more results than most people you know*. That's one of the requirements to qualify for an advanced food program.

There are a few others.

QUALIFYING FOR ADVANCED

1. Continuously kept a food journal for at least three months
2. Already hitting protein requirements
3. Have gotten results—women should be under 23% bodyfat; men should be under 14% bodyfat.

If you don't meet these requirements, stick to the basics. You need to work on The Eleven Habits, not advanced techniques.

So if it's all about the basics, why do we need advanced techniques at all?

We can't push the body into fewer calories forever. There's a point where it's beneficial to get a little more sophisticated, and that's where carbohydrate cycling comes in.

And there's a point where you have actually overdone the basics—you've done too much of a good thing. That's where smart refeeds come in.

The most advanced program we do is carbohydrate cycling. Carbohydrate cycling is where we manipulate the fourth variable.

For review, beginner and intermediate fat-loss clients work with three variables.

1. Quantity of food
2. Quality of food
3. Macronutrient ratios

Advanced fat-loss trainees add a fourth.

4. Macronutrient timing

The second advanced technique we're going to take a look at is a structured refeed. This is really about handling the problem of having dieted too hard for too long.

CARBOHYDRATE CYCLING

Carbohydrate cycling has been shown to be more effective for fat loss than simply adjusting quality and quantity of food. In other words, at the same amount of calories, you'll lose more fat with carbohydrate cycling. For advanced clients, it's a really powerful strategy for breaking through a plateau and getting to that next level of leanness.

So what is this carbohydrate cycling? Carbohydrate cycling means alternating between high-carb days and low-carb days.

I tend to note the days by what you *do* get to eat, so that means—

A low-carb day is actually a protein and fat day.
A high-carb day is actually a protein and carbs day.

Carbohydrate cycling gets good results, and a lot people seem to just like it. Even while it's a little more complex, there's something fun about the rotating days. And in a way it simplifies figuring out what you're going to eat.

For a 'no-carb' day, we're going to be in the neighborhood of 50 grams of carbohydrates per day. If someone wanted to argue a little higher—even up to 80 grams—I'd go for that too. Usually, anything less than 20% of total calories coming from carbs is considered low.

We start off with that as the low or 'no carbs' day: 50 grams of carbohydrates.

Then we look at protein. When we're doing carb cycling, I like clients to be in the neighborhood of one gram of protein per pound of target bodyweight. A little higher or lower could also work. I've started with less if people previously had much lower amounts of protein in their food journals. I might work them up, or if they were maintaining strength and muscle, I might not worry about it.

Then the rest sort of fills itself in—we fill in the rest of the energy from fat, up to the calorie requirement.

The high-carb day is also easy. Start with one gram of protein per pound of bodyweight, then fill in most of the remaining calories with carbs. A little fat here and there is fine.

Obviously, we use high-quality carbohydrates like quinoa, brown rice, sweet potatoes, fruit, and vegetables.

No-Carb Day
> Protein: One gram per pound of goal bodyweight
> Carbohydrates: 50 grams-ish, which you'll get from vegetables
> Fat: Fill in the rest of your calories
> Green leafy vegetables: Get as many as possible

High-Carb Day
> Protein: One gram per pound of goal bodyweight
> Carbohydrates: Fill in the rest of your calories
> Fat: As little as possible
> Green leafy vegetables: Get as many as possible

Working the numbers might initially seem cumbersome. What you'll find is it's actually very easy if you use a free online macronutrient calculator.

That being said, if you want to work it the old-fashioned way, all you need to know is that a gram of protein is four calories; one gram of carbohydrates is four calories, and one gram of fat is nine calories.

You shouldn't work this into your program (sadly, there's no protein and alcohol day), but for the record, one gram of alcohol is seven calories.

Now, let's get to the fun part and see what a week would look like.

BASIC CARB-CYCLING TEMPLATE				
NO CARB DAY	4 DAYS PER WEEK	PROTEIN	FAT	VEGETABLES
HIGH CARB DAY	2 DAYS PER WEEK	PROTEIN	CARBOHYDRATES	VEGETABLES
FREE DAY	1 DAY PER WEEK	FREE	FREE	FREE

AGGRESSIVE CARB-CYCLING TEMPLATE				
NO CARB DAY	5 DAYS PER WEEK	PROTEIN	FAT	VEGETABLES
HIGH CARB DAY	1 DAY PER WEEK	PROTEIN	CARBOHYDRATES	VEGETABLES
FREE DAY	1 DAY PER WEEK	FREE	FREE	FREE

RELAXED CARB-CYCLING TEMPLATE				
NO CARB DAY	3 DAYS PER WEEK	PROTEIN	FAT	VEGETABLES
HIGH CARB DAY	3 DAYS PER WEEK	PROTEIN	CARBOHYDRATES	VEGETABLES
FREE DAY	1 DAY PER WEEK	FREE	FREE	FREE

Ideally, you'd never have two high-carb days back to back.

I start with the *Basic Carb-Cycling Template*, and see how people respond. Mostly people do amazingly well on this. But as with everything I do, I modify from client feedback and results. Feedback and results are where we cut out the guesswork.

In terms of modifications, a lot of people can get great results on the more *Relaxed Carb-Cycling Template*. Since I'd be using this with an advanced client and we're trying to break through a plateau, we go straight for the jugular and use the *Basic Carb-Cycling Template*. It's always aggressive enough to get the results we want.

In my personal training career I've had three clients who responded so poorly to carbohydrates that we had to do an even more aggressive carbohydrate-cycling plan—we did five days low carb, one day high carb, and one free day. And out of nowhere they got magical results. This is the exception, not the rule, but it can happen.

As always, I start people on the absolute simplest plan possible. But when it comes to more complex plans, there's always a template. Ultimately your body is going to tell you exactly what you need in your meal plan.

When carbohydrate cycling, always try to put your hard and moderate strength training workouts on your high-carbohydrate days. It's totally okay to put the easy strength training workouts on a no-carbohydrate day.

Carbohydrate cycling works best when you confine all of your free meals to one day, which works inside of the plan as an extra high-carbohydrate day.

If because of social plans you needed to split this into three free meals during a week, you would put the free meals on high-carb days, and the free day would turn into another high-carb day.

The last thing to consider is what to do if you have to put a workout on a protein and fat day instead of a protein and carb day. That's fine once in a while. Just don't put that week's hard workout on a protein and fat day.

EXAMPLE WEEK—BASIC CARB CYCLING TEMPLATE

MONDAY	No Carb Day
TUESDAY	High Carb Day
WEDNESDAY	No Carb Day
THURSDAY	High Carb Day
FRIDAY	No Carb Day
SATURDAY	No Carb Day
SUNDAY	Free Day

REFEEDS: PERIODIZATION FOR YOUR DIET

If you have seasons of workouts, doesn't it make sense to have seasons of food? Sometimes it's summer, and sometimes it's winter. Can't help it…but summer comes around again. And that's the thing about workouts and food—you can't do summer all the time.

In the next section, we're going to talk about seasons of workouts. But there are seasons of food also. The most motivated, most driven clients are those who tend to over-diet. They either diet too hard for too long, or have had multiple bouts of hard dieting and have never fully recovered.

There's a time to *Bring It!* and there's a time to recover. A refeed is a time to recover from hard dieting.

The idea is this: Every week you're going to increase your food consumption by about a hundred calories per day. You'll stop when you get just above maintenance. You're going to build up very, very slowly.

Ideally, you'll add back some of the muscle you would have had if you hadn't been nearly starving all this time, and that, long term, will be a massive boost to your metabolism. Keep that in mind—on top of repairing your poor, hurt metabolism, we're going to add some muscle to boost it even further.

If you're using an online food journal, the estimates these give are close enough—you're probably going to be losing fat at your calorie goal for losing fat. And likewise, if you re-set it for maintenance, it will probably put you pretty close to maintenance.

For a refeed, expect to spend at least a month at maintenance calories. After that, you can reset to fat-loss goal calories again, and you'll find the whole process to be much, much easier.

The fun part is on the way back down, you'll reduce your calories by 200 calories per day and see if you start losing fat again. If not, in a week or two, reduce your calories by another 200 calories. What you'll probably find is that after your refeed, you can lose fat at a higher daily number of calories than before. This is a good thing. If we can have you leaner, fitter, sexier, stronger, and healthier at a higher caloric intake, that's awesome.

The biggest mistake most people make when they do a refeed is they drastically change the quality of the food. They start eating a bunch of crap and gain all fat. They create a quality problem.

And that's why I call this a *smart* refeed. A stupid refeed would be where you start eating a whole bunch of crap. We're going to increase calories. *We aren't going to decrease quality.*

If we remember that scale weight equals calories, we know that while you're doing a refeed, your scale weight will go up. Expect to gain up to five pounds of muscle and fat. Don't worry, we'll lose the fat again later…and keep the lean, sexy muscle.

As a failsafe, if you gain 10 pounds, consider that over your maintenance and stop increasing calories. Do two weeks to a month at maintenance, and then start making your way back down again.

But we also know that bodyfat percentage equals food quality and physical strength. So if you keep the quality on the awesome side, and keep working on strength during your refeed, you'll find a pretty solid gain of lean muscle. And this sexy, lean muscle will reward you with a much stronger, healthier, more powerful metabolism.

I repeat, a refeed does not mean eating a bunch of crap and fast food. A refeed is more *quality* food.

It all comes down to periodization, which is just a fancy word for having a long-term plan that includes up periods that are hard and down periods that are easier. Usually I just use the analogy of seasons: *Winter and Summer*.

Smart trainers always periodize their workout programs. If you've been going hard on your diet for a long time, you need to think about periodizing your food also.

Most people won't need to worry about refeeds. This is essentially a problem that occurs from doing too much right for too long. Going back to the qualifications, usually someone who needs a refeed is a woman who's been under 23% bodyfat for a very long time.

The first time I ever heard of strategic refeeds was in one of Lyle McDonald's books. Later, a YouTube video by Layne Norton had a big impact on the way I do refeeds, slowly easing into the increased caloric intake to minimize fat gain and maximize muscle gain.

That being said, I pretty much fumbled through client refeeds for most of my career until I found Leigh Peele. Leigh is *the expert* on strategic refeeds, and has had by far the biggest influence on how I now have clients do refeeds. I strongly recommend her books *Fat Loss Troubleshoot* and *Starve Mode* if you want a great step-by-step refeed plan.

WORKOUT PROGRAMS DURING YOUR REFEED

During a refeed you should set some sort of performance goal. Think of the extra food as fuel. Put away the scale for a while, and do something fun.

Going back to the analogy of seasons—while it's winter for your nutrition program, it can be summer for your strength and fitness. Or, in *Fat Loss Happens on Monday* terms, your food program would be on maintenance while you have a performance goal from the *Bring It!* program, found in the workout section later in the book.

Some goals you could chase during a refeed—
- Focus on the deadlift. Follow a powerlifting program.
- Focus on your pull-ups. Follow a really aggressive, dedicated pull-up program.
- Train for a Tactical Strength Challenge—deadlift, tactical pull-ups, five-minute snatch test.
- Train to run your first 5K, or to run a faster 5K.
- Train for a sprint triathlon.
- Train for a 5K mud or obstacle run.
- Work on a cool bodyweight skill from gymnastics, parkour, acrobatics, or yoga.
- Train for an SFG or RKC kettlebell instructor certification.
- Get an Olympic weightlifting coach and learn the clean & jerk and the snatch.

Any of these would be great options. And if you've been through the six phases of the *Pull Your Weight* program at least once, you'll have a great foundation of strength and conditioning from which to pursue any of these.

Most of these work really well on top of an abbreviated *Pull Your Weight* program. You could very easily do two days per week of whatever *Pull Your Weight* phase you're scheduled for, and spend three days per week training for a 5K. Or for a bodyweight skill. Or a deadlift program.

Whatever you do, watch out for too much overlap. If you do a deadlift program, you probably want to ditch the deadlifts from *Pull Your Weight*. If you're training for a 5K, you probably want to skip the interval training. And if you're working on a bodyweight skill like handstands, forearm-stands, crow, press-to-handstand, or straddle-planche, remove the pushing and pressing movements from *Pull Your Weight*. Two days of this and two days of that actually works well if you don't do competing movements.

On the flip side, something like training for an SFG or RKC certification will probably take a dedicated program. Training for a triathlon, even a sprint triathlon, will probably take most, if not all, of your workout time. And that's okay too—take a three-month season of training for something specific, and then come back to *Pull Your Weight*.

The bottom line is this: Take your head out of the losing-fat game as a reprieve. Bring up your calories and reset your metabolism. At the same time, focus any results-getting, type-A, or competitive leanings you have toward a strength or fitness goal.

ADVANCED DIETERS AND ONE CHANGE

People who are advanced should already have all The Eleven Habits cold. You don't need to worry about changing one habit per week.

It's been my experience that people who are already good at hitting macronutrient and calorie numbers can hit a new target if I give them one.

For example, if I switch someone who is dialed in with the calorie and macros goals over to carbohydrate cycling, she can usually do that in one week. Because she has all the other moving parts down, changing the macros is a smaller and easier change for an advanced client than adding general food preparation is for a beginner.

It makes sense if you think about sports: One of the differences between a pro athlete and an amateur is the pro has the basics ingrained at a subconscious level, freeing up attention for other things like strategy, field vision, and so on.

And that's the way it works with fat loss, too—advanced trainees should have The Eleven Habits mostly on autopilot. They should have enough attention freed up to make a different kind of change.

It's not that *One Change* doesn't apply to them. It's that their one change can be a bigger change than someone who is an intermediate or a beginner.

JOSH

CHAPTER 10

HOW TO GAUGE PROGRESS

HOW TO GAUGE PROGRESS

How to gauge progress is always a touchy subject, and for good reason. How you choose to gauge your progress determines how you're going to treat yourself, and whether or not you're going to be happy or sad about the changes to your body.

In the same way society and the media didn't teach you how to train well or eat properly for results, they also didn't teach you how to correctly gauge your progress.

Let's start at the most obvious spot—the scale. The scale is both deified by the public as the ultimate measure of success, as much as it's demonized by 'enlightened' trainers everywhere. Like everything, the truth is somewhere in the middle.

If you think back to where we talked about how scale weight equals calories consumed, and bodyfat percentage equals the quality of food…we know exactly what the scale means. Barring terrible hormonal issues or metabolic syndromes, for which you need to see a doctor, *If the scale is too high, you're eating too much.*

Where this starts to get fuzzy is this: Most women assume the scale is too high when it isn't. A woman who strength trains will probably be about 10 pounds heavier on the scale than she looks. All her friends will think she's 119 pounds, when really she's 130 pounds. Or whatever… you get the idea.

This doesn't happen just some of the time; *this happens all of the time.*

This leads into the muscle versus fat conversation.

1. Fat is the part that's jiggly. It takes up more space per pound than muscle does. That's why extra fat makes you look so much bigger.
2. Muscle is the part that's lean and tight. It takes up less space per pound than fat does. That's why people who have muscle look toned.

There is no long, lean muscle versus big, bulky muscle. There's just muscle or fat, and you get to choose which one you want more of.

SKINNY FAT AND THE MATRIX OF FAT VERSUS MUSCLE

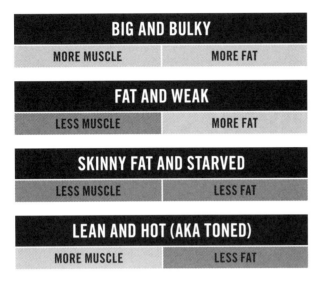

It should be obvious that the goal is to add muscle and not gain fat. But still, there are plenty of women who got sold on the super old-school 'muscle is bulky' idea. And hey, everyone thought that back in the '90s—it's not just you. But now we know better: There's only muscle or fat.

There's nothing magical called toned that is somehow neither of those. Likewise, we don't have long, lean muscle. Muscle is lean. Fat is bulky. If someone isn't long and lean, it's because of fat.

The toned look most women want is just less jiggly fat and more firm, tight muscle.

And for guys, this is why it takes so long if you want to get huge and jacked: Muscle takes up so little space. It takes a few pounds of muscle to take up the space a single pound of fat would have taken up.

PLEASE, I BEG YOU, LEARN FROM THESE CLICHÉS

When you see someone who looks hot, remember that looking hot means more muscle and less fat.

But people still don't get it. The most cliché thing in the world is a woman who's completely *skinny fat*, and thinks she needs to lose five pounds. In reality, she doesn't need to lose weight—remember the *skinny* part of skinny fat? The reason she doesn't look hot is because even though her scale weight is low, it's all fat and no muscle. The only way she can get the lean and toned look she wants is to gain a little muscle.

The second most cliché thing in the world is the guy who's 50 pounds overweight, but says he needs to go on a muscle-gain program. No…he'll look more muscular if he loses fat.

Girls always think the answer is to lose weight. Guys always think the answer is to gain muscle. News flash, again: The answer is in the middle for both of them. They both need the opposite of what they think they need if they want to look hot.

MEASURING RESULTS

Let's talk about measurements. Measuring your progress is something that's key to coaching yourself. If you measure your progress correctly, it can be a window into how well you're tracking.

Tracking in your food journal is going to tell you everything you need to know about how to become strategic about the future—what you're doing right and what you're doing wrong.

There are three things we track in terms of the results we're measuring.

- I want you to measure your scale weight.
- I want you to measure your bodyfat percentage, and I'll explain why in a minute.
- I want you to measure your circumference measurements with a tape measure—waist at the belly button level, hips at the biggest spot.

My preferred interval for taking all of these measurements is three weeks. In fact, I'd like for you to rotate through these measurements. One week measure your scale weight. The next week measure your bodyfat percentage. The week after, measure your circumference measurements. Then, start over with the first measurement.

A lot of people freak out when I talk about scale weight. On the flip side, there are a lot of people who are invested in scale weight more than they should be. My whole perspective on scale weight is that it's probably the least important measurement.

But scale weight does tell a story. It tells you, 'How much did I eat this week or this month?' or whatever interval you're measuring. It tells you, 'In this time interval, did the *quantity of food*—the calories—go up or down?' That's important to know.

Because the scale tells us about quantity of food consumed, it can be useful in terms of clarification about the numbers we get from the other measurements.

The next measurement is bodyfat percentage. I am a big fan of caliper measurements. If you can have someone else do it for you, I like the Durnin and Womersley method of caliper bodyfat measurements. The Durnin and Womersley method measures four sites: Biceps, triceps, subscapular, and iliac crest. Add up those four numbers, and plug the result into any of the dozens of body fat calculators available online when you google "Durnin and Womersley Body Fat Calculator."

If you're doing it on yourself, you can do the one-site measurement at the iliac crest. Just pinch some fat about ⅔ of the way from your belly button to your hip bone.

Essentially, you're just getting a millimeter number. If that number goes down, you know something good happened. If it goes up, you know you probably did something that was not effective.

That's how I like to measure bodyfat percentage. Even if you're doing the Durnin and Womersley method, I still like to get a measurement on the biggest or fattest spot of the stomach. It's not because it contributes in any way to an estimate of bodyfat percentage, it's probably the best way to track progress in that area.

Here are a couple of other thoughts about the caliper measurements—

- If you aren't used to doing this or you're not really good at it, take each measurement three times and average the three. I always take the stomach measurement three times and take an average because it's the most important. It's also the hardest to get an accurate number.
- The next thing about bodyfat percentage, especially with calipers, is to take the result with a grain of salt. There are a lot of things that can mess this up. It's a measurement that is *majorly prone to human error.*
- Even without human error, the results can be weirdly mercurial. Sometimes people can eat something and have a bad reaction and it will gauge weird. When you've just worked out, your skin might be a little too 'tough.' The fat literally will not be as slippery and it will gauge a little fatter than you normally are.

I don't stress too much about the bodyfat caliper test, but it's something I like to have. Just don't use it like it's the absolute truth; use it to see how things are trending over time.

If everything is rocking, we can see a 3% bodyfat change from month to month. If things are semi-rocking, we usually see a 2% bodyfat change. If we see a 1% change or less, there's something missing. We're doing something wrong in terms of quantity or quality, or possibly the ratios are contributing to this—or possibly the lack of preparation. We go back into the food log. We look for a strategy of what we can alter in the future.

If you want a really accurate bodyfat measurement, I'm a big fan of the DEXA scan. If there's a hospital in your area with a bone density wing, you can often get a DEXA scan for about $75. It's something worth looking into and is probably the most accurate bodyfat test available.

The last measurement is a really cool measurement because it's one of the easiest to get correct. It's hard to mess up the circumference measurements. With the circumference measurements, you basically just use a tape measure, wrap it around yourself, and get a measurement.

When I worked at 24 Hour Fitness, we started at the top and worked down. We did the neck, biceps, and wrists, although I don't know why we did the wrists. We even did the forearms. We did the stomach at the belly button level. We did the hips—basically the biggest spot around the butt. We did the thighs seven inches back from the knee. We did the calves as well. This would be one way to do it.

If you want to go a little more minimal, you can get a pretty good idea of what's going on from just the stomach and hips. Typically, we measure the stomach right at the belly button level. We don't go for the natural waist, which is the smallest spot, because that isn't where we store fat, so that's not as useful. If you're on the leaner side, the belly button is a good landmark for measuring your belly. If you're bigger, just measure the *biggest spot*.

Think about it like this: Whatever the biggest spot is, that's the spot you want to reduce, so that's what you should measure.

With the hips, we'll go around the butt at the biggest spot.

The most important thing with all these measurements is not to think of the measurement is 'the truth,' but to know you can measure it with some degree of accuracy, and track changes over time. You then get some information to work with to see if things are trending better or worse.

Remember, bodyfat percentage is always going to be the quality of food, plus the quality of your workouts. Scale weight is always going to be quantity of food.

Circumference measurements are probably the best combination. Circumference measurements are great because they even everything out.

SCALE WEIGHT	Quantity of food (calories)
YOUR BODYFAT PERCENTAGE	Quality of food and how strong you are
CIRCUMFERENCE MEASUREMENTS	Combination of quantity and quality of food

That being said, I never take any of these measures as the absolute truth.

One of the reasons that I like getting all three is because you're going to get funky measurements sometimes. Sometimes you're going to get a measurement that doesn't make sense. Don't stress about it! Just hang out. Wait a week and take the next measurement.

Then you can check in: *Does this next measurement say the same thing as the last measurement?*

If you get two measurements that say you're losing fat, believe them! If you get two measurements in a row that say you're gaining fat, believe them!

If you get two measurements that don't agree, hang out for a week and take another measurement. *Go with the two out of the three that agree.*

Look, if your bodyfat percentage measurements are all over the map, but your scale weight and circumference measurements are going down, you're losing fat. You just suck at taking bodyfat percentage measurements.

Or on the flip side, if your scale weight is staying the same, but your bodyfat percentage and circumference measurements are going down, that means you're gaining muscle and losing fat.

Now this should be obvious: If everything is going up—scale weight, circumference measurements, and bodyfat percentage—you're eating too many calories.

In general the measurements are either telling you things are working or things are not working. If we get one measurement where things aren't working, I don't typically stress out at that point unless the food journal is a total mess, and then I'll know things aren't working.

However, let's say we're doing everything right. The food journal looks great. You've been honest in the food journal. The quantity is right. The quality is right. The ratios are right. Everything is cool.

If we get a crazy measurement that makes it look like things aren't working, I don't stress out that first time. I wait another week and take a look at the next measurement. If the next measurement says things are still going backward, then I'll start taking a look. If it looks right in the food journal, then maybe the food journal is not accurate, and we go from there.

I just don't want you to break down into tears when you've done everything right, but when you measure that week, it comes back that you gained fat, your scale weight went up, or that the circumference measurements are up. For whatever reason, sometimes things just don't measure correctly that week, but *that's okay.* Just look for the trend over time. You want the trend over time to be going the right way. In general, you want most of the measurements going the right way.

This is the biggest thing to understand about measurements: On any *one day* they can be wrong. However, *over time they are the law.*

If over time everything is trending in one direction or the other, you'll know that things are either working or not working. Regardless of what you may perceive to be the right amount of food or the right quality of food, the measurements over time will let you know the reality.

The great thing about measurements is they're easy to count. You can see the hard numbers right there. Over the last three months, everything has been trending down. There have been times where it bumped up, but the trend is down. However, it could be that it's been a whole month and things have been trending backward, as though everything has been gaining and the results are backtracking. Maybe you're not really as tight as you think and you need to go back to your food journal to see if you missed something.

Here's one last thought: It's rare for people to deliberately lie in their food journals. The reality is it's easy to omit or forget things. It's almost like we're designed to forget things. Use measurements as a way to check yourself for where you may have been a little easier on yourself, omitted or forgot some things. This is everything you need to know about measurements.

BODYFAT PERCENTAGE IN DETAIL

Bodyfat percentage is a great way to measure progress if you have a reliable way to measure it.

I like using calipers to measure bodyfat percentage in my clients, but measuring with calipers is a skill and most people suck at it, even personal trainers. In fact, it's been years since I've seen a trainer do it correctly.

Hydrostatic weighing is uncomfortable because you need to be submerged underwater for a period of time, but it's accurate.

The DEXA scan is probably the best. It's accurate and it's easy—you lie there and get scanned. It's primarily a bone density test that secondarily gives an accurate bodyfat percentage reading.

People always ask about the electronic impedance scales. We used to say these weren't ever effective, but now they have versions that are reliable. The catch: The electronic impedance scales that are accurate cost between $10,000 and $20,000. You might be able to find an upscale health club that has one, but you aren't going to get one for personal use.

If you have access to any of these, the numbers can be useful. They're phenomenally useful in terms of knowing when to stop dieting. Truth be told, most people never feel 'perfect' no matter how lean they get. Bodyfat percentage is an awesome way to know you're lean enough and can move on to other things.

Part of this comes down to self-image and body dysmorphia. Relax, it's not just you; it's everyone. You don't see yourself exactly as you are. And you don't see yourself as everyone else sees you.

Trust me and trust the numbers—if you're a woman in the 18–23% bodyfat range, you can stop. You're hotter than 99% of the women in the world; you look awesome in a bikini, and you can wear whatever you want.

Men want you, and women want to be you. You're done.

The reason I give that range is because—here's a shocker—women have drastically different shapes, much more so than men. Guys basically always look hotter when they're leaner. Women don't. Some women look hotter at 23%, some look hotter at 18%, and some are in the middle.

In other words, if you're more suited to the super sporty lean look, that's hot and you should go with that. If you've got some of those great womanly curves, that's hot and you should hold on to some of those.

HERE'S MY REALITY BODYFAT SCALE—

Above 30% bodyfat: There's something to fix. For your health and for how you want to look, you really want to get leaner than 30%.

At 26% bodyfat: You're totally healthy, and even though TV tells us a woman who's at 26% bodyfat is average, the reality is most of America isn't healthy or average, and you're actually ahead of 80% of America.

At 23% bodyfat: You're really in shape now. You're officially a workout girl and you're ahead of 90% of the women in America. You're fit, lean, and there's nothing left to fix. Depending on your body type, you may find you're totally done at 23%.

At 21% bodyfat: You're super hot. You look great in clothes; you can wear whatever you want; you should feel great wearing a swimsuit. Coincidentally, right about here you should be able to do three chin-ups and deadlift your bodyweight three times.

At 19% bodyfat: You're a rock star. You look amazing in clothes; you can wear whatever you want. You can't wait for bikini season. You've officially won at leanness. Men want you, women want to be you, and you're the envy of all your friends. I'm only half joking about that last part.

For men, it's exactly the same sequence, but about 10% lower.

Above 22% bodyfat: There's something to fix. For your health and for how you want to look, you really want to get leaner than 22%.

At 17% bodyfat: You're totally healthy, and even though TV tells us a guy who's at 17% bodyfat is pretty average, the reality is most of America isn't healthy or average, and you're actually ahead of 80% of America.

At 14% bodyfat: You're really in shape now. You're officially a workout guy and you're ahead of 90% of the men in America. You're fit, lean, and there's nothing left to fix.

At 12% bodyfat: You're wicked lean. You look great in clothes; you can wear whatever you want, and you should feel great taking your shirt off at the pool. Coincidentally, right about here you should be doing 10 chin-ups and deadlifting one-and-a-half times your bodyweight three times.

At 9% bodyfat: You're a rock star. Most dudes will have a really flat stomach and abs at 9%. Women will swoon, guys will give you high-fives, and if you walk around with your shirt off long enough, you'll probably score a reality TV show.

CALIPERS, INTERNAL FAT, AND AGE

With caliper measurements, I never take age into account. But in reality, as you get older, you start to collect extra essential fat around your organs. While this doesn't change how you look, it would increase the bodyfat percentage reading you get from a DEXA scan or a hydrostatic bodyfat measurement.

According to the American Council on Exercise Bodyfat Percentage Chart, after age 20, men are going to add about 1% of internal fat every five years and women are going to add about 2% of internal bodyfat every five years.

YOU'RE ALREADY A ROCK STAR. THERE'S NOTHING LEFT TO FIX.

That's what I tell my female clients when they hit 19% bodyfat.

And this is really, really important. This is what we use bodyfat percentage measurements for—to give yourself a place where you can stop and say you got there.

Let me be more explicit: Bodyfat measurement is not a tool to see how far you have to go. *Bodyfat percentage is a tool so you know when you can stop.*

It's about how you talk to yourself.

> *You're already a rock star.*
> *There's nothing to left to fix.*

If I have a female client at 19% bodyfat, I let her know she's done. She's a rock star and she's hotter than 99% of the women in America. Okay…if you live in Malibu, take a trip through the middle of the country sometime.

I've helped female clients get down to 16% bodyfat or even 14% bodyfat, but I'm letting them know every single session that they're already rock stars; there's nothing to left to fix.

Really, getting down to 14% or 16% bodyfat as a woman is totally unnecessary. I'm kind of rocking the boat saying this, I know. There are a lot of fitness industry people telling you to get down to figure model bodyfat percentages, but that's crazy talk. Most clients don't even *want* to look like that.

But when I tell them they hit 19%, they look awesome and they're done, things change.

It's hard to accept.

Really. Some people have a hard time being done.

I actually start the process waaaaaaay before 19% bodyfat. Once a woman hits 26% bodyfat, I'm letting her know she's totally healthy, and even though TV tells us a woman who's at 26% bodyfat is average, the reality is she's ahead of 80% of America.

She should feel really good to be there. That being said, it's totally okay and normal and healthy to want to be a little leaner.

Then at 23% bodyfat, I'm letting her know she's really in shape now—she's officially a workout girl and she's ahead of 90% of the women in America. She's fit, lean, and there's nothing left to fix.

If she wants to be a rock star, we can get her to rock-star status, but she's already awesome.

At 21% bodyfat, a woman should know she's really ahead of the game. Women should relate to themselves as being really, really hot at 21% bodyfat, and should feel great about that.

Along with that, by this point my clients have completely transformed their relationships to fitness—they're stronger, healthier, doing pull-ups, deadlifting bodyweight, kicking ass, and relating to themselves as athletes.

At this point you have achieved rock-stardom. You're done.

We shift the context to fitness-related goals—whatever fun and cool things you've always wanted to be able to do—mud runs, training for a kettlebell certification, running 5Ks, doing a Tactical Strength Challenge…whatever is cool to you.

You may get leaner from here, but it's not necessary, and it's not the goal.

In the interest of transparency, years ago when I first came up with the bodyfat percentage scale above, I was really only training 'civilians.' Since then, I've done food coaching for a couple of fitness models and for tons of kettlebell instructors and personal trainers. These are people who are professionally expected to be a little leaner than the guidelines above, and may need to be within striking distance of getting super-human lean for a photo shoot—leaner than walking around on a day-to-day basis.

PHOTOSHOP, CELLULITE, AND YOU LOOKING BANGIN' IN REAL LIFE

There's a lot of controversy around what's possible, what you should shoot for, and what you're told you should look like.

There are two basic messages you're getting—
1. From the media: *You should look like this Photoshopped model.*
2. From most bloggers: *It's all Photoshopped and totally unrealistic.*

I, of course, rest in the middle.

I love to write about celebrity workouts and diets. I also love to see celebrity beach candids—we get to see what people really look like. Granted, you could also just go to your local gym and see what people really look like. The point is, the un-Photoshopped paparazzi shots of celebrities are really hot, and they may still have a little bit of fat on their thighs or butts. They may have a little more stomach than you thought they would.

Yes, in real life even models and actresses have cellulite.

I love seeing the articles where they show the celebrity Photoshopped and the celebrity in real life. Again, usually we discover the pre-Photoshop celebrity looks like a very fit real-life woman.

What you'll usually see without Photoshop, a celebrity may have a really flat, sexy, enviable stomach, but her waist, even without any extra fat, is still nowhere near as narrow as it was on that last magazine cover.

You may find the celebrity has a really flat, lean, and sexy stomach, or she's got really smooth, amazingly sexy cellulite-free thighs…but unless she's 20 years old or just finished temporarily starving herself for a photo shoot, she never has both.

What I want you to take away from this is that we can get you to the kind of really lean, hot, and sexy that happens in real life. Your friends and your significant other will all notice—because in real life it's even more striking.

But what's really sad is that you might not see it because you're comparing yourself to Photoshopped model images.

I always think of one female client who was insistent about getting down to 14% bodyfat because she wanted to lose every last bit of cellulite on her legs. And we got her down to 14% bodyfat, but she still had a little bit of cellulite and she was totally crushed. She had full-on eight-pack abs and other gym members asked if she was a model, but she was hung up on the literally four square inches of her body that weren't perfect.

It still makes me sad. It's the silliest thing ever, the way humans are wired. Everyone else sees and envies what's great about us, and we always see our flaws.

I've had so many female clients tell me something like, "My husband is so totally amazed with how great I look now!" or "My boyfriend says he can totally tell how much my body has changed and he loves it!"

This is usually when they get to 21–23% bodyfat.

Let me set that apart for emphasis: Usually female clients who start getting major compliments from their friends, family, and significant others are in the 21–23% bodyfat range.

This is nowhere near a Photoshopped-picture level.

I'm just saying, most guys seem to be really happy with realistic-looking women.

When I worked in a big gym, most of the clients I had were women who came up to me, pointed at one of my other clients, and asked, "What would it take to look like her?"

And the client they were pointing at was usually about 19% bodyfat and looked amazing. Often, they'd point at the clients who were at 14% bodyfat and say, "I don't want to get *that* lean."

I'm telling you, it's easy to see this on other people. It can be hard to see it on yourself.

To come full circle, even when you look *amazing*—when people in your life are telling you they can't believe how good you look—it won't look like the magazine covers.

And that's okay. Reality is a really great place to live.

DAN

CHAPTER 11

SETTING THE MIND TO THE GOAL

SETTING YOUR MIND TOWARD THE GOAL

It really comes down to this: Many of us—and my hand is raised up, too—have a record of failure when it comes to diet- and food-based approaches to fat loss. I always joke, "My doctor put me on a diet. It wasn't enough food, so now I'm on two diets."

There's no question *Fat Loss Happens on Monday* is a unique approach, but you may have a history of not succeeding that might have you sighing, 'Here I go again.'

But, this is not again.

This is going to be different. I want to encourage you to truly get your mind right before we venture on. We will use these five steps.

1) Examine your prepositions.
2) Think about your mission.
3) Hunt…finish the task.
4) It's just a problem.
5) Make it a MUST.

Goals and goal-setting are a crucial point of every single thing we do. Steve Ledbetter reminds us that if we have **one** goal, we have an 80% chance of succeeding at it. Sadly, if we have three, we have statistically the same chance of getting those three as compared to not setting any goals at all.

In other words, it doesn't look good.

My most common response to practically any question is, *What's your goal?*

Let's be clear about this from the beginning. Every second you spend thinking about your goal—the clarity of what you really want—is like chipping at a rich vein in a gold mine. Or, like I often tell my athlete clients, it's like stealing; it's so easy and obvious once you set your mind to a single task, you'll wonder why everybody doesn't do it.

Years ago, a friend of mine was spending a lot of time on the road selling whatever he was selling at the time. He took some good advice and decided to turn his travels into a mobile university, and began collecting audiobooks. At the time, these came in large boxes with dozens of cassettes inside. Part of the fun of a road trip was pulling out the right one and hoping to flip it to the correct side.

As he bought more and more tapes, he often gave me his overflow. When he gave me Earl Nightingale's *Lead the Field,* my life changed. Nightingale, a survivor of the attack on Pearl Harbor, was the pioneer of recorded motivational work. His website sums the key point.

> *"When he was 29, Earl's enlightenment had come to him as a bolt out of the blue while reading* Think and Grow Rich. *It came when he realized that the six words he read were the answer to the question he had been looking for: That we become what we think about."*

We become what we think about.

I want you to think about this…a lot.

My first hope for you is that you will succeed at many, most, or all of your goals in life. My concern is that many of us have achieved things we didn't want and certainly didn't expect when we were daydreaming in elementary school about what we wanted to be when we grew up.

In supporting your goals, I want to be a Nabi. The name comes from the Hebrew and is often translated into the term Prophet. That's fine, of course, but I want you to think about the difference between the two words, forthteller and fortuneteller.

A Nabi looks into the heart. Often, we see prophets of all types and stripes as fortunetellers. We put our money down and the fortuneteller flips the cards, reads the palm, and tells you your ship is just about to come in and you will find true love. That is not a forth-teller.

Forthtelling is the skill of a friend, family member, or mentor. You may have had this talk with Mom and Dad.

"Listen, if you keep on doing X, you'd better prepare for Y."

You know, it doesn't have to be negative here.

"Listen, if you keep on studying this hard, you had better prepare for graduation and success in college."

"Listen, if you keep on eating right and training, you had better prepare for a lifetime of health and wellness."

But we all know what I really mean. It's usually used as a threat about future events. Yet, we control that future through our choices today.

I often joke that the most disciplined people in the world are those who are going to start a diet tomorrow. Tomorrow, they will have the discipline to train, to eat only crunchy veggies, and to drink water.

Of course, it's not what you're going to eat that's the problem; *it's what you ate* that's the problem.

My job is not to predict your future. My job is to point, to illuminate, and to walk with you in this goal. Goal-setting is simply pointing yourself from here, Point A, to there, Point B. As you decide what your goal is, your B, I want you to do one more thing before moving into the specifics of fat loss or body composition.

I want you to examine your prepositions.

What?

During my education, one of my professors shared an insight from a rabbi that changed my vision of success in life: *Examine your prepositions.*

According to my wife, a preposition is anything a rabbit can do to a log. A rabbit can be *around, at, behind, below, beneath, beside, between, beyond, by, with, within, without*…a log.

The great question the rabbi poses is this: *What are **your** prepositions?*

Simply, who are you with, around, below, beside…and all the rest?

The more connections you have, the more likely you will achieve your goals. Your support system will be there cheering you on and helping you with things like meal prep and shopping, the most social of the important steps of body composition.

Think about this. Examine your prepositions.

You Might Not Get Your Goal. Sorry.

Lately, I've been beating this joke about the fitness industry to death.

This is treadmill.

This is how you walk on it.

Pay me money.

With the Big Box, 24/7 gym operations dominating the fitness landscape since the 1980s, many of us still think the standard of training is cardio and bodybuilding. Andrew Read notes that most gyms are based on the Noah's Ark model, two of everything.

You go to the front desk and some girl named Paris, a certified professional trainer, offers you a deal where you can train for a lifetime at $49.95 a month. They will tap your bank account until you change banks, which, by the way, we discovered is true.

Then, the gym prices dropped. Hard.

Training business expert Thomas Plummer told me that one place offered $1.99 a year—this is no misprint—to bring in people. Listen, if all you're doing as a gym is renting treadmills, the buyer will always go to the cheapest treadmill. If your goal is so vague and loose that 30 minutes of treadmilling three times a week is going to get you there, pay the man the two bucks a year.

In some cities, fitness boxes have become the second home of many street people, as the economics of a warm place with all the comforts of a spa for a few bucks a month is worth it.

I want you to rethink something before we move on. I think the *how of fitness* is really important. You need to learn to do things right and to do things in a proper manner.

But, what's your why? Why do you want to be fit or lean or perform better?

Remember, the answer to 'how' is very important. You can find the answer to 'how' throughout this book.

As Viktor Frankl noted in *Man's Search for Meaning* when he quoted Nietzsche, one of the best books of all time, "If you have a *why* to live, you can bear with any *how*." His survival from a Nazi concentration camp walks us through the most horrific moments of human history and gives us an insight into making the world a better place.

It was Frankl's insight about how you find your why that made me change my life. One learns the *why* in three ways.

Love
Suffering (sadly, this is the easiest)
Work

The word passion, which gets thrown around in sports all the time, comes from the root *pati,* which means to suffer. It's about love, sure, but it's really about suffering for love.

Like everyone, I have suffered and given up a lot for things I love. My discus career is the story of training four to seven hours a day and realizing I had to give up so much of life to do it. Was it worth it?

Today, I can look back and smile and say, "Absolutely."

I frequently bounce two thoughts around my head.

"The last human freedom is the ability to control our own thoughts."

~ Victor Frankl

"The highest stage of moral culture is when we recognize that we ought to control our thoughts."

~ Charles Darwin

There's no question in my mind that true fitness, in body, mind, and soul, comes from realizing that our own thoughts, our own wills, dominate our decision-making process. This is the *why* of things.

My favorite part of teaching has always been when we entered into epics. I was once asked to explain an epic, versus a story perhaps.

"Epics are big!"

Epics take on big stories and big topics. Generally, epics take on the big issues like love, and its great friends, lust, death, and God. Most of my favorite works are epics, from *Gilgamesh* and the Arthurian legends to *Dune* and *The Godfather. Gilgamesh,* which includes the story of the Flood, has its hero achieve immortality by the great walls he builds, yet he truly achieves immortality by the clay tablets his story was written upon.

Others find value in Woody Allen's great insight: *I don't want to achieve immortality through my work…I want to achieve it through not dying.*

Gilgamesh, like Beowulf by the way, wanted his name to be remembered forever. He achieved his goal. But, he didn't achieve it by swallowing the thistle of immortality or by his building of the great walls. He's remembered by those meager clay tablets.

That's what I want you to think about: What's *behind* your goals? That's something bigger.

That's what I call your mission.

You might not get your goal. Sorry. If it's a championship, others want it, too. If it's a fitness goal, your life, including past, present, and future, might conspire against you.

I want you to focus on something bigger than a goal: *your mission.*

And, let me warn you, the key to Life, the Universe, and Everything is this—

The mission is to keep the mission, the mission.

Your mission helps you do one big thing: *decide*. Decide comes from the same root as homicide, suicide and patricide—it means to cut or to kill. But, your mission also keeps your focus consistent.

Here is a fun test, and I know you've done this. You want to go to a movie; let's say *Gone with the Wind*. So you tell everyone, "Let's go to a movie." Everyone discusses what movie they may want to see. Edna hates Rhett, so she won't go to *GWTW*; Larry wants to see a comedy and Bill, a horror movie. An hour later, you find yourself sitting in a movie theater watching a French film about a clown who lost his button.

Welcome to the wrong way to decide things. Decide means to cut!

"I'm going to *Gone with the Wind*—who wishes to join me?"

I have a long, boring story about how I ended up sitting at a Cardinals-Giants game when we wanted to see the 49ers-Broncos game. Failure to decide leads to all kinds of plan changes and compromises.

How do you find your mission? *Find your story.*

At one of my workshops, a woman had discovered kettlebells and lost 100 pounds in a year. She told me, "I want to change lives now."

Yep, I would hire her.

There's a simple way I teach people to discover their stories. Like in geometry, you must first discover your givens.

What are your givens? Well, I always joke that to find them, get married and have kids. Do you celebrate Christmas? Do you open presents on Christmas Eve or Christmas Day? Do you rinse the glasses before you put them in the dishwasher?

My brother Phil had a girlfriend who thought our house was crazy because we left bathroom doors closed. Her reason: In her house, the bathroom was occupied if the door was closed. In our house, we locked the doors!

Which is right? It doesn't matter, but you might think someone is weird because he cuts his meat while holding the fork in his right hand.

Those crazy things we consider life's rules are usually just our givens.

The longer we're in any relationship, the more buttons we seem to have. I had a boss, a guy who didn't have kids, who thought the hardest thing to get across to parents was to not be like an elevator. He said to me, "I don't get it. Bobby says something, and Mom and Dad go to the third floor. Bobby tries to push my button and I have no idea what he is doing. So, I tell him exactly what to do and he does it."

These are your personal givens.

If I say, "That dress looks nice on you," and you respond with, "Why, do the others make me look fat?" my given is to leave this relationship as fast as I can.

There are some fun ways to discover your givens, or at least give you some insights into your givens. The fun part of this is to look at someone else's list! Very simply—

What are your top 10 favorite movies?
What are your top 10 favorite books?
What have been the top 10 best things in your life and the top 10 challenges?

My movie list is—

Patton
Star Trek II: The Wrath of Khan
Lawrence of Arabia
Star Wars
Field of Dreams
Animal House
The Three Musketeers (with Michael York)
Robin Hood (with Errol Flynn)
Brigadoon
How to Succeed in Business without Really Trying

It wasn't until I did this many times that I realized most of these stories have an element of David and Goliath or an underdog theme. My athletic career follows the theme of these movies.

Sean Greeley added a new question for me: *What are the 10 best meals you ever had?*

This fits perfectly with something I asked my daughters years ago. You go out to dinner and two of the three things are awful, but one is perfect. Choose!

Food
Service
Company

Both daughters got it right; they chose the company. When Sean shared this insight of best meals, I realized as I made my list, great dining experiences are all about the people, not the food.

I do this yearly, and I keep the lists. In 1989, I wrote, among others—

Top 10 1989

Pregnancy
Tiff hired by Eastern Airlines
Updates on home at 1700 South
Net worth on January 18, 1989: $4,145, with $63,500 in liabilities

Just for reference, today—

Kelly is now a first grade teacher, and a wife and mother.
Eastern shut down right after I wrote that.
We moved from the Blue Bungalow the next year.
We have a lot more net worth and have been debt-free for years.

It helps to do this so you can see if you're making progress in all areas of your life, sure. But you also get a hint about what you think is bigger than mere goal-setting.

Two generations of my students have done this assignment. My daughters went to school with kids whose parents did this project. One mom told me, "I was smarter at 18 than I am now!" The assignment is called *My Life is My Message*. Having parent and child look at a list of books or movies together is one of life's golden moments.

When you unpack this information, you get an insight into your *why* of life. Many think my mission statement is 'Never Let Go,' from T. H. White's *The Sword in the Stone*. Actually, though, it's 'Make a Difference.'

For every decision I make, I ask myself: *Will this make a difference?* If it broadens this happy blue orb a little bit, I'm inclined to say yes.

I have often heard that on our tombstones there will be two numbers and a dash in between the year of birth, the year of death and that little dash. The dash is all the time we have to make a difference.

Take some time to figure out your story. What brings you to this goal? Does it fit into a larger picture about your life's journey? Taking the time to do that is like being given a vein of pure gold to mine.

What are your givens about life?

The fun thing about sharing Top 10 lists is that you can peek inside your own head and see what's important to you. And, remember, if you meet someone who has never read 10 full books and you read that many in a month, this might be an issue down the line. Think about who sits at the table with you during your 10 best meal experiences—you might consider dining with them more often if you can.

You may want to share what you know.

> *"There is a thing called knowledge of the world, which people do not have until they are middle-aged. It is something which cannot be taught to younger people, because it is not logical and does not obey laws which are constant. It has no rules. Only in the long years which bring women to the middle of life, a sense of balance develops…when she is beginning to hate her used body, she suddenly finds that she can do it. She can go on living…"*
>
> ~ T. H. White, *The Once and Future King*

Your mission may last long after that second number on your tombstone.

You might not get your goal, but you might make a difference in the process.

Examine your prepositions.

Think about your mission.

DAN

CHAPTER 12

A SIMPLE WAY TO LOOK AT THE PROBLEMS WITH THE FITNESS INDUSTRY

While vacationing in Ireland, I had the great opportunity to spend a day touching stones. Yes, stones.

Ireland has tombs that are older than the pyramids of Egypt. There are rings of huge stones littered around the country that have only been appreciated again in recent decades. When you touch these stones, you literally touch the past 5,000 years.

My guide started talking about health and fitness and asked if I had ever read J. Stanton's book *The Gnoll Credo*. Of course, later I would, but at the time he pointed out the big three keys to the gnolls. Ah, what are gnolls? Half-human and half-hyenas who have an interesting way of viewing the world, so now you know.

Plan the Hunt
Hunt
Discuss the Hunt

If I could take a big red pen and circle the number one problem in the fitness industry, it would be that we don't follow those three points. Listen, I don't care what idiotic thing you're going to try, I honestly don't, from three-day liver cleanses to walking across the country (any country).

Plan it, do it, then talk about what you did right or wrong.

Let me make this clear: I don't really care what thing you're going to do—*just finish it*.

Rarely have I met a person who was going to do a 12-week program actually finish it. Most of the money-back guarantees for those TV workouts have the little caveat: *If you finish it and don't get the results, we will gladly return your money*. You know why?

No one does rule number two of the Gnoll Credo: Hunt.

The Navy divers I know have a simple concept that is practically the same.

Plan the Dive.
Dive the Plan.

As a trainer, I go along with any idea my clients come up with in magazines or office conversations.

A three-day juice fast? Sure!

Walk six hours a day? Sure!

Wear a weight vest around all day long? Of course!

Here's the key: *I insist they finish the whole program.*

Here's the why: Once you go through the pain and agony of one three-day fast, you're more likely to understand that doing something this hard (and, with some of these ideas, potentially dangerous) doesn't fit into the rest of your life.

Examine your prepositions…then ask if your friends and family really won't mind if you drink nothing but hot water and cayenne pepper for three days. Now, I will make you do it if I can, but you're going to learn a great lesson about life.

No matter what you decide to do, I am begging you to finish it.

There are smarter ways to do anything you wish to do, but part of learning is to make poor choices and follow them to the end. Oh, and *end them!* And never let them see the light of day again.

Examine your prepositions.

Think about your mission.

Hunt.

The other issue that puffs its ugly head in fitness is the *either/or* issue. Either you're in shape or not is a common idea we see a lot in TV ads. The best example is from the book—a book I like a lot—Covert Bailey's *Fit or Fat*.

So, here are the choices: You're EITHER fit OR you're fat!

It's the problem for many of us. I have been fit *and* fat in my life. I competed in the Highland Games for years and some of my competitors outweighed me by a hundred pounds or more. I let my weight slide up because HG implements weigh a lot and you need to counter them with whatever you can use. A big body counters better than a little one.

And, there have been times when I was not fit and not fat, not fit and fat, and, happily, times when fit and not fat. I'm sure, like the colors of the rainbow, we have all been shades of fit and fat throughout our lives.

Fit is simply the ability to do a task. As we march through our vision of a less-fat future, don't let yourself get too stuck in this *either/or* that dominates our landscape.

Either/or has us always looking for *the* answer, rather than trusting the simple, the logical, and the true.

If you have a fairly clear goal, the B of the journey of A to B and the goal has this wonderful ability to expand all areas of your life, there are people willing to help.

As part of the fitness industry, I want to talk about an issue that plagues many people as they strive forward to their health and fitness goals. Clarity on this point is crucial in seeing yourself getting to Point B.

If I have an issue with the fitness industry, it's simply this: We have turned a problem into a mystery. I'm sure these two words, problems and mysteries, may seem alike, but they're far different concepts. Given time, problems can be solved. Sherlock Holmes—I have a vast collection of Holmes material by the way—was a master problem-solver. Given a few clues, he could march backward and piece together something simple or something complex.

Normal people see, but we do not observe.

If I lose my car keys—let's say I throw them in the garbage—given enough time, energy, and money, we as a society could find them. If the president allots a trillion dollars to the effort and we have millions of volunteers picking through the landfill, we will find those keys. Losing my keys is simply a problem. There's a solution. That's a problem.

Mysteries are something else altogether. I think Gabriel Marcel says it best: *The difference between a problem and a mystery is that we are part of a mystery.*

Truly, some of the great questions of life are mysteries.

Why do I love this person and not that person?

Maybe a better question, why do people love me?
What happens after death?
Why do bad things happen to good people?
Why do people watch some of this stuff on television?

The last question will vex philosophers for the next few centuries. The great mysteries truly don't have an answer, not in this life anyway.

Don't try to challenge this too much. Don't grab a piece of paper and list why you love somebody. It will be bad for you if the person you love finds the list. Prepare yourself for the very loud question, "Why only 57 items?!"

Really, it's not a question you can answer well.

Here's the problem: We, in the fitness industry and throughout the Western world, have turned fat loss, fitness, and health into mysteries. I have done my best in the area of strength training to turn this around, and frankly the answer to "How do I get stronger?" starts with this: Lift weights.

But fat loss? I have read dozens of books, watched documentaries, and sat through workshops and lectures on the topic. The more I learned, the less I knew. Was it eating carbs at 10:00 at night or after lifting? I couldn't keep all of the contradictory information straight in my little head.

Then, one day there was a moment of total clarity. A professor of nutrition told me this after I was giving a lecture one day.

"Fat loss. Oh, that's easy. We just tie you to a tree and come back in three days and you lose 17 pounds."

Don't try this at home, folks.

I used to think fat loss was a mystery with the search for the right ratio of macronutrients or amino acids or timing of eating. Then, I learned about the lap band. The lap band is an invasive surgery where the surgeon places something akin to a rubber band around the stomach. It 'shrinks' the stomach and the patient loses up to 100 pounds in a year. Why? Literally, the device makes you eat less.

"Eat less, move more," the great *MAD TV* episode, is true.

The powerful reason for keeping fat loss and health and fitness as a mystery is financial. Trust me, if I can tap into those empty hurtful parts of your life and give you an answer for only $49.99, wait make that $39.99, you might reach for the phone (operators standing by) and give me your credit card information. I'm not sure of an area of your person that is concomitantly more public and personal than your body. The fitness industry often preys on this weakness.

Think *problem*, not mystery, when it comes to your goal of fat loss. This is where you'll succeed using *Fat Loss Happens on Monday*—change your mindset, and use Josh's tools.

Examine your prepositions.
Think about your mission.
Hunt.
It's just a problem.

Now, let's get into the keys to goal-setting.

Generally, I see the art of goal-setting breaking into three 'generations.' The problem is simple. Most of us know what to do.

Let me say that again: Nearly every reader will know the basic direction to fat loss. It's like telling people they need to put on a seatbelt or to stop smoking or to floss daily. I mean, we know that information, but sometimes we just can't find the floss.

I've discovered three generations of goal-setting that break down very easily into three ideas.

1. *Should*
2. *Could*
3. *Must*

There's certainly a value to each level, but success in life and lifting only occurs during the *must* phase of goal-setting. Let's go through each, one by one.

THE SHOULD PHASE

As we go through our first stages of life, we enter into a goal-setting phase I call the *should phase*.

- You should go to a nice college.
- You should get a job.
- You should mow the lawn.

It all suggests a better approach to what you're doing. Most of us live in the shadow of *should*. I went to a workshop and the speaker kept repeating, "Don't should on yourself." It was funny…the first time—but she did make a good point.

The *should* approach to goal-setting is where most of us live as adults.

- I should lose a couple of pounds.
- I should get to the gym a little more often.
- I should try to keep an eye on my eating.

Basically, this approach is worthless. The person accepts the issue, then lets the problem slide past him as he reaches for the TV clicker and some chips. If you're reading this, you probably are beyond *should*, but I bet you know a lot of people in your life who live in *should*.

THE COULD PHASE

The *could* phase is the beginning of the path to success. The concept behind *could* includes the belief and the knowledge that one might possibly be successful in taking these steps. Generally, when people start using *could*, they seem to have a basic understanding of the path ahead of them.

In fact, they may even know the destination.

- You know, I could lose a couple of pounds. I could do the low-carb thing.
- You know, I could get to the gym a little more often. I could go right after work.
- You know, I could keep a little better eye on my diet.

Knowledge is power in the *could* stage. You know what to do, but just don't seem to find the power to do it.

And you know what? Not one thing I've written so far matters, because to be truly great, you've got to make your goals *musts*.

And that, my friends, is the key to success in sports and training.

THE MUST PHASE

The single best piece of diet advice I ever heard came from peak-performance consultant Anthony Robbins. Robbins got this advice from one of his clients. It's called the Alpo Diet. Invite a dozen friends over to your house. Tell them that by the end of the month you're going to lose 10 pounds. Tell them if you don't, you'll eat a can of Alpo in front of them.

For the next week, every time you feel the urge to take a piece of chocolate from the cubicle next to you, reread the contents of the Alpo can. If someone offers you something smothered in goo, open the Alpo can and take a good deep sniff.

You see, this is the crux of goal-setting: Rarely do people improve because of the pleasure of the goal; rather *it's pain that sets them on a goal*.

This method has become very popular. There's a website where you make a bet with the world that you will do your goal or the website will automatically send money to an organization you despise.

Just between us, we all have a list, right?

When I sit down with someone who has a goal, I use a simple, four-square chart. I ask them to fill in the four boxes.

- What pleasure will you get if you do get your goals?
- What pain will you get if you don't get your goals?

You know, those are the obvious two, but it's these next two questions that make the difference.

- What pain will you get if you do get your goals? (Be sure to reread that!)
- What pleasure will get if you don't get your goals?

I've worked with dozens of athletes using this chart and the remarkable thing about all of this work is that few athletes have much to say about the pleasure of getting their goals. 'It would be nice to be an Olympian' certainly doesn't stir the imagination as much as 'I'd have to eat a can of dog food if I fail.'

Pain drives most goals!

A guy might say 'I can't run a mile.' If I tell him his child is roped to the railroad tracks a mile away and he had to get there in less than eight minutes, he might run that mile! The temporary issues of heartrate increases and sweating are inconsequential vis-à-vis the pain of hurting or losing a child.

But does accomplishing a goal cause pain?

Oh, no question about that! Think about how many high school seniors will accept a college sports scholarship and then sneak away after less than a week of practice. The new level of competition causes obvious problems, but even smaller goals have issues.

- Losing fat often means buying new clothes.
- Becoming part of the Top 10 of anything often leads to the question, "When will you be number one?"
- The diploma issue: Now I have a nice piece of paper, but no job and no idea of what to do!

Okay, so now you see that achieving a goal can cause pain. But can a person experience pleasure from not reaching a goal? Obviously, the pleasure we get from failure must be greater than the successful completion of a goal, otherwise (and I'm trying to be nice) there wouldn't be anyone available to appear on those daytime television shows with subjects like 'people who date their cousin's pets.'

Many of us know people who have forsaken a worthy goal for romance. For the record, I can understand why someone would trade making love for making weight for wrestling, but we have to at least realize this is part of the issue with achieving goals.

There are wonderful things that can get in the way of accomplishment, so in a sense failing can be pleasurable. If you know this, you may be able to recognize and avoid it if you truly want to reach your goals.

Sadly, pain motivates most people much better than pleasure. Sorry, but it's true.

MAKING MUSTS

So, how do you make things a must? A couple of ideas—

- First, put it out there: Tell people what you want to do and enlist their help. Talk to people who have done what you're attempting. Let them know what you want to do.
- Second, grab the Alpo or whatever will stimulate you to do or not do what you have to do or not do. What in your life would bring you enormous pain? Here's an idea: If you don't lose those 10 pounds, your parent/spouse/friend sends in your application, signed and sealed, to join the Marine Corps or the French Foreign Legion. I can guarantee those 10 pounds will come off in bootcamp.
- Next, and this is an odd one, start acting like you've already achieved the goal. Hit the beach like you lost those 10 pounds or buy new clothes with the finished goal in mind. Start acting like you've accomplished something and, often before you know it, you've accomplished it.

When you succeed or fail, generally it comes back to the question that's plagued actors for a century: *What's my motivation?*

Sniff some dog food along the way and see if that helps!

Examine your prepositions.

Think about your mission.

Hunt…finish the task.

It's just a problem.

Make it a *must*.

JOSH

CHAPTER 13

ONE CHANGE REVIEW

Man, I love systems. My favorite thing in the world is developing fat-loss systems and testing them out on my clients.

And yet…I rarely follow them *exactly*. These are templates to work from, a starting place.

Take carbohydrate cycling, for example. I use that system to give my clients a recommendation, to the gram. But even though the recommendation calculates out to an exact number of grams of protein, carbs, and fat, it's not like they're expected to hit that exactly. It's just a general guideline. I don't really care if they're plus or minus 10%. It's a target to aim for.

And that's the way I feel about all of these systems. I'm giving you the systems I use to coach, but you may find that some parts work better than others. And that's how reality works.

You may find the meal-planning apps have a bigger impact on your results than meal-tracking apps. Or you may find you need both.

You may find implementing the habits one at a time works better than going meal by meal. Or you may find going meal by meal works, and the single habits don't. Or you might use both, like it's written here.

We're giving you the whole tool kit. Which tools work best for you is more individual than we like to admit in a book.

The *only* thing I would keep as a hard and fast rule is to do your food planning and preparation before your first workout of the week.

EASY FAT LOSS, HARD FAT LOSS

> *"Once you accept how hard it is to lose fat, it becomes easy."*
>
> ~ Craig Ballantyne,
> Turbulence Training

It could just be the clients I've had in the past, but it seems like the workouts were never the issue. I'd get them doing the right workouts, on the right program with the right movements. And that would be handled.

Then we'd get the food right. But the food was a battleground. The food was where we needed to make the biggest difference.

In other words, for most people, the workouts are the easy part and the food is the hard part.

> *"Training is the easy part. Get the easy part right."*
>
> ~ Vince Anderson,
> professional mountaineer and guide

Granted, Vince was talking about mountain bike racing, where staying healthy and uninjured was the hard part and training was the easy part. But I couldn't help extrapolating that quote for fat loss.

That quote stuck with me—it could be used as a way to sum up this entire book: *The food is the hard part, and that should be the focus.*

But the training—easy part—has to be correctly handled also.

And that leads into our next section: *Pull Your Weight*.

ONE CHANGE CHEAT SHEET

1. Only change one habit per week.
2. Only change one meal per week.
3. Making the change stick is more important than making more changes.
4. Preparing and cooking your food are the most important 'workouts' of the week.
5. Keep a food journal.
6. Scale weight equals calories consumed.
7. Bodyfat percentage (leanness) equals quality of food plus strength.
8. Getting the food right earns you easier workouts.

PULL YOUR WEIGHT

TO EVERYTHING THERE IS A SEASON ~ THE BYRDS

To every thing there is a season, and a time to every purpose under the heaven:

A time to be born, and a time to die; a time to plant, and a time to reap that which is planted;

A time to kill, and a time to heal; a time to break down, and a time to build up;

A time to weep, and a time to laugh; a time to mourn, and a time to dance;

A time to cast away stones, and a time to gather stones together; a time to embrace, and a time to refrain from embracing;

A time to get, and a time to lose; a time to keep, and a time to cast away;

A time to rend, and a time to sew; a time to keep silence, and a time to speak;

A time to love, and a time to hate; a time of war, and a time of peace.

~ Ecclesiastes 3:1-8

JOSH

CHAPTER 14

SEASONS OF TRAINING

The average workout girl or guy never thinks about their workout as being part of a season. If you take a look at professional athletes in any sport, there's an in-season and an off-season. College athletes have an in-season and an off-season. High school athletes play different sports each season.

Actors and actresses lean up for movies, and ease off between movies. This is their in-season and off-season. Similarly, rock stars lean up for tours, and ease off between tours. Victoria's Secret models talk about locking down their diets for the annual fashion show.

All of the workout programs you can purchase in books or DVDs are typically in-season workout programs. And they work great for that.

There are 30-day programs, 12-week programs—tons of great short-term programs.

Unfortunately, they suck for long-term results. You do a 12-week program, then you stop, and you get fat again. Or, you keep doing it longer than 12 weeks, and you get hurt. You're trying to be in-season all the time.

Either way, the programs on the market are *really hard* and *really short-term*.

Except no one who's really hot does hard workouts and hard diets *all the time*. In fact, most of the time, people who are rock-star hot do easier workouts and easier diets most of the time, and then they *Bring it!* a few times per year, either for an event or a challenge.

They're always within striking distance, slowly bringing up their strength on the easy workouts, slowly getting a little leaner each month with small changes.

This is what Dan was talking about earlier when he wrote about park-bench and bus-bench workouts.

The stronger you are, the easier it is to stay lean and hot.

The workouts we do in the *Pull Your Weight* program are what we would call park-bench workouts.

You're going to pick up a rep or two every week. After you've picked up enough reps, you can jump to the next level. That's it—small moves.

The people who consistently pick up a rep or two per week have enormous results at the end of six months or a year.

If there's any magic to how I train my personal training clients, this is it. They make really small progress, all the time, a couple reps per week…massive progress in months. They're entirely new people in a couple years. Every month, every year, fat loss gets easier—because they're stronger.

And that's all you need to do.

If you can pick up a couple reps per week, that's all it takes to transform your body long-term. Want a faster metabolism a year from now? Pick up a rep or two each workout. Move up to heavier kettlebells or harder bodyweight exercises over the next year.

A year from now, you'll be stronger and have a faster metabolism. You'll be leaner at any given bodyweight, and you'll get to eat more food.

This is the smart path.

THIS ONE TIME, AT BRAZILIAN JIU JITSU CAMP

When I was at jiu jitsu camp in Brazil for two months, I worked out six hours per day, five days per week. I was on vacation—I had nothing to worry about and no stress outside of my workouts. All I had to do was work out and have fun.

I got lean, strong, and felt amazing on six-hour workouts. It was unbelievable.

Back home in real life, with all of my work and family commitments, a two-hour workout will destroy me if it's on a week day. There's just too much other stress.

It's all about how much stress you already have in your life.

Without normal life stress, I could thrive under almost unlimited workout stress.

That's part of why many people don't respond well to the workouts they've been doing—they already have a lot of stress in their lives. Adding crushing workouts on top becomes way too much stress and it kills them.

You don't want to do 100% intensity workouts all the time. It just doesn't work in real life.

STRESS MAKES YOU FAT

Too much stress makes you fat. It increases adrenaline and cortisol; you don't process food well and you store more fat.

Adrenaline and cortisol are designed to shut down most of the body's biggest functions, such as digestion, and divert all bodily power to the eyes and ears and heart so you're primed and ready to run away from a tiger.

And if you were running away from a tiger, you really wouldn't care if your lunch digested well—you'd just want to run away.

But we don't have tigers that we run from for just a minute. We have bosses and bills and kids getting sick and *all kinds of lower-level stresses all day long*.

The **medium** and **easy** workouts in *Fat Loss Happens on Monday* will actually reduce stress.

If you're a busy person, you'll find you respond better to *Fat Loss Happens on Monday* than any workout program you have done before.

In a one-minute tiger attack, adrenaline and cortisol will save your life.

In day-to-day, 24/7 stress, adrenaline and cortisol will make you fat. Cycle your workouts between easy, medium, and hard.

JOSH

CHAPTER 15

THE EIGHT MOVEMENTS

We're going to change gears here and talk about how to train for fat loss.

Fat-loss workouts should always be made up of big movement patterns: pushing movements, pulling movements, squatting movements, and hip-hinging movements. The bigger the movement, the better.

You can probably think of a lot of examples of these movements in the gym and out. For this program, you're going to use eight movements that really lend themselves to home workouts: a bodyweight push, pull, and squat. A deadlift. And a kettlebell push, pull, squat, and swing.

Group One: Mostly Bodyweight
1. Pushups and appropriate regressions or progressions
2. Pull-ups, full range of motion, partial range of motion, and hangs
3. Bodyweight, split-stance squatting movements—lunges, split-squats, and single-leg squats
4. Deadlifts or single-leg deadlifts

Group Two: Kettlebell Work
1. Kettlebell military presses, one or two kettlebells
2. Kettlebell rows, one kettlebell
3. Kettlebell front squats, one or two kettlebells
4. Kettlebell swings, one or two kettlebells

Essentially we have two groups of pushing, pulling, squatting, and hip-hinging movements. We use pushing, pulling, squatting, and hip-hinging movements with bodyweight, and also with kettlebells.

These are what we could call big-bang movements—every one of these movements requires groups of muscles firing, bracing and stabilization at the core, and a focus on technique and coordination. All of these are components of very effective fat-loss movements.

You can do this entire program at home with some kettlebells. Most of the people I've trained using this program have found they needed to invest in heavier kettlebells in a fairly short time. That's a good thing—I hope it happens to you. It means you're getting some real work done, and you're starting to make progress.

WHY BODYWEIGHT MOVES ARE AWESOME FOR FAT LOSS

Bodyweight workouts are some of the most awesome fat-loss workouts in existence. The best thing about bodyweight workouts is that you can do them anywhere—at home, at the gym, traveling. You can get an unbelievable fat-loss workout anywhere, without any special equipment.

Bodyweight training is significantly more intense than working out with machines—more full body, more core, more stability, more body awareness. You're going to have a more intense fat-loss workout and as a total by-product, you'll move better, have better body awareness, and become a better athlete—or find your inner athlete for the first time.

Just like with kettlebell workouts: More work means more fat loss.

The biggest mistake people make with bodyweight workouts is they just do the same squats and pushups forever. They don't realize there's a whole world of progressive movement.

And if you can *progress the movement*—have a variety of beginner, intermediate, and advanced movements—that means you can do different kinds of workouts, everything from strength endurance, to circuits, and even strength workouts…all with just your body.

Progression is key. With dumbbells or kettlebells, to make it harder you just use heavier weights. With your body—obviously you can't just get a heavier body to make it harder, or a lighter body to make it easier. We need to be able to progress the difficulty of the exercises themselves. And that's what I've provided for you—a simple progression for each of the three movements.

Just like with the kettlebells, regardless of your level, you're going to get what you came for. And we never forget—no matter how cool or fun or tough bodyweight training is, you actually came here to get wicked lean.

That's what we're going to do.

Food is for the scale, and workouts are for getting lean and tight. Remember the table of results:

SCALE WEIGHT	Quantity of food you eat (calories)
YOUR BODYFAT PERCENTAGE	Quality of food you eat and how strong you are
CIRCUMFERENCE MEASUREMENTS	Combination of quantity *and* quality of food

We know what makes a person get smaller on the scale, and we know what makes a body leaner and tighter.

The goal of your workout isn't to get smaller on the scale. The goal of your workout is to get leaner and tighter, to make the jiggly bits less jiggly.

If you can reconcile yourself to the fact that scale weight is 100% food, you're going to save yourself a lot of struggle and frustration. Don't let anyone try to muddy this or make it more complicated.

And don't fool yourself into thinking you can out work the food. You can't. There aren't enough hours in the day to work your way past too much food.

This might be worth printing out and putting on your refrigerator: *Scale weight is from calories consumed. Bodyfat percentage is strength plus quality of food.* I don't want you to forget this.

Now that we know food is for the scale, and workouts are for getting lean, let's get to this business of working out.

FAT-LOSS STRENGTH STANDARDS

If you're a woman who can do three pull-ups and three deadlifts with bodyweight, your problem is food, not workouts.

If you're a man who can do 10 pull-ups and three deadlifts with 1.5 times your bodyweight, your problem is food, not workouts.

> **WOMEN'S STRENGTH STANDARD**
> THREE CHIN-UPS
> AND THREE DEADLIFTS WITH YOUR BODYWEIGHT

> **MEN'S STRENGTH STANDARD**
> TEN CHIN-UPS
> AND THREE DEADLIFTS WITH 1.5 TIMES YOUR BODYWEIGHT

If you can meet these strength standards, and you don't have the body you want, then your problem is food, not workouts.

TWO KETTLEBELLS ARE BETTER THAN ONE

More work in less time means better fat-loss results and more time to spend on the rest of your life. Let's recap that: More work will get you more results. But more time *isn't* the same as more work. The benefit of two kettlebells is that you can get *more work* done in *less time*.

With one kettlebell, we get more stabilization and more core effort—actually 40% more according to EMG testing—and with two kettlebells, we get more total work and more fat loss.

Can we get the best of both worlds? Of course. With two uneven kettlebells, we get to do both at the same time. It's an amazingly elegant way to have your borscht and eat it too. I got the idea from Pavel Tsatsouline's book and DVD set called *Return of the Kettlebell*. If you don't already know, Pavel brought the kettlebell revolution to the West, and he's the Chief Instructor at the SFG Instructor Certification, which you can find at strongfirst.com.

Most people start kettlebell lifting with one kettlebell. But most instructors do a lot of two-kettlebell workouts. And most kettlebell instructors have bangin' bodies.

At the Denver Kettlebell Bootcamp, the beginners class was always done with one kettlebell, and the advanced class always used two.

This programming will work for both beginner, intermediate, and advanced workout folks. And in that way, this may be the only two-kettlebell book that has something for everyone. Regardless of your level, you're going to get what you came for. But no matter how cool or fun or tough kettlebell lifting is, you actually came here to get wicked lean.

We've got multiple levels we're going to work through, and progression is remarkably simple.

Let's take a look at the Women's Military Press Progression as an example:

MILITARY PRESS PROGRESSION—WOMEN	
EASIER	ONE-KETTLEBELL PUSH PRESS, 8KG
	ONE-KETTLEBELL MILITARY PRESS, 8KG
	TWO-KETTLEBELL MILITARY PRESS, 8KG+8KG
	ONE-KETTLEBELL MILITARY PRESS, 12KG
	TWO-KETTLEBELL MILITARY PRESS, 12KG+8KG
	TWO-KETTLEBELL MILITARY PRESS, 12KG+12KG
	ONE-KETTLEBELL MILITARY PRESS, 16KG
	TWO-KETTLEBELL MILITARY PRESS, 16KG+12KG
HARDER	TWO-KETTLEBELL MILITARY PRESS, 16KG+16KG

*Note: All other progressions are listed later.

There's no hurry to rush through the levels, and really there's *nowhere to get*. You don't win a prize when you get to the end.

I will say this, though—The strongest people are always the hottest.

Take any two men or women at the same bodyweight—the stronger one will be leaner.

Your scale weight is given by the amount of food that you eat. Your bodyfat percentage—how lean and tight your body is—is given by how strong you are, and the quality of the food you eat.

I repeat it (again) because it's just that simple…and that important.

WHAT IF I DON'T HAVE THAT MANY KETTLEBELLS?

No problem. I actually didn't assume you did. You can skip any step you'd like or need to. I listed all the steps for illustration purposes. Ideally, you'd make the smallest possible jumps, which, even with all these kettlebells, are still pretty big jumps!

I have clients who work out at kettlebell gyms that have all of these, plus the half-steps, like 14- and 18-kilogram kettlebells. That's awesome. But it isn't necessary.

The large rep ranges from 6 to 12 reps in the metabolic phase help you bridge the gap between the kettlebells you have. If you have an 8-kilogram kettlebell and two 12-kilogram kettlebells, those three are enough for 90% of female clients for a long time. Likewise, many guys could get by with a 16-kilogram kettlebell and two 20-kilogram kettlebells for a while.

Besides the big jumps in reps to help with gaps between kettlebells, also feel free to use unevenly weighted pairs of kettlebells. Just be sure to brace your abs and butt, and keep shoulders and hips square during the movements.

Whatever you have, use that. You could actually start this program with one kettlebell and a doorway pull-up bar. Add a kettlebell every other paycheck—it isn't that much more than a gym membership, and once you have six, you've got a home gym for life.

Speaking of gyms, in the olden days kettlebells used to be hard to find, but now it's extremely rare to find a gym that doesn't have at least a dozen of them.

HOME DEADLIFTS WITH KETTLEBELLS?

About half the people reading this are going to be working out at home with bodyweight and kettlebells, and won't have a barbell at home. So how do you hit the deadlift standard without a barbell?

Mike Boyle, world-famous strength coach and author of *Advances in Functional Training*, has been a big proponent of single-leg training over barbell training. When I saw him speak at a recent Perform Better Summit, he talked about how he does lots of barbell work with younger athletes. But as people get older, he moves away from two-leg barbell exercises, and into doing mostly or entirely single-leg exercises.

He's found that within six weeks, most of his athletes can do more work on one leg than they can do if he took a two-leg exercise and divided the weight in half.

In other words, if there's a woman who can do a 150-pound deadlift, she should be able to work up to doing *more* than 75 pounds on each leg for single-leg deadlifts.

Mike calls this bilateral deficit. He essentially says with two-leg exercises, we aren't getting the workout we could be getting, because people can get stronger on each leg than they can on two.

What this means for you: If you're a woman who is working out with kettlebells and you need to hit the deadlift standard, you want to work up to single-leg deadlifting half your bodyweight on each leg.

And if you're a man, you'd work up to three-quarters of your bodyweight on each leg.

Women's Single-Leg Deadlift Standard

Three deadlifts with half your bodyweight each leg

Men's Single-Leg Deadlift Standard

Three deadlifts with three-quarters of your bodyweight each leg

DAN

CHAPTER 16

GET OFF MY BACK

I have a mental image for clarity when it comes to setting problems apart from mysteries. Years ago, my wife Tiffini came home from work with a book, Charles Coonradt's *The Game of Work*.

At the time, I was still working as a high school teacher. We had run through a period of several principals I found tough to follow. My mantra for leadership is 'Lead me, follow me, or get out of my way.'

Coonradt perfectly explained my problem.

> *"Another common field of play in business is shaped like an amoeba—a random, globular shape. It describes the employee's understanding of what he or she thinks is expected, and the only problem is that it wiggles and jiggles and changes shape. When something goes wrong that the employee didn't think was his or her responsibility, sure enough, someone points it out as his or her responsibility on the amoeba."*

This reflects what I often see in the area of nutrition. As I popped open my computer recently, I saw a famous name in the fitness industry link to a site that was anti-Paleo diet. Paleo dieting is the notion that one should eat like a hunter-gatherer from 10,000 years ago: meat, fish, veggies, fruits in season, water, and lots of walking around in nature.

The article stated that what I just wrote was wrong. This is the amoeba in the fitness industry—just when you thought you found the right thing to eat for breakfast, you were told breakfast was bad for you!

Coonradt recommends, from the sporting world, to imagine work like a field of play. There are out of bounds, and that could be from stealing from the cash register to inappropriate sexual behaviors. His great insight is that we march upward from what he calls the safety zone (helpful coach and humble athlete) to what I think is his great insight, *Get Off My Back*, to, finally, *Paydirt*.

The safety zone as a strength coach is what this whole book is about: What is a reasonable but safe and sound approach to fitness that can last a lifetime? What is the least one can do to get the most benefit?

GOMB, *Get Off My Back*, is something akin to what I learned from Coach Maughan at Utah State.

If he had an athlete who would lift weights three days a week and show up to practice five days a week through the fall and winter, he honestly didn't push, pull, or beat this athlete into doing more. The mantra here was little and often over the long haul, which is exactly what Josh has been writing about.

Training intelligently for four years trumps these occasional bouts of lunatic high-intensity training that can lead to injuries, illness, and stagnation. In Coonradt's world, one needs to find measurements to help employees know they're on track and doing a good job. If they're meeting those standards, well, GOMB!

I think we need those same things in fitness and in health like we do so naturally in sports. Every single year of both high school and college, I threw the discus farther. My standard was to improve at least 20 feet a year. It amazes me to write this as it's so clear, so obvious, that I easily followed this simple formula. Sure, in college, it was tough to add that much, but in my worst years, I still got very close. GOMB.

Josh tells us about some standards, and if you're strong enough to do them, the quality of your food is your issue. Getting stronger, although it certainly has merits, isn't going to help you until you nail down the food shopping, food prep, and food journal.

That's enough. GOMB.

One of the most common questions I receive is when is enough, enough? This ties into Tim Ferriss's elusive search for the minimum effective dose that answers the question: *What is the least I need to do to get the benefit?*

Humans can survive a little poison, but there's a threshold. In more positive terms, there's a point where the benefits of doing something emerge and it's our task to find that level, note it, and share it with others.

If all I need is at this level, well then, GOMB, I'm doing it.

This is the wonderful concept called hormesis. This means that light exposure to toxins, or really any kind of stress, gives the system a chance to adapt favorably. Recently, we've seen a return to the idea of letting kids play in the dirt and go to school without putting on a hazmat suit, with pounds of hand sanitizer dripping off their limbs, so they get a chance to build their immune systems.

Mithridatism is the next big step where people willfully expose themselves to poisons and toxins. We see this famously in *The Princess Bride* when Wesley, the Man in Black, tells us after choosing a cup with poison in it, "They were both poisoned. I spent the last few years building up an immunity to iocane powder."

Coonradt's final idea of *Paydirt* is where we often get stuck in the fitness industry. It has its place: We all want to have six-pack abs, finish a marathon, and compete as a gymnast, Olympic lifter, and martial artist…all in one weekend.

Take a lot of photos as it's hard to make that a lifestyle. I applaud it—in fact, I love it, but it's just not sustainable for most of us.

Certainly, at times in your year and in your life, push yourself to the wall and try to win the golden ring. But it's also reasonable to keep yourself in good shape, good health, and good company with less than pure insanity.

The take-away: Shysters want fitness, health, and fat loss to look like an amoeba…a constantly changing shape. Josh and I are offering you the chance to get off your own back here with honest information, resources, and planning.

In addition, we're offering you a chance to really light it up every so often.

Is it too simple?

GOMB!

JOSH

CHAPTER 17

YOU GOTTA GET REAL

If the problem is food, stop chasing new workouts. You're just spinning your wheels.

If the problem is that you aren't strong enough, you need to work on both, food and workouts.

Most people in the gym aren't strong enough to do all of these workouts at the heaviest kettlebell weights or the hardest bodyweight progressions. And for most people it could take years to get there.

Go ahead and get started now. Work on the food at the same time you're edging yourself toward these standards.

In fact, if you lock down the food, you may find yourself at the body you want long before you reach the higher levels of kettlebell weights and bodyweight progressions. The strength standards of the deadlifts and pull-ups are kind of in the middle of the progressions we've given you.

It doesn't take superhuman strength—just enough. Remember, it really *is* about the food.

As long as you work on the food and work on your strength, you're going to get a little leaner, more confident, and sexier every week.

And that's the game we're playing.

A LOT OF THE WORKOUTS ARE MEDIUM OR EASY

You've got to be wondering how you're going to get the rock-star body you've always wanted doing this many **easy** workouts.

After all, we've been conditioned by *The Biggest Loser* and *P90X* to believe that fat-loss workouts have to be really, really hard.

In fact, we desperately want to believe hard fat-loss workouts are the answer…so we don't have to go to work on our food.

MEDIUM AND EASY WORKOUTS EQUAL LONG-TERM FAT LOSS

If you get real about the food, you'll understand there's really no need to throttle yourself all the time with your workouts.

In fact, throttling yourself all the time is a bad idea just because it's unsustainable. You can only go 100% balls-out for a month or two. After that, it leads to burnout, dropout, struggle, backward results, or injury.

In my early fat-loss e-books, I used to say intensity is the number one factor in a fat-loss workout. And in the **short term,** it is.

For an eight-week blast like the *Bring It!* program, make it intense. And you should do an eight-week blast twice per year.

In the long term, you want to do a lot of medium and easy…build things up over time. In the long term, consistency trumps intensity every time.

> *"And in those simple, beautiful movements, I remembered what was really important in training; that consistency trumps intensity, all the time… that intensity is born from consistency…that one cannot force it. We have to lay in wait for it, patiently, instinctively, calmly, and be ready to grab it when Grace lays it down in front of us."*
>
> ~ Mark Reifkind, Master SFG Instructor

FAT-LOSS GURUS ARE IGNORANT AND THEY'RE SCARED

You've been throttled from fat-loss workouts so many times before because the trainers or fat-loss gurus didn't really know what they were doing…so they just kicked your ass.

In fact, they hoped you were so drowning in puke and sweat that you wouldn't notice if you didn't get results. After all, it was a hard workout.

> *"Both science and experience of the strongest people in the world have proved that you have no business training 'on the nerve,' at least not on a regular basis. Yet the 'high intensity' fad keeps coming back under different guises. It may sound tough, but in my humble opinion, it is tougher to measure your strength with pounds or reps than with puke or volume."*
>
> ~ Pavel Tsatsouline, SFG Chief Instructor

To repurpose Pavel's quote, it's smarter to measure your fat-loss workouts by bodyfat percentage than with sweat or soreness.

If you know what it takes for fat loss, you do those things. You must reduce calories, you must get stronger in your kettlebell workouts, and you must eat better-quality food.

DAN

CHAPTER 18

THE BASIC BASICS

Chip Conrad from BodyTribe has a very simple model for constructing a training program. At birth, your first physical movement challenge was three-fold.

How to Stand
How to Sit
How to Crawl

The key to understanding movement is seeing the flow between these three initial challenges. If you master crawling and standing, you're certainly on your way to walking.

Many of the programs designed for people over 30 skip this insight. That's why it's always wise to have the basic fundamental human movements in your training. Simply mixing a swing, a goblet squat, and a pushup in some variation will bring you right back to your first years of life. If you mix and match things well, it will become dance-like in its flow.

The devil, as always, is in the details.

Can you do more than this? Of course! Can you use machines, ropes, bells of every sort and fashion, mats, rocks, anvils, or tires? Sure. The answer to most *can you* questions in fitness are yes, clearly.

Can you lift light and get strong? That's a good question. Years ago I experimented with the idea of using light to moderate weights with very tight rest periods. For example, on big moves like the front squat or the overhead squat, I did three sets of eight repetitions with only one minute of rest. The idea was to let the fatigue build-up of the first two sets impact the third.

Did it work? Yes, in fact, I was staggered to find this prepared me better for Olympic lifting meets than my standard idea of doing heavy front squats in sets of two or three.

But I never missed a rep doing this program.

My sets were low and I remained fresh. My body liked the fact that I wasn't being crushed all the time and rewarded me with happy efforts on the lifting platform.

Should you move the barbell, for example, fast or slow? Should you do really high reps or low?

The truth is this: *It all works.*

It always has and it always will.

Years ago, I read Terry Todd's work explaining the need to vary reps over a few months. So, I did a month of 20–25 reps, a month of 8–12, and finished with a month of 5–8 reps. In hindsight, I don't know why I didn't keep doing it because I made excellent progress with my body composition. It didn't help me with my performance as much as doing singles and doubles did, but one can easily see how these three months of following Todd's insights would be great for anyone.

In case you missed the point: It works because it all works.

So, how does it work?

How does this work? If 'this' is strength training, all we know is this: *To get stronger, lift weights.*

Any and all clarity beyond that is suspect!

This question or my lack of understanding of how any of this works is the fundamental principle of my coaching career.

So, let us return to our basic point about my overarching principle. It's fine that we don't know how it works, if it works. Remember, we must follow the evidence, no matter where it leads.

> *"How often have I said to you that when you have eliminated the impossible, whatever remains, however improbable, must be the truth?"*
>
> ~ Sherlock Holmes, *The Sign of the Four*

JOSH

CHAPTER 19

HOW TO MAKE A FAT-LOSS PROGRAM THAT WORKS LONG TERM

Cycles, seasons, wheels of plans—it's a big plan that's broken into smaller chunks.

We've got two cycles of training—these are like seasons.

Then in each season we've got three phases—these phases are like months.

Each month of training has a weekly workout cycle.

Each week has a cycle, each month has a cycle, and the cycle of alternating the two cycles is the program. Each builds to a peak in terms of workout volume, and then starts over in the next cycle.

Each season of training has a different emphasis and style.

Each month of training has a different, specific training adaptation it targets.

Each week of training builds from easy at the beginning of each month to hard at the end.

Each week has easier days and harder days.

Let's take a look.

Our first cycle of training looks like this—

> Phase One: **Metabolic** (12 reps per set)
> Phase Two: **Endurance** (20 reps per set)
> Phase Three: **Strength** (6 reps per set)

Our second cycle of training looks like this—

> Phase Four: **Metabolic/Endurance/Strength** (12 reps, 20 reps, 6 reps)
> Phase Five: **Stronger Metabolic/Endurance/Strength** (8 reps, 15 reps, 5 reps)
> Phase Six: **Volume** (two moves per workout, more sets per move)

Each season has three months, and each cycle has three phases. Each cycle has a design.

The first cycle is called alternating periodization, where we work on one fitness quality each month—*either metabolic, endurance, or strength*—and then we change it.

We milk each repetition range (sets of 12, sets of 20, or sets of 6) for as much fat loss as we can. Usually we can get about four weeks of fat-loss results out of any given repetition range, and then we change.

The second cycle is called undulating periodization, where you work on multiple fitness qualities at the same time. This can extend the results, getting life out of each phase, because you're only exposed to each repetition-range once per week. Since the movements alternate two different days, you actually only get exposed to each individual workout once every two weeks. And that's why undulating periodization phases can continue to work for fat-loss results for six weeks, or even longer.

Both cycles are part of one cohesive program: The three phases of the first cycle set you up for the first two phases of the second cycle.

The sixth phase is a totally different training stimulus, working on volume. We use the same exercises, but with a slightly more advanced split. It's a smart same-but-different transition from the first two phases: Same movements, similar rep range, but it works up to *twice as much volume* per movement.

Each phase in each of the cycles is different enough that you've got access to renewed fat-loss results with each change.

And both cycles are different enough from each other that you could alternate between the two forever, and continue to progress.

WHY THIS ISN'T LIKE EVERY OTHER PROGRAM

Most fat-loss programs aren't smart enough to have reps that change every month, nor do they work on different fitness qualities at different times. They only change the exercises, which is so 1995.

Actually, it's just uneducated. But now you know better, and you can chuck those old workouts in the shredder.

If I had an aspiration for the fitness industry, it would be that more trainers would put together programs of cycles containing multiple phases. Long-term programs should supplant the idea of workouts.

I have to thank the National Academy of Sports Medicine for introducing me to alternating periodization and undulating periodization back in 2004. Other major influences in fat-loss periodization came in 2006, seeing Alwyn Cosgrove's *Afterburn* and *Afterburn II* programs, Craig Ballantyne's *Turbulence Training*, and then later the *Results Fitness Program Design Manual*. Somewhere around then I started playing with alternating periodization for beginner and intermediate clients, and undulating periodization for advanced clients.

This is a little different than the programs written by trainers who are good at this kind of multi-phase, multi-cycle approach to fat loss. If there's one argument that could be made against this program, it's that the monthly rep changes are too big in the first three phases.

> *Phase One: 12 reps per set*
> *Phase Two: 20 reps per set*
> *Phase Three: 6 reps per set*

This program is kind of renegade in that it makes such *huge* jumps between rep ranges. I'll have to blame that on starting off as a National Academy of Sports Medicine (NASM) trainer. When we changed phases, you knew you'd changed phases. To be fair, NASM included half-step phases, but I never used them.

Most of the trainers who are on point with changing rep ranges on a monthly basis are usually too concerned with not losing some of the strength or endurance adaptation from the previous phase.

The three phases we're cycling through are completely distinct adaptations.

> Phase One: 12 reps—*Metabolic*
> Phase Two: 20 reps—*Endurance*
> Phase Three: 6 reps—*Strength*

Normally, you'd be concerned you'd lose the metabolic adaptation when you go so far to the endurance end of the spectrum, and then you'd lose your endurance adaptation when you go to the far end of the strength spectrum.

It's true, you will…*but what if we don't care about losing that strength adaptation? What if we only care about fat loss?*

Usually, a really good fat-loss program looks like this—

> *Phase One: 15 reps*
> *Phase Two: 10 reps*
> *Phase Three: 12 reps*
> *Phase Four: 8 reps*

That's exactly what the smart fat-loss trainers are doing: Making small changes, keeping it kind of in the same world. They change enough that it works for fat loss, but are really making the absolute smallest change possible. It's really intelligent, and I totally respect that.

In fact, they're hitting similar adaptations.

> *Phase One: 15 reps—Metabolic-Endurance*
> *Phase Two: 10 reps—Metabolic*
> *Phase Three: 12 reps—Metabolic*
> *Phase Four: 8 reps—Metabolic-Strength*

It makes a lot of sense to do that—essentially moving around within the metabolic rep range. It's genius to move around in that rep range, especially if you have *a large palette of movements* and the movements you're doing change every phase. The more other moving parts there are in the workout program, the less you want to change rep ranges.

That's great—but it's not what I do.

One note on movements versus sets and reps: You never stall on fat-loss results due to not changing movements—*you stall because of not changing sets and reps.*

The only time I ever have people change movements is either when they move to a harder or easier version of a bodyweight exercise, or when they get bored. From a fat-loss standpoint, movement changes make no difference at all.

Over the last 10 years, I've always done bigger rep swings than that. For the RKC Blog, I wrote a program like this for strength trainers who wanted to break out of the five-rep strength range and do some legit fat-loss workouts.

> *Phase One: 15 reps—Metabolic-Endurance*
> *Phase Two: 5 reps—Strength*
> *Phase Three: 20 reps—Endurance*
> *Phase Four: 8 reps—Strength-Metabolic*

And then, the most common program I've done with my clients over the last 10 years is this—

> *Phase One: 2x20 reps—Endurance*
> *Phase Two: 5x5 reps—Strength*
> *Phase Three: 3x15 reps—Metabolic-Endurance*
> *Phase Four: 4x8 reps—Metabolic-Strength*
> *Phase Five: 3x12 reps—Metabolic*

That's the way I think about it: Starting at both extremes and then working back toward the middle. In theory, the first three phases should be too far apart to work. But it's worked really well for my clients.

While the sequence above is how I engineered it and how I think about it, it's not how I actually run it. I almost always start with 3x12, so it looks like this—

> *Phase One: 3x12 reps—Metabolic*
> *Phase Two: 2x20 reps—Endurance*
> *Phase Three: 5x5 reps—Strength*
> *Phase Four: 3x15 reps—Metabolic-Endurance*
> *Phase Five: 4x8 reps—Metabolic-Strength*

Since I don't really care about maintaining strength in any given rep range, we can make bigger jumps. Even though I want you to hit the pull-up and deadlift goals, that's only in service to hitting your fat-loss goals.

In other words, *fat loss comes first.*

Strength is only a goal because it will help you with fat loss. Don't get those confused. As Dan always says, "One goal at a time."

What I've found is if we aren't changing the movements every phase, we can get away with much bigger changes in rep ranges.

Given that we're using the same eight movements for the entire program, which by itself is a complete departure from other fat-loss programs, we can make a jump from metabolic focus in one phase to endurance the next.

If you look at the first three phases of my normal five-phase cycle—

> *Phase One: 12 reps—Metabolic*
> *Phase Two: 20 reps—Endurance*
> *Phase Three: 5 reps—Strength*
> *Phase Four: 15 reps—Metabolic-Endurance*
> *Phase Five: 8 reps—Metabolic-Strength*

It sure does look an awful lot like this program, doesn't it?

> *Phase One: 12 reps—Metabolic*
> *Phase Two: 20 reps—Endurance*
> *Phase Three: 6 reps—Strength*

That gives you a little window into my thinking in designing programs like this.

A case could be made for adding two more phases to this cycle, a 15-rep metabolic-endurance phase and an 8-rep metabolic-strength phase. But I didn't.

Again, since we aren't changing the movements every phase, we don't need those middle phases to bridge the gap. We get bigger changes, a bigger metabolic disturbance while keeping continuity with the same movements.

It works really well. There's no question when you go from the 12 metabolic reps to the 20 endurance reps, or from 20 endurance reps to the 6 strength reps, you know you're working a completely different adaptation.

This isn't the best way to get super strong. It's the best way to get *lean*.

BONUS: STRENGTH IN THE SECOND CYCLE

This program isn't really set up to get you to your first pull-up by the end of the first phase. You'll find though, if you're willing to put fat loss first in the first cycle, you'll have an easier time getting that pull-up later. Losing bodyweight is one of the fastest ways to make pull-ups easier. And if you've lost bodyfat percentage, your strength-to-weight ratio has increased, making pull-ups easier.

In fact, that might be one of the clues to why I chose pull-ups for the strength standard: They're a strength move that *directly* rewards having a low bodyfat percentage. In other words, the hotter you look, the better you're going to be at pull-ups.

If you're interested in strength as much as fat loss, you'll be rewarded in the second cycle, where you'll go from the four-week strength phase into two more phases that include a strength day.

From the strength phase to the metabolic/endurance/strength phase to the stronger metabolic/endurance/strength phase, you'll have 16 weeks of consecutive strength work to make a real breakthrough in pull-ups or deadlifts, or whatever is fun for you.

> *Phase Four: 6 reps—***Strength**
> *Phase Five: 12 reps, 20 reps, 6 reps—*Metabolic/Endurance/**Strength**
> *Phase Six: 10 reps, 15 reps, 5 reps—*Stronger Metabolic/Endurance/**Strength**

Those multi-adaptation phases in the second cycle are in the program because *they're the absolute best possible fat-loss program you could do.*

Secondarily, the research is pretty clear that they're awesome for strength. I mention that because of how much things have changed in the last few years. Ten years ago none of my clients cared about strength until I convinced them it would get them hotter bodies. Now, some of the leanest clients who come to me are worried about what's going to happen to their deadlift one-rep max during the endurance phase!

The program hasn't changed, but the public perspective has turned a full 180.

In the first cycle, we put fat loss first, at the expense of maximum strength. In the second cycle, you get lucky because it turns out that the best possible program for fat loss works really well for strength also.

SOLVING THE ADVANCED FAT-LOSS WORKOUT PROBLEM

We know the most powerful training program for fat loss is a multi-adaptation phase. This is where one day you hit metabolic, one day you hit endurance, and another day you hit strength. You have one day of each, every week. The fancy name for that is undulating periodization.

The biggest issue with the plan is it's completely unwieldy for intermediate workout folks, and sometimes it's even a lot to manage for advanced trainees. For beginners, it's usually not even an option. It's too hard to set up, and it's too hard to track.

We fix that issue by giving you *a whole month* at each of those rep ranges. You don't have to figure out what weight of kettlebell or which pushup progression to use in that rep range, because you have a whole month to figure that out.

Simple, elegant, easy.

On top of that, we find that again, since we're using the same eight movements through the entire program, you're really only managing the three rep ranges you already know. Where most fat-loss programs make things unnecessarily complex by adding a completely different set of movements on top, we're staying the course with the same eight simple, big-bang exercises that produce the most results.

That's the other reason we skip some of the intermediate rep ranges. By using the same rep ranges and the same movements, we can skip ahead to a very advanced fat-loss program. You don't need to wait nine months to do a multi-adaptation phase, because we completely set up for it in the first three phases.

Just use the three months of workout journals from your first three months of workouts to lean on. You'll have had three months of becoming completely familiar with yourself and your abilities in those three rep ranges before getting to the fairly advanced task of doing all three at the same time.

This whole program is set up to give you the absolute best results from a fairly advanced fat-loss workout program, but have each phase set up the next in such a way that it occurs very simply.

I'm giving you all the background here for fun, and for those who are interested. In reality, you can just do each workout, day by day, and get all of the results without ever worrying about *why* it works.

The First Cycle of the *Pull Your Weight* Program

Phase One: *Metabolic (12 reps per set)*
Phase Two: *Endurance (20 reps per set)*
Phase Three: *Strength (6 reps per set)*

The Second Cycle of the *Pull Your Weight* Program

Phase Four: *Metabolic/Endurance/Strength (12, 20, 6 reps per set)*
Phase Five: *Stronger Metabolic/Endurance/Strength (8, 15, 5 reps per set)*
Phase Six: *Volume Phase (fewer movements, more total reps per move)*

JOSH

CHAPTER 20

HOW THE MOVEMENT PROGRESSIONS WORK

Every movement listed in the workouts has a progression. It's up to you to find the appropriate progression of each movement for your current fitness level, and for the particular set and repetition range.

If you have no idea where to start, start at the beginning—start with the first progression of every movement. If you max out the rep range for that workout, move up to the next movement in the progression. If you've been working out awhile, you probably already have a feel for where to start.

For example, in the metabolic phase, which is 6–12 repetitions per set, if you can do 12 repetitions, move up to the next harder progression. If you can't do 6 repetitions, move down to the next easier move in the progression. It's that simple.

These progressions start very, very easy, and they get very, very hard. There is a right progression of each movement for each person's fitness level.

I decided to go into more detail and spell out every step of the progressions, including kettlebell weights, because there was a fair amount of confusion in previous programs I've written. This should make it super clear. Every possible step is here.

This doesn't mean you need to do each step and every combination of kettlebells in the progression. But if you have enough kettlebells to progress this way, this would be the easiest and smoothest transition between steps.

You'll find detailed exercise descriptions and photos in the exercise section beginning on page 235.

PUSHUP PROGRESSION	
EASIER	PUSHUP, KNEES
	PUSHUP PLANK—FIVE SECONDS
	PUSHUP, FULL DOWN, KNEES UP
	PUSHUP, ½
	PUSHUP
	SINGLE-LEG PUSHUP
	SPIDERMAN PUSHUP
	ARCHER PUSHUP
	PUSHUP, BAND RESISTED
HARDER	PUSHUP, WEIGHTED VEST

PULL-UP PROGRESSION	
EASIER	*RESISTANCE BANDS CAN BE USED TO ASSIST AT EVERY LEVEL*
	PULL-UP HANG—THREE SECONDS
	PULL-UP HANG, ACTIVE SHOULDERS—THREE SECONDS
	CHIN-UP, TOP HOLD—ONE SECOND
	CHIN-UP NEGATIVE—THREE SECONDS
	CHIN-UP, ¼
	CHIN-UP, ½
	CHIN-UP, ¾
	CHIN-UP
	PULL-UP
HARDER	PULL-UP, TACTICAL

SINGLE-LEG DEADLIFT PROGRESSION—WOMEN	
EASIER	STICK DEADLIFT DRILL
	KETTLEBELL ROMANIAN DEADLIFT, 8KG+8KG
	KETTLEBELL ROMANIAN DEADLIFT, 12KG+12KG
	ASSISTANCE HOLD SINGLE-LEG, OPPOSITE-HAND DEADLIFT, 8KG
	ASSISTANCE HOLD SINGLE-LEG, OPPOSITE-HAND DEADLIFT, 12KG
	SINGLE-LEG, OPPOSITE HAND DEADLIFT, 8KG
	SINGLE-LEG, OPPOSITE HAND DEADLIFT, 12KG
	SINGLE-LEG, OPPOSITE HAND DEADLIFT, 16KG
	TWO-KETTLEBELL SINGLE-LEG DEADLIFT, 8KG+8KG
	TWO-KETTLEBELL SINGLE-LEG DEADLIFT, 12KG+12KG
	TWO-KETTLEBELL SINGLE-LEG DEADLIFT, 16KG+16KG
	TWO-KETTLEBELL SINGLE-LEG DEADLIFT, 20KG+20KG
HARDER	TWO-KETTLEBELL SINGLE-LEG DEADLIFT, 24KG+24KG

SINGLE-LEG DEADLIFT PROGRESSION—MEN	
EASIER	STICK DEADLIFT DRILL
	DEADLIFT, ROMANIAN, 16KG+16KG
	DEADLIFT, ROMANIAN, 20KG+20KG
	DEADLIFT, SINGLE-LEG ASSISTED, 16KG
	DEADLIFT, SINGLE-LEG ASSISTED, 20KG
	DEADLIFT, SINGLE-LEG, OPPOSITE-HAND, 16KG
	DEADLIFT, SINGLE-LEG, OPPOSITE-HAND, 20KG
	DEADLIFT, SINGLE-LEG, OPPOSITE-HAND, 24KG
	DEADLIFT, SINGLE-LEG, TWO-KETTLEBELL, 16KG+16KG
	DEADLIFT, SINGLE-LEG, TWO-KETTLEBELL, 20KG+20KG
	DEADLIFT, SINGLE-LEG, TWO-KETTLEBELL, 24KG+24KG
	DEADLIFT, SINGLE-LEG, TWO-KETTLEBELL, 28KG+28KG
HARDER	DEADLIFT, SINGLE-LEG, TWO-KETTLEBELL, 32KG+32KG

BARBELL DEADLIFT PROGRESSION	
EASIER	STICK DEADLIFT DRILL
	DEADLIFT, ROMANIAN
HARDER	BARBELL DEADLIFT

The barbell deadlift progression is the least complex. Once you work up to the barbell deadlift, it's just a matter of adding weight to the bar.

MILITARY PRESS PROGRESSION—WOMEN	
EASIER	ONE-KETTLEBELL PUSH PRESS, 8KG
	ONE-KETTLEBELL MILITARY PRESS, 8KG
	TWO-KETTLEBELL MILITARY PRESS, 8KG+8KG
	ONE-KETTLEBELL MILITARY PRESS, 12KG
	TWO-KETTLEBELL MILITARY PRESS, 12KG+8KG
	TWO-KETTLEBELL MILITARY PRESS, 12KG+12KG
	ONE-KETTLEBELL MILITARY PRESS, 16KG
	TWO-KETTLEBELL MILITARY PRESS, 16KG+12KG
HARDER	TWO-KETTLEBELL MILITARY PRESS, 16KG+16KG

MILITARY PRESS PROGRESSION—MEN	
EASIER	ONE-KETTLEBELL PUSH PRESS, 16KG
	ONE-KETTLEBELL MILITARY PRESS, 16KG
	TWO-KETTLEBELL MILITARY PRESS, 16KG+16KG
	ONE-KETTLEBELL MILITARY PRESS, 20KG
	TWO-KETTLEBELL MILITARY PRESS, 20KG+16KG
	TWO-KETTLEBELL MILITARY PRESS, 20KG+20KG
	ONE-KETTLEBELL MILITARY PRESS, 24KG
	TWO-KETTLEBELL MILITARY PRESS, 24KG+20KG
HARDER	TWO-KETTLEBELL MILITARY PRESS, 24KG+24KG

TWO-KETTLEBELL SWING PROGRESSION—WOMEN

EASIER	STICK DEADLIFT DRILL
	DEADLIFT, ROMANIAN, 8KG+8KG
	DEADLIFT, ROMANIAN, 12KG+12KG
	ONE-KETTLEBELL SWING, 8KG
	ONE-KETTLEBELL SWING, 12KG
	TWO-KETTLEBELL SWING, 8KG+8KG
	TWO-KETTLEBELL SWING, 12KG+12KG
HARDER	TWO-KETTLEBELL SWING, 16KG+16KG

TWO-KETTLEBELL SWING PROGRESSION—MEN

EASIER	STICK DEADLIFT DRILL
	DEADLIFT, ROMANIAN, 16KG+16KG
	DEADLIFT, ROMANIAN, 20KG+20KG
	ONE-KETTLEBELL SWING, 16KG
	ONE-KETTLEBELL SWING, 20KG
	TWO-KETTLEBELL SWING, 16KG+16KG
	TWO-KETTLEBELL SWING, 20KG+20KG
HARDER	TWO-KETTLEBELL SWING, 24KG+24KG

LUNGE & SPLIT-SQUAT PROGRESSION—WOMEN

EASIER	BODYWEIGHT SQUAT
	SPLIT-SQUAT
	LUNGE, WALKING
	SPLIT-SQUAT, REAR-FOOT-ELEVATED
	SPLIT-SQUAT, REAR-FOOT-ELEVATED, 8KG+8KG
	SPLIT-SQUAT, REAR-FOOT-ELEVATED, 12KG+12KG
	SPLIT-SQUAT, REAR-FOOT-ELEVATED, 16KG+16KG
	LUNGE, AIRBORNE
	LUNGE, AIRBORNE, 8KG
	LUNGE, AIRBORNE, 12KG
	LUNGE, AIRBORNE, 16KG
	PISTOL SQUAT, BOX ASSISTED, 8KG
	PISTOL SQUAT, BOX ASSISTED, 12KG
	PISTOL SQUAT, BOX ASSISTED, 16KG
	PISTOL SQUAT, 8KG
	PISTOL SQUAT, 12KG
HARDER	PISTOL SQUAT, 16KG

LUNGE & SPLIT-SQUAT PROGRESSION—MEN	
EASIER	BODYWEIGHT SQUAT
	SPLIT-SQUAT
	LUNGE
	LUNGE, WALKING
	SPLIT-SQUAT, REAR-FOOT-ELEVATED
	SPLIT-SQUAT, REAR-FOOT-ELEVATED, 16KG+16KG
	SPLIT-SQUAT, REAR-FOOT-ELEVATED, 20KG+20KG
	SPLIT-SQUAT, REAR-FOOT-ELEVATED, 24KG+24KG
	LUNGE, AIRBORNE
	LUNGE, AIRBORNE, 16KG
	LUNGE, AIRBORNE, 20KG
	LUNGE, AIRBORNE, 24KG
	PISTOL SQUAT, BOX ASSISTED, 16KG
	PISTOL SQUAT, BOX ASSISTED, 20KG
	PISTOL SQUAT, BOX ASSISTED, 24KG
	PISTOL SQUAT, 16KG
	PISTOL SQUAT, 20KG
HARDER	PISTOL SQUAT, 24KG

KETTLEBELL SQUAT PROGRESSION—WOMEN	
EASIER	GOBLET SQUAT, 8KG
	GOBLET SQUAT, 12KG
	GOBLET SQUAT, 16KG
	TWO-KETTLEBELL SQUAT, 8KG+8KG
	TWO-KETTLEBELL SQUAT, 12KG+8KG
	TWO-KETTLEBELL SQUAT, 12KG+12KG
	TWO-KETTLEBELL SQUAT, 16KG+12KG
	TWO-KETTLEBELL SQUAT, 16KG+16KG
	REAR-FOOT-ELEVATED SPLIT-SQUAT WITH TWO KETTLEBELLS, 8KG+8KG
	REAR-FOOT-ELEVATED SPLIT-SQUAT WITH TWO KETTLEBELLS, 12KG+12KG
	REAR-FOOT-ELEVATED SPLIT-SQUAT WITH TWO KETTLEBELLS, 16KG+16KG
	TWO-KETTLEBELL SQUAT, 20KG+20KG
HARDER	TWO-KETTLEBELL SQUAT, 24KG+24KG

KETTLEBELL SQUAT PROGRESSION—MEN

EASIER	GOBLET SQUAT, 16KG
	GOBLET SQUAT, 20KG
	GOBLET SQUAT, 24KG
	TWO-KETTLEBELL SQUAT, 16KG+16KG
	TWO-KETTLEBELL SQUAT, 20KG+16KG
	TWO-KETTLEBELL SQUAT, 20KG+20KG
	TWO-KETTLEBELL SQUAT, 24KG+20KG
	TWO-KETTLEBELL SQUAT, 24KG+24KG
	REAR-FOOT-ELEVATED SPLIT-SQUAT WITH TWO KETTLEBELLS, 16KG+16KG
	REAR-FOOT-ELEVATED SPLIT-SQUAT WITH TWO KETTLEBELLS, 20KG+20KG
	REAR-FOOT-ELEVATED SPLIT-SQUAT WITH TWO KETTLEBELLS, 24KG+24KG
	TWO-KETTLEBELL SQUAT, 28KG+28KG
HARDER	TWO-KETTLEBELL SQUAT, 32KG+32KG

The trick with the squats is that I'd like you to be able to keep progressing with the two-kettlebell squat, but really strong clients are going to work their way past the kettlebells they own. That's where progressing to the rear-foot-elevated split-squats comes in. Moving to the split-squat pattern is the easiest way to keep progressing in strength in lieu of heavier kettlebells.

PLANK PROGRESSION

EASIER	FOREARM PLANK
	TALL PLANK
	SINGLE-LEG PLANK
HARDER	SHOULDER-TAP PLANK

HIP BRIDGE/SIDE PLANK PROGRESSION

EASIER	HIP BRIDGE
	OPPOSITE-ARM, OPPOSITE-LEG RAISE
	SINGLE-LEG HIP BRIDGE
HARDER	SIDE PLANK

THE ORIGINAL BODYWEIGHT WORKOUT DAY

The first version of this program was stylistically cool. It was essentially a two-kettlebell workout day alternating with a bodyweight and deadlift workout day.

The kettlebell progressions were to just move to heavier kettlebells. The bodyweight progressions moved to more difficult movements.

It looked really cool. The only thing is, in real life if we had kettlebells to work with, I would have you smooth out the transition from one bodyweight exercise to the next by loading them with kettlebells, especially the lunges and split-squats.

And if we could, instead of progressing the pushups to a one-arm pushup such as the original program shown below, I'd progress to a weighted vest pushup. With my in-person clients, that's what I do.

These progressions shifted from a cool stylistic template to a more useable and realistic template.

ORIGINAL BODYWEIGHT LUNGE & SPLIT-SQUAT PROGRESSION	
EASIER	BODYWEIGHT SQUAT
	SPLIT-SQUAT
	LUNGE
	WALKING LUNGE
	REAR-FOOT-ELEVATED SPLIT-SQUAT
	AIRBORNE LUNGE
	PISTOL SQUAT, TO A BOX
HARDER	PISTOL SQUAT, BUTT TO ANKLES

ORIGINAL BODYWEIGHT PUSHUP PROGRESSION	
EASIER	KNEE PUSHUP
	FIVE-SECOND PUSHUP PLANK
	PUSHUP DOWN, KNEE-PUSHUP UP
	PARTIAL PUSHUP—HALFWAY DOWN
	PUSHUP
	SINGLE-LEG PUSHUP
	SPIDERMAN PUSHUP
	WINDSHIELD WIPER PUSHUP
	ARCHER PUSHUP
HARDER	ONE-ARM PUSHUP

TO INFINITY AND BEYOND!

As I write this, I have clients who have far exceeded the heaviest weights listed in this program. I have a guy doing the whole program with two 32-kilogram kettlebells, and rowing a 40-kilogram kettlebell. And I have a few ladies doing the program with double 18-kilogram kettlebells, double 20-kilogram kettlebells, and occasionally a single 24-kilogram kettlebell. These are kettlebell instructors or hard-core do-it-yourself-ers who train themselves like instructors.

You don't need to stop when you get to the end of these progressions. Feel free to get as strong and awesome as you want. It seems to hold—the stronger you get, the easier it is to stay lean.

That being said, even my strongest clients get most of their results from their food journals. And if you're so strong that you far exceed this program and you're still soft around the middle, that's another indicator that your issue is food, not workouts.

JOSH

CHAPTER 21

METABOLIC PHASE WORKOUTS

METABOLIC PHASE OUTLINE

	METABOLIC PHASE			
WEEK ONE	FOOD JOURNAL REVIEW, PLANNING, PREPARATION, COOKING			
	2 SETS	6–12 REPS	MEDIUM	KETTLEBELL
	1 SET	6–12 REPS	EASY	DEADLIFT AND BODYWEIGHT
	1 SET	6–12 REPS	EASY	KETTLEBELL
WEEK TWO	FOOD JOURNAL REVIEW, PLANNING, PREPARATION, COOKING			
	3 SETS	6–12 REPS	MEDIUM	DEADLIFT AND BODYWEIGHT
	2 SETS	6–12 REPS	MEDIUM	KETTLEBELL
	1 SETS	6–12 REPS	EASY	DEADLIFT AND BODYWEIGHT
WEEK THREE	FOOD JOURNAL REVIEW, PLANNING, PREPARATION, COOKING			
	4 SETS	6–12 REPS	HARD	KETTLEBELL
	3 SETS	6–12 REPS	MEDIUM	DEADLIFT AND BODYWEIGHT
	2 SETS	6–12 REPS	EASY	KETTLEBELL
WEEK FOUR	FOOD JOURNAL REVIEW, PLANNING, PREPARATION, COOKING			
	4 SETS	6–12 REPS	HARD	DEADLIFT AND BODYWEIGHT
	3 SETS	6–12 REPS	MEDIUM	KETTLEBELL
	3 SETS	6–12 REPS	MEDIUM	DEADLIFT AND BODYWEIGHT

Exercise descriptions start on page 235.

METABOLIC PHASE AND PULL-UPS

You might not be able to do any pull-up bar hangs, and will do bent-over rows instead. That's totally cool.

If you can do a few three-second bar hangs, do as many as you can, and then fill in the rest of the reps with kettlebell bent-over rows.

If you can do at least six reps of three-second bar hangs, that's awesome. If you start with six hangs, and work your way up to 12 hangs per set, that's great progress.

If you can do chin-up negatives or partial chin-ups, you're a total ninja. YouTube makes it look like everyone is a badass and can do a million chin-ups. But I'm telling you right now, if you can do sets of 6–12 *partial* chin-ups, you're doing super awesome.

METABOLIC PHASE WEEK ONE
Sunday and/or Monday

FOOD	JOURNAL REVIEW	PLANNING	PREPARATION	COOKING

Tuesday—Medium

Remember: *If you have no idea where to start, start at the beginning—start with the first progression of every movement.*

SUPERSET ONE	MOVEMENT	SETS	REPETITIONS
	TWO-KETTLEBELL MILITARY PRESS	2	6–12
	TWO-KETTLEBELL SWING	2	6–12

SUPERSET TWO	MOVEMENT	SETS	REPETITIONS
	ONE-KETTLEBELL ROW	2	6–12
	TWO-KETTLEBELL FRONT SQUAT	2	6–12

Thursday—Easy

SUPERSET ONE	MOVEMENT	SETS	REPETITIONS
	DEADLIFT	1	6–12
	PUSHUP PROGRESSION	1	6–12

SUPERSET TWO	MOVEMENT	SETS	REPETITIONS
	PULL-UP PROGRESSION	1	6–12
	LUNGE OR SPLIT-SQUAT PROGRESSION	1	6–12

METABOLIC PHASE WORKOUTS

INTERVAL TRAINING	MOVEMENT	INTERVAL	DURATION
	ONE-KETTLEBELL SWING	20 SECONDS WORK, 40 SECONDS REST	4 MINUTES

Saturday—Easy

SUPERSET ONE	MOVEMENT	SETS	REPETITIONS
	TWO-KETTLEBELL MILITARY PRESS	1	6–12
	TWO-KETTLEBELL SWING	1	6–12

SUPERSET TWO	MOVEMENT	SETS	REPETITIONS
	ONE-KETTLEBELL ROW	1	6–12
	TWO-KETTLEBELL FRONT SQUAT	1	6–12

INTERVAL TRAINING	MOVEMENT	INTERVAL	DURATION
	ONE-KETTLEBELL SWING	20 SECONDS WORK, 40 SECONDS REST	5 MINUTES

METABOLIC PHASE WEEK TWO

Sunday and/or Monday

FOOD	JOURNAL REVIEW	PLANNING	PREPARATION	COOKING

Tuesday—Medium

SUPERSET ONE	MOVEMENT	SETS	REPETITIONS
	PULL-UP PROGRESSION	3	6–12
	LUNGE OR SPLIT-SQUAT PROGRESSION	3	6–12

SUPERSET TWO	MOVEMENT	SETS	REPETITIONS
	DEADLIFT	3	6–12
	PUSHUP PROGRESSION	3	6–12

Thursday—Easy

SUPERSET ONE	MOVEMENT	SETS	REPETITIONS
	TWO-KETTLEBELL MILITARY PRESS	2	6–12
	TWO-KETTLEBELL SWING	2	6–12

SUPERSET TWO	MOVEMENT	SETS	REPETITIONS
	ONE-KETTLEBELL ROW	2	6–12
	TWO-KETTLEBELL FRONT SQUAT	2	6–12

INTERVAL TRAINING	MOVEMENT	INTERVAL	DURATION
	ONE-KETTLEBELL SWING	20 SECONDS WORK, 40 SECONDS REST	6 MINUTES

Saturday—Easy

SUPERSET ONE	MOVEMENT	SETS	REPETITIONS
	DEADLIFT	1	6–12
	PUSHUP PROGRESSION	1	6–12

SUPERSET TWO	MOVEMENT	SETS	REPETITIONS
	PULL-UP PROGRESSION	1	6–12
	LUNGE OR SPLIT-SQUAT PROGRESSION	1	6–12

INTERVAL TRAINING	MOVEMENT	INTERVAL	DURATION
	ONE-KETTLEBELL SWING	20 SECONDS WORK, 40 SECONDS REST	7 MINUTES

METABOLIC PHASE WEEK THREE

Sunday and/or Monday

FOOD	JOURNAL REVIEW	PLANNING	PREPARATION	COOKING

Tuesday—Hard

SUPERSET ONE	MOVEMENT	SETS	REPETITIONS
	TWO-KETTLEBELL MILITARY PRESS	4	6–12
	TWO-KETTLEBELL SWING	4	6–12

SUPERSET TWO	MOVEMENT	SETS	REPETITIONS
	ONE-KETTLEBELL ROW	4	6–12
	TWO-KETTLEBELL FRONT SQUAT	4	6–12

Thursday—Medium

SUPERSET ONE	MOVEMENT	SETS	REPETITIONS
	PULL-UP PROGRESSION	3	6–12
	LUNGE OR SPLIT-SQUAT PROGRESSION	3	6–12

SUPERSET TWO	MOVEMENT	SETS	REPETITIONS
	DEADLIFT	3	6–12
	PUSHUP PROGRESSION	3	6–12

INTERVAL TRAINING	MOVEMENT	INTERVAL	DURATION
	ONE-KETTLEBELL SWING	20 SECONDS WORK, 40 SECONDS REST	8 MINUTES

Saturday—Easy

SUPERSET ONE	MOVEMENT	SETS	REPETITIONS
	TWO-KETTLEBELL MILITARY PRESS	2	6–12
	TWO-KETTLEBELL SWING	2	6–12

SUPERSET TWO	MOVEMENT	SETS	REPETITIONS
	ONE-KETTLEBELL ROW	2	6–12
	TWO-KETTLEBELL FRONT SQUAT	2	6–12

INTERVAL TRAINING	MOVEMENT	INTERVAL	DURATION
	ONE-KETTLEBELL SWING	20 SECONDS WORK, 40 SECONDS REST	9 MINUTES

METABOLIC PHASE WEEK FOUR

Sunday and/or Monday

FOOD	JOURNAL REVIEW	PLANNING	PREPARATION	COOKING

Tuesday—Hard

SUPERSET ONE	MOVEMENT	SETS	REPETITIONS
	DEADLIFT	4	6–12
	PUSHUP PROGRESSION	4	6–12

SUPERSET TWO	MOVEMENT	SETS	REPETITIONS
	PULL-UP PROGRESSION	4	6–12
	LUNGE OR SPLIT-SQUAT PROGRESSION	4	6–12

Thursday—Medium

SUPERSET ONE	MOVEMENT	SETS	REPETITIONS
	TWO-KETTLEBELL MILITARY PRESS	3	6–12
	TWO-KETTLEBELL SWING	3	6–12

SUPERSET TWO	MOVEMENT	SETS	REPETITIONS
	ONE-KETTLEBELL ROW	3	6–12
	TWO-KETTLEBELL FRONT SQUAT	3	6–12

INTERVAL TRAINING	MOVEMENT	INTERVAL	DURATION
	ONE-KETTLEBELL SWING	20 SECONDS WORK, 40 SECONDS REST	10 MINUTES

Saturday—Medium

SUPERSET ONE	MOVEMENT	SETS	REPETITIONS
	PULL-UP PROGRESSION	3	6–12
	LUNGE OR SPLIT-SQUAT PROGRESSION	3	6–12

SUPERSET TWO	MOVEMENT	SETS	REPETITIONS
	DEADLIFT	3	6–12
	PUSHUP PROGRESSION	3	6–12

INTERVAL TRAINING	MOVEMENT	INTERVAL	DURATION
	ONE-KETTLEBELL SWING	20 SECONDS WORK, 40 SECONDS REST	10 MINUTES

JOSH

CHAPTER 22

ENDURANCE PHASE WORKOUTS

ENDURANCE PHASE OUTLINE

	ENDURANCE PHASE			
WEEK ONE	FOOD JOURNAL REVIEW, PLANNING, PREPARATION, COOKING			
	2 SETS	10–20 REPS	MEDIUM	SWINGS AND BODYWEIGHT
	1 SET	10–20 REPS	EASY	KETTLEBELL
	1 SET	10–20 REPS	EASY	SWINGS AND BODYWEIGHT
WEEK TWO	FOOD JOURNAL REVIEW, PLANNING, PREPARATION, COOKING			
	3 SETS	10–20 REPS	HARD	KETTLEBELL
	2 SETS	10–20 REPS	MEDIUM	SWINGS AND BODYWEIGHT
	1 SET	10–20 REPS	EASY	KETTLEBELL
WEEK THREE	FOOD JOURNAL REVIEW, PLANNING, PREPARATION, COOKING			
	3 SETS	10–20 REPS	HARD	SWINGS AND BODYWEIGHT
	2 SETS	10–20 REPS	MEDIUM	KETTLEBELL
	2 SETS	10–20 REPS	MEDIUM	SWINGS AND BODYWEIGHT
WEEK FOUR	FOOD JOURNAL REVIEW, PLANNING, PREPARATION, COOKING			
	3 SETS	10–20 REPS	HARD	KETTLEBELL
	3 SETS	10–20 REPS	HARD	SWINGS AND BODYWEIGHT
	3 SETS	10–20 REPS	HARD	KETTLEBELL

Exercise descriptions start on page 235.

ENDURANCE PHASE AND PULL-UPS

As before, you might not be able to do any bar hangs, and will be doing bent-over rows instead. That's totally cool.

If you can only do a few three-second hangs, do as many as you can, and then fill in the rest of the reps with kettlebell bent-over rows. This kind of drop set is a great way to work into getting stronger on the pull-up bar, and to eventually hit the pulling reps you're looking for.

If you can do at least 10 reps of three-second hangs, that's killer. Start with 10 hangs, and work your way up to 15 hangs per set—that's awesome progress.

If you get to where 20 hangs feels easy, you can move up to 10 reps of the one-second flexed-arm hold at the top.

If you can do chin-up negatives or partial chins, you're a total ninja. If you can do sets of 10–20 partial pull-ups, you're really at the top echelon of fat-loss clients.

THE ENDURANCE PHASE AND MILITARY PRESSES

Doing the military presses in the endurance phase might be a bear for you, even with only one kettlebell, using your lightest one.

Granted, there's a pretty huge range in the endurance phase, from 10 reps to 20 reps, and that will help. But that's still more overhead strength than most beginners and even some intermediates will have.

The easiest solution would be to just do your military presses with an appropriately weighted dumbbell if you have one. I trained people for a decade in gyms, and there's no shame in my game: We'd just grab the right weight.

And even when I did in-home training, I'd always have some lighter dumbbells to bridge the gap to that first kettlebell. Almost everyone who did Turkish getups started with a 5-pound dumbbell, then moved up to 10 pounds, then 15 pounds, then to that 18-pound kettlebell, and then on the way moving up with kettlebells.

But let's say you're working out at home, and you don't have any dumbbells. You've got a few kettlebells, but your lightest kettlebell is too heavy. We'll go to the old-school Russian military's system.

The Russian military issued only one kettlebell weight: 53 pounds, and people had to come up with creative ways of making that one weight feel heavier or lighter. They designed a progression, just like our pushup progression.

The overhead pressing progression for a kettlebell that was too heavy went like this—

CLASSIC MILITARY PRESS PROGRESSION	
EASIER	KETTLEBELL PUSH JERK
	KETTLEBELL PUSH PRESS
	KETTLEBELL PUSH PRESS UP, SLOW LOWERING DOWN
HARDER	KETTLEBELL MILITARY PRESS

We're going to skip the push jerk. Love it as I do—it's fun—it's got a timing component that's a little tricky, and it's completely unnecessary for our purposes. The push press, on the other hand, is easy to learn and should be enough to make that too-heavy kettlebell easier to get overhead.

A push press is kind of like if you were trying to cheat on a military press. You sit into a little mini-squat, and then try to jump the weight up. Basically you're getting a little help from your legs.

And a little help goes a long way. You should be able to work in the 10–20-rep range with help from your legs in a push press.

The 'push press up to military press down' is exactly what it sounds like: Do a push press to get the weight up, then go slow and tight like a military press on the way down. This is a great half-step to the full military press. When your 20-rep push presses get easy, this is the next progression.

WHY YOU DON'T NEED TO HATE THE ENDURANCE PHASE

The endurance phase really is a lot of reps. But it's also a great phase, and you can love it as much as the others.

There's a common error that leaves people absolutely dreading it: *They start too heavy.* On all of the phases in the first cycle, I recommend starting too light, and moving up in weight after you've maxed out all of the reps. That goes double for the endurance phase.

If you're at all unsure where to start, in each progression start two levels down from where you were in the metabolic phase. Worst-case scenario: You max out all the sets and reps every workout, and move to the next progression…a couple of times in a row.

By the end of the second week, you'll have settled into the right progressions and kettlebell weights for each exercise, and will have started to adapt to higher-rep endurance training. You'll get everything you need out of this phase, without being crushed and without dreading the workouts.

Like all the phases in the first cycle, week three should be challenging and week four should be hard. This will be just in time for it to come back around to an easy week one of the strength phase.

WHY AREN'T THERE ANY DEADLIFTS IN THE ENDURANCE PHASE?

In the endurance phase, deadlifts are replaced with double-kettlebell swings. The other side of the coin is that there aren't any double swings in the strength phase. They've been replaced with deadlifts.

It's a simple matter of the right tool for the job. You'll get more out of doing double swings for higher reps, and it's a little safer. For whatever reason, form seems to come apart on high-rep deadlift sets.

And in the strength phase, you're going to be deadlifting the whole time. Deadlifts are perfect for low-rep sets. We're really going to take advantage of that in the strength phase.

This is another reason we're doing the big jumps from phase to phase. We're just not messing around. When we do endurance, we do endurance, and when we do strength, we do strength. The metabolic phase is the only one of the first three phases that has both deadlifts and double swings, depending on the day.

In the second cycle, given that phases can span multiple rep ranges—where you might have a metabolic day, an endurance day, and a strength day all in one week—we will see deadlifts on the strength day and double swings on the endurance day.

ENDURANCE PHASE WEEK ONE
Sunday and/or Monday

FOOD	JOURNAL REVIEW	PLANNING	PREPARATION	COOKING

Tuesday—Medium

	MOVEMENT	SETS	REPETITIONS
SUPERSET ONE	PULL-UP PROGRESSION	2	10–20
	LUNGE OR SPLIT-SQUAT PROGRESSION	2	10–20

SUPERSET TWO	MOVEMENT	SETS	REPETITIONS
	TWO-KETTLEBELL SWING	2	10–20
	PUSHUP PROGRESSION	2	10–20

Thursday—Easy

SUPERSET ONE	MOVEMENT	SETS	REPETITIONS
	TWO-KETTLEBELL MILITARY PRESS	1	10–20
	TWO-KETTLEBELL SWING	1	10–20

SUPERSET TWO	MOVEMENT	SETS	REPETITIONS
	ONE-KETTLEBELL ROW	1	10–20
	TWO-KETTLEBELL FRONT SQUAT	1	10–20

INTERVAL TRAINING	MOVEMENT	INTERVAL	DURATION
	ONE-KETTLEBELL SWING	30 SECONDS WORK, 60 SECONDS REST	4.5 MINUTES

Saturday—Easy

SUPERSET ONE	MOVEMENT	SETS	REPETITIONS
	PULL-UP PROGRESSION	1	10–20
	LUNGE OR SPLIT-SQUAT PROGRESSION	1	10–20

SUPERSET TWO	MOVEMENT	SETS	REPETITIONS
	TWO-KETTLEBELL SWING	1	10–20
	PUSHUP PROGRESSION	1	10–20

INTERVAL TRAINING	MOVEMENT	INTERVAL	DURATION
	ONE-KETTLEBELL SWING	30 SECONDS WORK, 60 SECONDS REST	6 MINUTES

ENDURANCE WEEK TWO

Sunday and/or Monday

| FOOD | JOURNAL REVIEW | PLANNING | PREPARATION | COOKING |

Tuesday—Medium

SUPERSET ONE	MOVEMENT	SETS	REPETITIONS
	TWO-KETTLEBELL MILITARY PRESS	3	10–20
	TWO-KETTLEBELL SWING	3	10–20

SUPERSET TWO	MOVEMENT	SETS	REPETITIONS
	ONE-KETTLEBELL ROW	3	10–20
	TWO-KETTLEBELL FRONT SQUAT	3	10–20

Wednesday—Medium

SUPERSET ONE	MOVEMENT	SETS	REPETITIONS
	PULL-UP PROGRESSION	2	10–20
	LUNGE OR SPLIT-SQUAT PROGRESSION	2	10–20

SUPERSET TWO	MOVEMENT	SETS	REPETITIONS
	TWO-KETTLEBELL SWING	2	10–20
	PUSHUP PROGRESSION	2	10–20

INTERVAL TRAINING	MOVEMENT	INTERVAL	DURATION
	ONE-KETTLEBELL SWING	30 SECONDS WORK, 60 SECONDS REST	7.5 MINUTES

Saturday—Easy

SUPERSET ONE	MOVEMENT	SETS	REPETITIONS
	TWO-KETTLEBELL MILITARY PRESS	1	10–20
	TWO-KETTLEBELL SWING	1	10–20

SUPERSET TWO	MOVEMENT	SETS	REPETITIONS
	ONE-KETTLEBELL ROW	1	10–20
	TWO-KETTLEBELL FRONT SQUAT	1	10–20

INTERVAL TRAINING	MOVEMENT	INTERVAL	DURATION
	ONE-KETTLEBELL SWING	30 SECONDS WORK, 60 SECONDS REST	9 MINUTES

ENDURANCE PHASE WEEK THREE

Sunday and/or Monday

| FOOD | JOURNAL REVIEW | PLANNING | PREPARATION | COOKING |

Tuesday—Hard

SUPERSET ONE	MOVEMENT	SETS	REPETITIONS
	PULL-UP PROGRESSION	3	10–20
	LUNGE OR SPLIT-SQUAT PROGRESSION	3	10–20

SUPERSET TWO	MOVEMENT	SETS	REPETITIONS
	TWO-KETTLEBELL SWING	3	10–20
	PUSHUP PROGRESSION	3	10–20

ENDURANCE PHASE WORKOUTS

Thursday—Medium

SUPERSET ONE	MOVEMENT	SETS	REPETITIONS
	TWO-KETTLEBELL MILITARY PRESS	2	10–20
	TWO-KETTLEBELL SWING	2	10–20

SUPERSET TWO	MOVEMENT	SETS	REPETITIONS
	ONE-KETTLEBELL ROW	2	10–20
	TWO-KETTLEBELL FRONT SQUAT	2	10–20

INTERVAL TRAINING	MOVEMENT	INTERVAL	DURATION
	ONE-KETTLEBELL SWING	30 SECONDS WORK, 60 SECONDS REST	10.5 MINUTES

Saturday—Medium

SUPERSET ONE	MOVEMENT	SETS	REPETITIONS
	PULL-UP PROGRESSION	2	10–20
	LUNGE OR SPLIT-SQUAT PROGRESSION	2	10–20

SUPERSET TWO	MOVEMENT	SETS	REPETITIONS
	TWO-KETTLEBELL SWING	2	10–20
	PUSHUP PROGRESSION	2	10–20

INTERVAL TRAINING	MOVEMENT	INTERVAL	DURATION
	ONE-KETTLEBELL SWING	30 SECONDS WORK, 60 SECONDS REST	12 MINUTES

ENDURANCE PHASE WEEK FOUR

Sunday and/or Monday

| FOOD | JOURNAL REVIEW | PLANNING | PREPARATION | COOKING |

Tuesday—Hard

SUPERSET ONE	MOVEMENT	SETS	REPETITIONS
	TWO-KETTLEBELL MILITARY PRESS	3	10–20
	TWO-KETTLEBELL SWING	3	10–20

SUPERSET TWO	MOVEMENT	SETS	REPETITIONS
	ONE-KETTLEBELL ROW	3	10–20
	TWO-KETTLEBELL FRONT SQUAT	3	10–20

Thursday—Hard

SUPERSET ONE	MOVEMENT	SETS	REPETITIONS
	PULL-UP PROGRESSION	3	10–20
	LUNGE OR SPLIT-SQUAT PROGRESSION	3	10–20

SUPERSET TWO	MOVEMENT	SETS	REPETITIONS
	TWO-KETTLEBELL SWING	3	10–20
	PUSHUP PROGRESSION	3	10–20

INTERVAL TRAINING	MOVEMENT	INTERVAL	DURATION
	ONE-KETTLEBELL SWING	30 SECONDS WORK, 60 SECONDS REST	13.5 MINUTES

Saturday—Medium

SUPERSET ONE	MOVEMENT	SETS	REPETITIONS
	TWO-KETTLEBELL MILITARY PRESS	3	10–20
	TWO-KETTLEBELL SWING	3	10–20

SUPERSET TWO	MOVEMENT	SETS	REPETITIONS
	ONE-KETTLEBELL ROW	3	10–20
	TWO-KETTLEBELL FRONT SQUAT	3	10–20

INTERVAL TRAINING	MOVEMENT	INTERVAL	DURATION
	ONE-KETTLEBELL SWING	30 SECONDS WORK, 60 SECONDS REST	15 MINUTES

JOSH

CHAPTER 23

STRENGTH PHASE WORKOUTS

STRENGTH PHASE OUTLINE

	STRENGTH PHASE			
WEEK ONE	FOOD JOURNAL REVIEW, PLANNING, PREPARATION, COOKING			
	3 SETS	2–6 REPS	MEDIUM	KETTLEBELL
	2 SETS	2–6 REPS	EASY	DEADLIFT AND BODYWEIGHT
	1 SET	2–6 REPS	EASY	KETTLEBELL
WEEK TWO	FOOD JOURNAL REVIEW, PLANNING, PREPARATION, COOKING			
	4 SETS	2–6 REPS	MEDIUM	DEADLIFT AND BODYWEIGHT
	3 SETS	2–6 REPS	MEDIUM	KETTLEBELL
	2 SETS	2–6 REPS	EASY	DEADLIFT AND BODYWEIGHT
WEEK THREE	FOOD JOURNAL REVIEW, PLANNING, PREPARATION, COOKING			
	5 SETS	2–6 REPS	HARD	KETTLEBELL
	4 SETS	2–6 REPS	MEDIUM	DEADLIFT AND BODYWEIGHT
	3 SETS	2–6 REPS	MEDIUM	KETTLEBELL
WEEK FOUR	FOOD JOURNAL REVIEW, PLANNING, PREPARATION, COOKING			
	5 SETS	2–6 REPS	HARD	DEADLIFT AND BODYWEIGHT
	5 SETS	2–6 REPS	HARD	KETTLEBELL
	4 SETS	2–6 REPS	MEDIUM	DEADLIFT AND BODYWEIGHT

Exercise descriptions start on page 235.

THE STRENGTH PHASE AND PUSHUPS

A lot of people have never done bodyweight exercises like pushups for strength. This phase might be the first time you've ever done full pushups from your toes. Others might be working from full pushups in the endurance phase to now doing Spiderman or archer pushups.

Stronger people may use a weighted vest for pushups. Or, if you're really a strength monster, you may find yourself doing Spiderman pushups wearing a weighted vest.

A weight vest might not be the first thing most people think of when it comes to putting together a home gym, but it's by far the best way to add resistance to bodyweight exercises like pushups, pull-ups, and lunges. If you're in the kind of shape where archer pushups are easy, you'll get a lot of mileage out of a weight vest.

Band-resisted pushups are a great, easy, and cheap half-step between making normal pushups harder, and spending the money on a weighted vest.

I used to have my pushup progressions end at one-arm pushups. And while I think they're super cool, I've very rarely used them with my fat-loss clients. I've had tons of clients progress to doing pushups with a weight vest, and only three who actually worked up to one-arm pushups.

I may be committing kettlebell trainer heresy, but I like to stick to what I actually have my fat-loss clients do. And what they do is a lot of two-arm pushups: Spiderman pushups, archer pushups, band-resisted pushups, and weighted-vest pushups.

THE STRENGTH PHASE AND KETTLEBELL FRONT SQUATS

Some really strong people might run into this problem: Your heaviest kettlebells aren't heavy enough for the kettlebell front squats in this phase. You have four options.

1. Buy heavier kettlebells.
2. If you have access to a barbell, do barbell front squats instead of kettlebell front squats.
3. One-and-a-half reps: From the top of the kettlebell front squat, go all the way down. Come halfway up, then go back down. Then all the way back up. In other words, you're doing a full rep, then an extra half-rep at the bottom of the movement for every rep listed in the workout.
4. Do two-kettlebell rear-foot-elevated split-squats instead. This is one of those great home-gym workarounds. It's amazing how much harder it is going from two legs to one leg.

STRENGTH PHASE AND DEADLIFTS

The strength phase doesn't have any two-kettlebell swings; it only has deadlifts.

This is the only phase in the whole program where I'm going to specify some days that you'll do single-leg deadlifts instead of barbell deadlifts. Barbell deadlifts every workout would be really rough, and I'd rather you switch it up.

In the metabolic phase, I'm assuming if you work out in a gym, you're doing barbell deadlifts, and if you work out at home you're doing single-leg deadlifts.

In the strength phase, even if you work out in a gym and have access to barbells, you should alternate workouts between deadlifts and single-leg deadlifts. If you train at home and only do single-leg deadlifts every workout, that's totally fine.

GETTING TO YOUR FIRST PULL-UP

In the intermediate stages of pull-ups, it's going to be all about pull-up negatives and partial pull-ups.

The positive of a pull-up would be pulling yourself up, which may still be too hard at this point. The negative of a pull-up would be lowering yourself down.

With pull-up negatives, you start at the top and slowly lower yourself down, 3 seconds per negative.

Partial pull-ups are both actions—the pulling and the lowering…the positive and the negative, but only for *a part* of the movement.

In quarter-rep partial pull-ups, start at the top, lower yourself down four to six inches, and then pull yourself back up.

For half-pull-ups, you might lower yourself down 12 inches and pull yourself back up. You get the idea.

¼, ½, AND ¾ PULL-UPS ARE THE MOST CRUCIAL PULL-UP STEPS

The partial pull-ups are an often-overlooked, but amazing way to work into full pull-ups.

This is actually how gymnasts work into really hard skills, doing the movement, but making it easier by shortening the range of motion.

There's nothing magic about partial pull-ups—quarter-, half- or three-quarter pull-ups. In reality, you could start with a one-inch partial pull-up. In a couple weeks, do a two-inch partial pull-up—that's progress. The trick is that you're slowly working your way down, farther into the movement.

When you get a half pull-up, that's a massive accomplishment!

You can do the workouts and really rock out, doing exactly the amount of pull-up that's right for you.

You don't win a prize when you get to full pull-ups. As awesome as they are, the important thing is to use the exact right move for where you are right now.

STRENGTH PHASE: WEEK ONE

Sunday and/or Monday

FOOD	JOURNAL REVIEW	PLANNING	PREPARATION	COOKING

Tuesday—Medium

	MOVEMENT	SETS	REPETITIONS
SUPERSET ONE	TWO-KETTLEBELL MILITARY PRESS	3	2–6
	SINGLE-LEG DEADLIFT	3	2–6

	MOVEMENT	SETS	REPETITIONS
SUPERSET TWO	ONE-KETTLEBELL ROW	3	2–6
	TWO-KETTLEBELL FRONT SQUAT	3	2–6

Thursday—Easy

	MOVEMENT	SETS	REPETITIONS
SUPERSET ONE	PULL-UP PROGRESSION	2	2–6
	LUNGE OR SPLIT-SQUAT PROGRESSION	2	2–6

SUPERSET TWO	MOVEMENT	SETS	REPETITIONS
	DEADLIFT	2	2–6
	PUSHUP PROGRESSION	2	2–6

INTERVAL TRAINING	MOVEMENT	INTERVAL	DURATION
	ONE-KETTLEBELL SWING	30 SECONDS WORK, 30 SECONDS REST	4 MINUTES

Saturday—Easy

SUPERSET ONE	MOVEMENT	SETS	REPETITIONS
	TWO-KETTLEBELL MILITARY PRESS	1	2–6
	SINGLE-LEG DEADLIFT	1	2–6

SUPERSET TWO	MOVEMENT	SETS	REPETITIONS
	ONE-KETTLEBELL ROW	1	2–6
	TWO-KETTLEBELL FRONT SQUAT	1	2–6

INTERVAL TRAINING	MOVEMENT	INTERVAL	DURATION
	ONE-KETTLEBELL SWING	30 SECONDS WORK, 30 SECONDS REST	5 MINUTES

STRENGTH PHASE: WEEK TWO

Sunday and/or Monday

FOOD	JOURNAL REVIEW	PLANNING	PREPARATION	COOKING

Tuesday—Medium

SUPERSET ONE	MOVEMENT	SETS	REPETITIONS
	PULL-UP PROGRESSION	4	2–6
	LUNGE OR SPLIT-SQUAT PROGRESSION	4	2–6

STRENGTH PHASE WORKOUTS

SUPERSET TWO	MOVEMENT	SETS	REPETITIONS
	DEADLIFT	4	2–6
	PUSHUP PROGRESSION	4	2–6

Thursday—Medium

SUPERSET ONE	MOVEMENT	SETS	REPETITIONS
	TWO-KETTLEBELL MILITARY PRESS	3	2–6
	SINGLE-LEG DEADLIFT	3	2–6

SUPERSET TWO	MOVEMENT	SETS	REPETITIONS
	ONE-KETTLEBELL ROW	3	2–6
	TWO-KETTLEBELL FRONT SQUAT	3	2–6

INTERVAL TRAINING	MOVEMENT	INTERVAL	DURATION
	ONE-KETTLEBELL SWING	30 SECONDS WORK, 30 SECONDS REST	6 MINUTES

Saturday—Easy

SUPERSET ONE	MOVEMENT	SETS	REPETITIONS
	PULL-UP PROGRESSION	2	2–6
	LUNGE OR SPLIT-SQUAT PROGRESSION	2	2–6

SUPERSET TWO	MOVEMENT	SETS	REPETITIONS
	DEADLIFT	2	2–6
	PUSHUP PROGRESSION	2	2–6

INTERVAL TRAINING	MOVEMENT	INTERVAL	DURATION
	ONE-KETTLEBELL SWING	30 SECONDS WORK, 30 SECONDS REST	7 MINUTES

STRENGTH PHASE: WEEK THREE

Sunday and/or Monday

| FOOD | JOURNAL REVIEW | PLANNING | PREPARATION | COOKING |

Tuesday—Hard

SUPERSET ONE	MOVEMENT	SETS	REPETITIONS
	TWO-KETTLEBELL MILITARY PRESS	5	2–6
	SINGLE-LEG DEADLIFT	5	2–6

SUPERSET TWO	MOVEMENT	SETS	REPETITIONS
	ONE-KETTLEBELL ROW	5	2–6
	TWO-KETTLEBELL FRONT SQUAT	5	2–6

Thursday—Medium

SUPERSET ONE	MOVEMENT	SETS	REPETITIONS
	PULL-UP PROGRESSION	4	2–6
	LUNGE OR SPLIT-SQUAT PROGRESSION	4	2–6

SUPERSET TWO	MOVEMENT	SETS	REPETITIONS
	DEADLIFT	4	2–6
	PUSHUP PROGRESSION	4	2–6

INTERVAL TRAINING	MOVEMENT	INTERVAL	DURATION
	ONE-KETTLEBELL SWING	30 SECONDS WORK, 30 SECONDS REST	8 MINUTES

Saturday—Easy

SUPERSET ONE	MOVEMENT	SETS	REPETITIONS
	TWO-KETTLEBELL MILITARY PRESS	3	2–6
	SINGLE-LEG DEADLIFT	3	2–6

STRENGTH PHASE WORKOUTS

SUPERSET TWO	MOVEMENT	SETS	REPETITIONS
	ONE-KETTLEBELL ROW	3	2–6
	TWO-KETTLEBELL FRONT SQUAT	3	2–6

INTERVAL TRAINING	MOVEMENT	INTERVAL	DURATION
	ONE-KETTLEBELL SWING	30 SECONDS WORK, 30 SECONDS REST	9 MINUTES

STRENGTH PHASE: WEEK FOUR

Sunday and/or Monday

FOOD	JOURNAL REVIEW	PLANNING	PREPARATION	COOKING

Tuesday—Hard

SUPERSET ONE	MOVEMENT	SETS	REPETITIONS
	PULL-UP PROGRESSION	5	2–6
	LUNGE OR SPLIT-SQUAT PROGRESSION	5	2–6

SUPERSET TWO	MOVEMENT	SETS	REPETITIONS
	DEADLIFT	5	2–6
	PUSHUP PROGRESSION	5	2–6

Thursday—Medium

SUPERSET ONE	MOVEMENT	SETS	REPETITIONS
	TWO-KETTLEBELL MILITARY PRESS	5	2–6
	SINGLE-LEG DEADLIFT	5	2–6

SUPERSET TWO	MOVEMENT	SETS	REPETITIONS
	ONE-KETTLEBELL ROW	5	2–6
	TWO-KETTLEBELL FRONT SQUAT	5	2–6

INTERVAL TRAINING	MOVEMENT	INTERVAL	DURATION
	ONE-KETTLEBELL SWING	30 SECONDS WORK, 30 SECONDS REST	10 MINUTES

Saturday—Medium

SUPERSET ONE	MOVEMENT	SETS	REPETITIONS
	PULL-UP PROGRESSION	4	2–6
	LUNGE OR SPLIT-SQUAT PROGRESSION	4	2–6

SUPERSET TWO	MOVEMENT	SETS	REPETITIONS
	DEADLIFT	4	2–6
	PUSHUP PROGRESSION	4	2–6

INTERVAL TRAINING	MOVEMENT	INTERVAL	DURATION
	ONE-KETTLEBELL SWINGS	30 SECONDS WORK, 30 SECONDS REST	10 MINUTES

JOSH

CHAPTER 24

THE METABOLIC/ENDURANCE/STRENGTH PHASE

Undulating periodization—working on multiple qualities in multiple rep ranges in the same phase—can be super effective for both fat loss and strength when it's done well.

Unfortunately, it's almost never done well.

With the current trend of muscle confusion and random workouts, people give lip service to working in multiple rep ranges. In reality, they're just shot-gunning whatever they think of. This is distinct from actually working on a rep range—to track it and get better at it.

There are so many misnomers. People say you never want to adapt to your workouts, but nothing could be further from the truth. You totally want to adapt to your workouts—*and the adaptation we want is called fat loss and muscle gain.*

The problem is actually when *you stop adapting.*

When you stop adapting to your workouts, that's when we need to change up the sets and reps. That's why every four to six weeks in this program, we've got a new set and rep range. We give you the time to adapt, to lose fat, and *then we change it.*

And that's exactly what we've got going in this multiple rep range phase. If you're intermediate to advanced in your training, you can get even better fat loss with a multiple rep range phase, and you can continue to get results for longer.

That's why we've extended this phase to six weeks.

Setting Up the Metabolic/Endurance/Strength Phase

For people who haven't trained this way, this can be cumbersome at first. The biggest question is, "How do I know which kettlebell or bodyweight progression to use for each day?"

It's no accident that for the undulating periodization phase you're using the same three rep ranges you've been using. The first three phases literally set up the fourth phase.

This simplifies figuring out what weights to start with—start with whichever kettlebell or bodyweight progression you used when you did that specific phase.

For the metabolic day, start with what you were using in the metabolic phase, for the endurance day, start with what you were using in the endurance phase, and for the strength day, use what you just finished using in the strength phase.

Yes, you're going to be using totally different weights for the strength day than you use for the endurance day. Again, you should have a pretty good feel for what to use, given you've previously had a full phase with each of these rep ranges.

Next, the stronger metabolic/endurance/strength phase (10 reps, 15 reps, 5 reps) shouldn't be too hard to set up right after the first metabolic/endurance/strength phase (12 reps, 20 reps, 6 reps). Everything is going to be just a little bit heavier.

METABOLIC/ENDURANCE/STRENGTH PHASE WORKOUTS

Metabolic/Endurance/Strength Phase Outline

	METABOLIC/ENDURANCE/STRENGTH PHASE			
WEEK ONE	FOOD JOURNAL REVIEW, PLANNING, PREPARATION, COOKING			
	1 SET	6–12 REPS	EASY	KETTLEBELL
	1 SET	10–20 REPS	EASY	SWING AND BODYWEIGHT
	2 SETS	2–6 REPS	EASY	DEADLIFT AND KETTLEBELL
WEEK TWO	FOOD JOURNAL REVIEW, PLANNING, PREPARATION, COOKING			
	2 SETS	6–12 REPS	MEDIUM	DEADLIFT AND BODYWEIGHT
	2 SETS	10–20 REPS	MEDIUM	KETTLEBELL
	3 SETS	2–6 REPS	MEDIUM	DEADLIFT AND BODYWEIGHT
WEEK THREE	FOOD JOURNAL REVIEW, PLANNING, PREPARATION, COOKING			
	3 SETS	6–12 REPS	MEDIUM	KETTLEBELL
	2 SETS	10–20 REPS	MEDIUM	SWING AND BODYWEIGHT
	4 SETS	2–6 REPS	MEDIUM	DEADLIFT AND KETTLEBELL
WEEK FOUR	FOOD JOURNAL REVIEW, PLANNING, PREPARATION, COOKING			
	3 SETS	6–12 REPS	MEDIUM	DEADLIFT AND BODYWEIGHT
	2 SETS	10–20 REPS	MEDIUM	KETTLEBELL
	4 SETS	2–6 REPS	MEDIUM	DEADLIFT AND BODYWEIGHT
WEEK FIVE	FOOD JOURNAL REVIEW, PLANNING, PREPARATION, COOKING			
	4 SETS	6–12 REPS	HARD	KETTLEBELL
	2 SETS	10–20 REPS	MEDIUM	SWING AND BODYWEIGHT
	5 SETS	2–6 REPS	HARD	DEADLIFT AND KETTLEBELL
WEEK SIX	FOOD JOURNAL REVIEW, PLANNING, PREPARATION, COOKING			
	4 SETS	6–12 REPS	HARD	DEADLIFT AND BODYWEIGHT
	3 SETS	10–20 REPS	HARD	KETTLEBELL
	5 SETS	2–6 REPS	HARD	DEADLIFT AND BODYWEIGHT

Exercise descriptions start on page 235.

METABOLIC/ENDURANCE/STRENGTH PHASE WEEK ONE

Sunday and/or Monday

| FOOD | JOURNAL REVIEW | PLANNING | PREPARATION | COOKING |

Tuesday—Easy

SUPERSET ONE	MOVEMENT	SETS	REPETITIONS
	TWO-KETTLEBELL MILITARY PRESS	1	6–12
	TWO-KETTLEBELL SWING	1	6–12

SUPERSET TWO	MOVEMENT	SETS	REPETITIONS
	ONE-KETTLEBELL ROW	1	6–12
	TWO-KETTLEBELL FRONT SQUAT	1	6–12

Thursday—Easy

SUPERSET ONE	MOVEMENT	SETS	REPETITIONS
	TWO-KETTLEBELL SWING	1	10–20
	PUSHUP PROGRESSION	1	10–20

SUPERSET TWO	MOVEMENT	SETS	REPETITIONS
	PULL-UP PROGRESSION	1	10–20
	LUNGE OR SPLIT-SQUAT PROGRESSION	1	10–20

INTERVAL TRAINING	MOVEMENT	INTERVAL	DURATION
	ONE-KETTLEBELL SWING	60 SECONDS WORK, 120 SECONDS REST	6 MINUTES

Saturday—Easy

SUPERSET ONE	MOVEMENT	SETS	REPETITIONS
	TWO-KETTLEBELL MILITARY PRESS	2	2–6
	DEADLIFT	2	2–6

SUPERSET TWO	MOVEMENT	SETS	REPETITIONS
	ONE-KETTLEBELL ROW	2	2–6
	TWO-KETTLEBELL FRONT SQUAT	2	2–6

INTERVAL TRAINING	MOVEMENT	INTERVAL	DURATION
	ONE-KETTLEBELL SWING	60 SECONDS WORK, 120 SECONDS REST	6 MINUTES

METABOLIC/ENDURANCE/STRENGTH PHASE WEEK TWO

Sunday and/or Monday

FOOD	JOURNAL REVIEW	PLANNING	PREPARATION	COOKING

Tuesday—Medium

SUPERSET ONE	MOVEMENT	SETS	REPETITIONS
	DEADLIFT	3	6–12
	PUSHUP PROGRESSION	3	6–12

SUPERSET TWO	MOVEMENT	SETS	REPETITIONS
	PULL-UP PROGRESSION	3	6–12
	LUNGE OR SPLIT-SQUAT PROGRESSION	3	6–12

Thursday—Medium

SUPERSET ONE	MOVEMENT	SETS	REPETITIONS
	TWO-KETTLEBELL MILITARY PRESS	2	10–20
	TWO-KETTLEBELL SWING	2	10–20

SUPERSET TWO	MOVEMENT	SETS	REPETITIONS
	ONE-KETTLEBELL ROW	2	10–20
	TWO-KETTLEBELL FRONT SQUAT	2	10–20

THE METABOLIC/ENDURANCE/STRENGTH PHASE

INTERVAL TRAINING	MOVEMENT	INTERVAL	DURATION
	ONE-KETTLEBELL SWING	60 SECONDS WORK, 120 SECONDS REST	9 MINUTES

Saturday—Medium

SUPERSET ONE	MOVEMENT	SETS	REPETITIONS
	DEADLIFT	3	2–6
	PUSHUP PROGRESSION	3	2–6

SUPERSET TWO	MOVEMENT	SETS	REPETITIONS
	PULL-UP PROGRESSION	3	2–6
	LUNGE OR SPLIT-SQUAT PROGRESSION	3	2–6

INTERVAL TRAINING	MOVEMENT	INTERVAL	DURATION
	ONE-KETTLEBELL SWING	60 SECONDS WORK, 120 SECONDS REST	9 MINUTES

METABOLIC/ENDURANCE/STRENGTH PHASE WEEK THREE

Sunday and/or Monday

FOOD	JOURNAL REVIEW	PLANNING	PREPARATION	COOKING

Tuesday—Medium

SUPERSET ONE	MOVEMENT	SETS	REPETITIONS
	TWO-KETTLEBELL MILITARY PRESS	3	6–12
	TWO-KETTLEBELL SWING	3	6–12

SUPERSET TWO	MOVEMENT	SETS	REPETITIONS
	ONE-KETTLEBELL ROW	3	6–12
	TWO-KETTLEBELL FRONT SQUAT	3	6–12

Thursday—Medium

SUPERSET ONE	MOVEMENT	SETS	REPETITIONS
	TWO-KETTLEBELL SWING	2	10–20
	PUSHUP PROGRESSION	2	10–20

SUPERSET TWO	MOVEMENT	SETS	REPETITIONS
	PULL-UP PROGRESSION	2	10–20
	LUNGE OR SPLIT-SQUAT PROGRESSION	2	10–20

INTERVAL TRAINING	MOVEMENT	INTERVAL	DURATION
	ONE-KETTLEBELL SWING	60 SECONDS WORK, 120 SECONDS REST	12 MINUTES

Saturday—Medium

SUPERSET ONE	MOVEMENT	SETS	REPETITIONS
	TWO-KETTLEBELL MILITARY PRESS	4	2–6
	DEADLIFT	4	2–6

SUPERSET TWO	MOVEMENT	SETS	REPETITIONS
	ONE-KETTLEBELL ROW	4	2–6
	TWO-KETTLEBELL FRONT SQUAT	4	2–6

INTERVAL TRAINING	MOVEMENT	INTERVAL	DURATION
	ONE-KETTLEBELL SWING	60 SECONDS WORK, 120 SECONDS REST	12 MINUTES

METABOLIC/ENDURANCE/STRENGTH PHASE WEEK FOUR

Sunday and/or Monday

| FOOD | JOURNAL REVIEW | PLANNING | PREPARATION | COOKING |

Tuesday—Medium

SUPERSET ONE	MOVEMENT	SETS	REPETITIONS
	DEADLIFT	3	6–12
	PUSHUP PROGRESSION	3	6–12

SUPERSET TWO	MOVEMENT	SETS	REPETITIONS
	PULL-UP PROGRESSION	3	6–12
	LUNGE OR SPLIT-SQUAT PROGRESSION	3	6–12

Thursday—Medium

SUPERSET ONE	MOVEMENT	SETS	REPETITIONS
	TWO-KETTLEBELL MILITARY PRESS	2	10–20
	TWO-KETTLEBELL SWING	2	10–20

SUPERSET TWO	MOVEMENT	SETS	REPETITIONS
	ONE-KETTLEBELL ROW	2	10–20
	TWO-KETTLEBELL FRONT SQUAT	2	10–20

INTERVAL TRAINING	MOVEMENT	INTERVAL	DURATION
	ONE-KETTLEBELL SWING	60 SECONDS WORK, 120 SECONDS REST	9 MINUTES

Saturday—Medium

SUPERSET ONE	MOVEMENT	SETS	REPETITIONS
	DEADLIFT	4	2–6
	PUSHUP PROGRESSION	4	2–6

SUPERSET TWO	MOVEMENT	SETS	REPETITIONS
	PULL-UP PROGRESSION	4	2–6
	LUNGE OR SPLIT-SQUAT PROGRESSION	4	2–6

INTERVAL TRAINING	MOVEMENT	INTERVAL	DURATION
	ONE-KETTLEBELL SWING	60 SECONDS WORK, 120 SECONDS REST	9 MINUTES

METABOLIC/ENDURANCE/STRENGTH PHASE WEEK FIVE

Sunday and/or Monday

FOOD	JOURNAL REVIEW	PLANNING	PREPARATION	COOKING

Tuesday—Hard

SUPERSET ONE	MOVEMENT	SETS	REPETITIONS
	TWO-KETTLEBELL MILITARY PRESS	4	6–12
	TWO-KETTLEBELL SWING	4	6–12

SUPERSET TWO	MOVEMENT	SETS	REPETITIONS
	ONE-KETTLEBELL ROW	4	6–12
	TWO-KETTLEBELL FRONT SQUAT	4	6–12

Thursday—Medium

SUPERSET ONE	MOVEMENT	SETS	REPETITIONS
	TWO-KETTLEBELL SWING	2	10–20
	PUSHUP PROGRESSION	2	10–20

THE METABOLIC/ENDURANCE/STRENGTH PHASE

SUPERSET TWO	MOVEMENT	SETS	REPETITIONS
	PULL-UP PROGRESSION	2	10–20
	LUNGE OR SPLIT-SQUAT PROGRESSION	2	10–20

INTERVAL TRAINING	MOVEMENT	INTERVAL	DURATION
	ONE-KETTLEBELL SWING	60 SECONDS WORK, 120 SECONDS REST	12 MINUTES

Saturday—Hard

SUPERSET ONE	MOVEMENT	SETS	REPETITIONS
	TWO-KETTLEBELL MILITARY PRESS	5	2–6
	DEADLIFT	5	2–6

SUPERSET TWO	MOVEMENT	SETS	REPETITIONS
	ONE-KETTLEBELL ROW	5	2–6
	TWO-KETTLEBELL FRONT SQUAT	5	2–6

INTERVAL TRAINING	MOVEMENT	INTERVAL	DURATION
	ONE-KETTLEBELL SWING	60 SECONDS WORK, 120 SECONDS REST	12 MINUTES

METABOLIC/ENDURANCE/STRENGTH WEEK SIX

Sunday and/or Monday

FOOD	JOURNAL REVIEW	PLANNING	PREPARATION	COOKING

Tuesday—Hard

SUPERSET ONE	MOVEMENT	SETS	REPETITIONS
	DEADLIFT	4	6–12
	PUSHUP PROGRESSION	4	6–12

SUPERSET TWO	MOVEMENT	SETS	REPETITIONS
	PULL-UP PROGRESSION	4	6–12
	LUNGE OR SPLIT-SQUAT PROGRESSION	4	6–12

Thursday—Hard

SUPERSET ONE	MOVEMENT	SETS	REPETITIONS
	TWO-KETTLEBELL MILITARY PRESS	3	10–20
	TWO-KETTLEBELL SWING	3	10–20

SUPERSET TWO	MOVEMENT	SETS	REPETITIONS
	ONE-KETTLEBELL ROW	3	10–20
	TWO-KETTLEBELL FRONT SQUAT	3	10–20

INTERVAL TRAINING	MOVEMENT	INTERVAL	DURATION
	ONE-KETTLEBELL SWING	60 SECONDS WORK, 120 SECONDS REST	15 MINUTES

Saturday—Hard

SUPERSET ONE	MOVEMENT	SETS	REPETITIONS
	DEADLIFT	5	2–6
	PUSHUP PROGRESSION	5	2–6

SUPERSET TWO	MOVEMENT	SETS	REPETITIONS
	PULL-UP PROGRESSION	5	2–6
	LUNGE OR SPLIT-SQUAT PROGRESSION	5	2–6

INTERVAL TRAINING	MOVEMENT	INTERVAL	DURATION
	ONE-KETTLEBELL SWING	60 SECONDS WORK, 120 SECONDS REST	15 MINUTES

STRONGER METABOLIC/ENDURANCE/STRENGTH PHASE WORKOUTS

Stronger Metabolic/Endurance/Strength Phase Outline

	STRONGER METABOLIC/ENDURANCE/STRENGTH PHASE			
WEEK ONE	FOOD JOURNAL REVIEW, PLANNING, PREPARATION, COOKING			
	1 SET	4–8 REPS	EASY	KETTLEBELL
	1 SET	8–15 REPS	EASY	SWING AND BODYWEIGHT
	2 SETS	1–5 REPS	EASY	DEADLIFT AND KETTLEBELL
WEEK TWO	FOOD JOURNAL REVIEW, PLANNING, PREPARATION, COOKING			
	2 SETS	4–8 REPS	MEDIUM	DEADLIFT AND BODYWEIGHT
	2 SETS	8–15 REPS	MEDIUM	KETTLEBELL
	3 SETS	1–5 REPS	MEDIUM	DEADLIFT AND BODYWEIGHT
WEEK THREE	FOOD JOURNAL REVIEW, PLANNING, PREPARATION, COOKING			
	3 SETS	4–8 REPS	MEDIUM	KETTLEBELL
	2 SETS	8–15 REPS	MEDIUM	SWING AND BODYWEIGHT
	4 SETS	1–5 REPS	MEDIUM	DEADLIFT AND KETTLEBELL
WEEK FOUR	FOOD JOURNAL REVIEW, PLANNING, PREPARATION, COOKING			
	3 SETS	4–8 REPS	MEDIUM	DEADLIFT AND BODYWEIGHT
	2 SETS	8–15 REPS	MEDIUM	KETTLEBELL
	4 SETS	1–5 REPS	MEDIUM	DEADLIFT AND BODYWEIGHT
WEEK FIVE	FOOD JOURNAL REVIEW, PLANNING, PREPARATION, COOKING			
	4 SETS	4–8 REPS	HARD	KETTLEBELL
	2 SETS	8–15 REPS	MEDIUM	SWING AND BODYWEIGHT
	5 SETS	1–5 REPS	HARD	DEADLIFT AND KETTLEBELL
WEEK SIX	FOOD JOURNAL REVIEW, PLANNING, PREPARATION, COOKING			
	4 SETS	4–8 REPS	HARD	DEADLIFT AND BODYWEIGHT
	3 SETS	8–15 REPS	HARD	KETTLEBELL
	5 SETS	1–5 REPS	HARD	DEADLIFT AND BODYWEIGHT

Exercise descriptions start on page 235.

STRONGER METABOLIC/ENDURANCE/STRENGTH PHASE WEEK ONE

Sunday and/or Monday

| FOOD | JOURNAL REVIEW | PLANNING | PREPARATION | COOKING |

Tuesday—Easy

SUPERSET ONE	MOVEMENT	SETS	REPETITIONS
	TWO-KETTLEBELL MILITARY PRESS	1	4–8
	TWO-KETTLEBELL SWING	1	4–8

SUPERSET TWO	MOVEMENT	SETS	REPETITIONS
	ONE-KETTLEBELL ROW	1	4–8
	TWO-KETTLEBELL FRONT SQUAT	1	4–8

Thursday—Easy

SUPERSET ONE	MOVEMENT	SETS	REPETITIONS
	TWO-KETTLEBELL SWING	1	8–15
	PUSHUP PROGRESSION	1	8–15

SUPERSET TWO	MOVEMENT	SETS	REPETITIONS
	PULL-UP PROGRESSION	1	8–15
	LUNGE OR SPLIT-SQUAT PROGRESSION	1	8–15

INTERVAL TRAINING	MOVEMENT	INTERVAL	DURATION
	ONE-KETTLEBELL SWING	30 SECONDS WORK, 30 SECONDS REST	2 MINUTES

Saturday—Easy

SUPERSET ONE	MOVEMENT	SETS	REPETITIONS
	TWO-KETTLEBELL MILITARY PRESS	2	1–5
	DEADLIFT	2	1–5

THE METABOLIC/ENDURANCE/STRENGTH PHASE

SUPERSET TWO	MOVEMENT	SETS	REPETITIONS
	ONE-KETTLEBELL ROW	2	1–5
	TWO-KETTLEBELL FRONT SQUAT	2	1–5

INTERVAL TRAINING	MOVEMENT	INTERVAL	DURATION
	ONE-KETTLEBELL SWING	30 SECONDS WORK, 30 SECONDS REST	3 MINUTES

STRONGER METABOLIC/ENDURANCE/STRENGTH PHASE WEEK TWO

Sunday and/or Monday

FOOD	JOURNAL REVIEW	PLANNING	PREPARATION	COOKING

Tuesday—Medium

SUPERSET ONE	MOVEMENT	SETS	REPETITIONS
	DEADLIFT	3	4–8
	PUSHUP PROGRESSION	3	4–8

SUPERSET TWO	MOVEMENT	SETS	REPETITIONS
	PULL-UP PROGRESSION	3	4–8
	LUNGE OR SPLIT-SQUAT PROGRESSION	3	4–8

Thursday—Medium

SUPERSET ONE	MOVEMENT	SETS	REPETITIONS
	TWO-KETTLEBELL MILITARY PRESS	2	8–15
	TWO-KETTLEBELL SWING	2	8–15

SUPERSET TWO	MOVEMENT	SETS	REPETITIONS
	ONE-KETTLEBELL ROW	2	8–15
	TWO-KETTLEBELL FRONT SQUAT	2	8–15

INTERVAL TRAINING	MOVEMENT	INTERVAL	DURATION
	ONE-KETTLEBELL SWING	30 SECONDS WORK, 30 SECONDS REST	4 MINUTES

Saturday—Medium

SUPERSET ONE	MOVEMENT	SETS	REPETITIONS
	DEADLIFT	3	1–5
	PUSHUP PROGRESSION	3	1–5

SUPERSET TWO	MOVEMENT	SETS	REPETITIONS
	PULL-UP PROGRESSION	3	1–5
	LUNGE OR SPLIT-SQUAT PROGRESSION	3	1–5

INTERVAL TRAINING	MOVEMENT	INTERVAL	DURATION
	ONE-KETTLEBELL SWING	30 SECONDS WORK, 30 SECONDS REST	5 MINUTES

STRONGER METABOLIC/ENDURANCE/STRENGTH PHASE WEEK THREE

Sunday and/or Monday

FOOD	JOURNAL REVIEW	PLANNING	PREPARATION	COOKING

Tuesday—Medium

SUPERSET ONE	MOVEMENT	SETS	REPETITIONS
	TWO-KETTLEBELL MILITARY PRESS	3	4–8
	TWO-KETTLEBELL SWING	3	4–8

SUPERSET TWO	MOVEMENT	SETS	REPETITIONS
	ONE-KETTLEBELL ROW	3	4–8
	TWO-KETTLEBELL FRONT SQUAT	3	4–8

THE METABOLIC/ENDURANCE/STRENGTH PHASE

Thursday—Medium

SUPERSET ONE	MOVEMENT	SETS	REPETITIONS
	TWO-KETTLEBELL SWING	2	8–15
	PUSHUP PROGRESSION	2	8–15

SUPERSET TWO	MOVEMENT	SETS	REPETITIONS
	PULL-UP PROGRESSION	2	8–15
	LUNGE OR SPLIT-SQUAT PROGRESSION	2	8–15

INTERVAL TRAINING	MOVEMENT	INTERVAL	DURATION
	ONE-KETTLEBELL SWING	30 SECONDS WORK, 30 SECONDS REST	6 MINUTES

Saturday—Medium

SUPERSET ONE	MOVEMENT	SETS	REPETITIONS
	TWO-KETTLEBELL MILITARY PRESS	4	1–5
	DEADLIFT	4	1–5

SUPERSET TWO	MOVEMENT	SETS	REPETITIONS
	ONE-KETTLEBELL ROW	4	1–5
	TWO-KETTLEBELL FRONT SQUAT	4	1–5

INTERVAL TRAINING	MOVEMENT	INTERVAL	DURATION
	ONE-KETTLEBELL SWING	30 SECONDS WORK, 30 SECONDS REST	7 MINUTES

STRONGER METABOLIC/ENDURANCE/STRENGTH PHASE WEEK FOUR

Sunday and/or Monday

| FOOD | JOURNAL REVIEW | PLANNING | PREPARATION | COOKING |

Tuesday—Medium

SUPERSET ONE	MOVEMENT	SETS	REPETITIONS
	DEADLIFT	3	4–8
	PUSHUP PROGRESSION	3	4–8

SUPERSET TWO	MOVEMENT	SETS	REPETITIONS
	PULL-UP PROGRESSION	3	4–8
	LUNGE OR SPLIT-SQUAT PROGRESSION	3	4–8

Thursday—Medium

SUPERSET ONE	MOVEMENT	SETS	REPETITIONS
	TWO-KETTLEBELL MILITARY PRESS	2	8–15
	TWO-KETTLEBELL SWING	2	8–15

SUPERSET TWO	MOVEMENT	SETS	REPETITIONS
	ONE-KETTLEBELL ROW	2	8–15
	TWO-KETTLEBELL FRONT SQUAT	2	8–15

INTERVAL TRAINING	MOVEMENT	INTERVAL	DURATION
	ONE-KETTLEBELL SWING	30 SECONDS WORK, 30 SECONDS REST	8 MINUTES

Saturday—Medium

SUPERSET ONE	MOVEMENT	SETS	REPETITIONS
	DEADLIFT	4	1–5
	PUSHUP PROGRESSION	4	1–5

SUPERSET TWO	MOVEMENT	SETS	REPETITIONS
	PULL-UP PROGRESSION	4	1–5
	LUNGE OR SPLIT-SQUAT PROGRESSION	4	1–5

INTERVAL TRAINING	MOVEMENT	INTERVAL	DURATION
	ONE-KETTLEBELL SWING	30 SECONDS WORK, 30 SECONDS REST	8 MINUTES

STRONGER METABOLIC/ENDURANCE/STRENGTH PHASE WEEK FIVE

Sunday and/or Monday

FOOD	JOURNAL REVIEW	PLANNING	PREPARATION	COOKING

Tuesday—Hard

SUPERSET ONE	MOVEMENT	SETS	REPETITIONS
	TWO-KETTLEBELL MILITARY PRESS	4	4–8
	TWO-KETTLEBELL SWING	4	4–8

SUPERSET TWO	MOVEMENT	SETS	REPETITIONS
	ONE-KETTLEBELL ROW	4	4–8
	TWO-KETTLEBELL FRONT SQUAT	4	4–8

Thursday—Medium

SUPERSET ONE	MOVEMENT	SETS	REPETITIONS
	TWO-KETTLEBELL SWING	2	8–15
	PUSHUP PROGRESSION	2	8–15

SUPERSET TWO	MOVEMENT	SETS	REPETITIONS
	PULL-UP PROGRESSION	2	8–15
	LUNGE OR SPLIT-SQUAT PROGRESSION	2	8–15

INTERVAL TRAINING	MOVEMENT	INTERVAL	DURATION
	ONE-KETTLEBELL SWING	30 SECONDS WORK, 30 SECONDS REST	9 MINUTES

Saturday—Hard

SUPERSET ONE	MOVEMENT	SETS	REPETITIONS
	TWO-KETTLEBELL MILITARY PRESS	5	1–5
	DEADLIFT	5	1–5

SUPERSET TWO	MOVEMENT	SETS	REPETITIONS
	ONE-KETTLEBELL ROW	5	1–5
	TWO-KETTLEBELL FRONT SQUAT	5	1–5

INTERVAL TRAINING	MOVEMENT	INTERVAL	DURATION
	ONE-KETTLEBELL SWING	30 SECONDS WORK, 30 SECONDS REST	9 MINUTES

STRONGER METABOLIC/ENDURANCE/STRENGTH PHASE WEEK SIX

Sunday and/or Monday

FOOD	JOURNAL REVIEW	PLANNING	PREPARATION	COOKING

Tuesday—Hard

SUPERSET ONE	MOVEMENT	SETS	REPETITIONS
	DEADLIFT	4	4–8
	PUSHUP PROGRESSION	4	4–8

SUPERSET TWO	MOVEMENT	SETS	REPETITIONS
	PULL-UP PROGRESSION	4	4–8
	LUNGE OR SPLIT-SQUAT PROGRESSION	4	4–8

THE METABOLIC/ENDURANCE/STRENGTH PHASE

Thursday—Hard

SUPERSET ONE

MOVEMENT	SETS	REPETITIONS
TWO-KETTLEBELL MILITARY PRESS	3	8–15
TWO-KETTLEBELL SWING	3	8–15

SUPERSET TWO

MOVEMENT	SETS	REPETITIONS
ONE-KETTLEBELL ROW	3	8–15
TWO-KETTLEBELL FRONT SQUAT	3	8–15

INTERVAL TRAINING

MOVEMENT	INTERVAL	DURATION
ONE-KETTLEBELL SWING	30 SECONDS WORK, 30 SECONDS REST	10 MINUTES

Saturday—Hard

SUPERSET ONE

MOVEMENT	SETS	REPETITIONS
DEADLIFT	5	1–5
PUSHUP PROGRESSION	5	1–5

SUPERSET TWO

MOVEMENT	SETS	REPETITIONS
PULL-UP PROGRESSION	5	1–5
LUNGE OR SPLIT-SQUAT PROGRESSION	5	1–5

INTERVAL TRAINING

MOVEMENT	INTERVAL	DURATION
ONE-KETTLEBELL SWING	30 SECONDS WORK, 30 SECONDS REST	10 MINUTES

VOLUME PHASE WORKOUTS
Volume Phase Outline

	VOLUME PHASE			
WEEK ONE	FOOD JOURNAL REVIEW, PLANNING, PREPARATION, COOKING			
	4 SETS	5–10 REPS	MEDIUM	KETTLEBELL PRESS AND SWING
	3 SETS	5–10 REPS	EASY	KETTLEBELL SQUAT AND ROW
	2 SETS	5–10 REPS	EASY	DEADLIFT AND PUSHUP
WEEK TWO	FOOD JOURNAL REVIEW, PLANNING, PREPARATION, COOKING			
	5 SETS	5–10 REPS	MEDIUM	PULL-UP AND LUNGE, SPLIT-SQUAT
	4 SETS	5–10 REPS	MEDIUM	KETTLEBELL PRESS AND SWING
	3 SETS	5–10 REPS	EASY	KETTLEBELL SQUAT AND ROW
WEEK THREE	FOOD JOURNAL REVIEW, PLANNING, PREPARATION, COOKING			
	6 SETS	5–10 REPS	MEDIUM	DEADLIFT AND PUSHUP
	5 SETS	5–10 REPS	MEDIUM	PULL-UP AND LUNGE, SPLIT-SQUAT
	4 SETS	5–10 REPS	MEDIUM	KETTLEBELL PRESS AND SWING
WEEK FOUR	FOOD JOURNAL REVIEW, PLANNING, PREPARATION, COOKING			
	7 SETS	5–10 REPS	HARD	KETTLEBELL SQUAT AND ROW
	6 SETS	5–10 REPS	MEDIUM	DEADLIFT AND PUSHUP
	5 SETS	5–10 REPS	MEDIUM	PULL-UP AND LUNGE, SPLIT-SQUAT
WEEK FIVE	FOOD JOURNAL REVIEW, PLANNING, PREPARATION, COOKING			
	8 SETS	5–10 REPS	HARD	PULL-UP AND LUNGE, SPLIT-SQUAT
	7 SETS	5–10 REPS	HARD	KETTLEBELL PRESS AND SWING
	6 SETS	5–10 REPS	MEDIUM	KETTLEBELL SQUAT AND ROW
WEEK SIX	FOOD JOURNAL REVIEW, PLANNING, PREPARATION, COOKING			
	8 SETS	5–10 REPS	HARD	DEADLIFT AND PUSHUP
	7 SETS	5–10 REPS	HARD	PULL-UP AND LUNGE, SPLIT-SQUAT
	6 SETS	5–10 REPS	MEDIUM	KETTLEBELL PRESS AND SWING

Exercise descriptions start on page 235.

HOW THE VOLUME PHASE IS DIFFERENT

The volume phase plays by slightly different rules than the previous five phases. Where the other phases have four movements per workout and two to five sets per movement, this phase only has two movements per workout, and ramps up to eight sets per movement. You'll be doing fewer moves per day, but you're doing a lot more of them.

The volume phase is only about how many total reps we can get per movement in each workout.

It's worth mentioning, the easiest way to completely hate the volume phase is to use kettlebells that are too heavy, or bodyweight progressions that are too hard.

In this phase *I really urge you to start too light*. Go ahead and max out all your reps for each set, and then move up.

THE METABOLIC/ENDURANCE/STRENGTH PHASE

The volume of work—the total number of sets and reps—is going to ramp up really fast. Depending on what kettlebell weights and bodyweight exercises you start with, you may find yourself needing to drop to lighter kettlebells or easier bodyweight exercises to keep hitting all the sets.

First off, there's unlimited rest—literally rest as much as you want. It's pretty normal to rest less at the beginning of each workout and more at the end.

Just get all the sets, keep your form right, and get some work done. This phase is going to be very challenging just by the sheer volume of sets and reps there are in the workout.

VOLUME PHASE WEEK ONE

Sunday and/or Monday

FOOD	JOURNAL REVIEW	PLANNING	PREPARATION	COOKING

Tuesday—Medium

SUPERSET	MOVEMENT	SETS	REPETITIONS
	TWO-KETTLEBELL MILITARY PRESS	4	5–10
	TWO-KETTLEBELL SWING	4	10–20

Thursday—Easy

SUPERSET	MOVEMENT	SETS	REPETITIONS
	TWO-KETTLEBELL SQUAT	3	5–10
	TWO-KETTLEBELL BENT-OVER ROW	3	5–10

INTERVAL TRAINING	MOVEMENT	INTERVAL	DURATION
	ONE-KETTLEBELL SWING	60 SECONDS WORK, 90 SECONDS REST	5 MINUTES

Saturday—Easy

SUPERSET	MOVEMENT	SETS	REPETITIONS
	DEADLIFT	2	1–5
	PUSHUP PROGRESSION	2	5–10

INTERVAL TRAINING	MOVEMENT	INTERVAL	DURATION
	ONE-KETTLEBELL SWING	60 SECONDS WORK, 90 SECONDS REST	5 MINUTES

VOLUME PHASE WEEK TWO

Sunday and/or Monday

| FOOD | JOURNAL REVIEW | PLANNING | PREPARATION | COOKING |

Tuesday—Medium

SUPERSET	MOVEMENT	SETS	REPETITIONS
	PULL-UP PROGRESSION	5	1–5
	LUNGE OR SPLIT-SQUAT PROGRESSION	5	5–10

Thursday—Medium

SUPERSET	MOVEMENT	SETS	REPETITIONS
	TWO-KETTLEBELL MILITARY PRESS	4	5–10
	TWO-KETTLEBELL SWING	4	10–20

INTERVAL TRAINING	MOVEMENT	INTERVAL	DURATION
	ONE-KETTLEBELL SWING	60 SECONDS WORK, 90 SECONDS REST	7.5 MINUTES

Saturday—Easy

SUPERSET	MOVEMENT	SETS	REPETITIONS
	TWO-KETTLEBELL SQUAT	3	5–10
	TWO-KETTLEBELL BENT-OVER ROW	3	5–10

INTERVAL TRAINING	MOVEMENT	INTERVAL	DURATION
	ONE-KETTLEBELL SWING	60 SECONDS WORK, 90 SECONDS REST	7.5 MINUTES

VOLUME PHASE WEEK THREE

Sunday and/or Monday

| FOOD | JOURNAL REVIEW | PLANNING | PREPARATION | COOKING |

Tuesday—Medium

SUPERSET	MOVEMENT	SETS	REPETITIONS
	DEADLIFT	6	1–5
	PUSHUP PROGRESSION	6	5–10

Thursday—Medium

SUPERSET	MOVEMENT	SETS	REPETITIONS
	PULL-UP PROGRESSION	5	1–5
	LUNGE OR SPLIT-SQUAT PROGRESSION	5	5–10

INTERVAL TRAINING	MOVEMENT	INTERVAL	DURATION
	ONE-KETTLEBELL SWING	60 SECONDS WORK, 90 SECONDS REST	10 MINUTES

Saturday—Medium

SUPERSET	MOVEMENT	SETS	REPETITIONS
	TWO-KETTLEBELL MILITARY PRESS	4	5–10
	TWO-KETTLEBELL SWING	4	10–20

INTERVAL TRAINING	MOVEMENT	INTERVAL	DURATION
	ONE-KETTLEBELL SWING	60 SECONDS WORK, 90 SECONDS REST	10 MINUTES

VOLUME PHASE WEEK FOUR

Sunday and/or Monday

FOOD	JOURNAL REVIEW	PLANNING	PREPARATION	COOKING

Tuesday—Hard

SUPERSET	MOVEMENT	SETS	REPETITIONS
	TWO-KETTLEBELL SQUAT	7	5–10
	TWO-KETTLEBELL BENT-OVER ROW	7	5–10

Thursday—Medium

SUPERSET	MOVEMENT	SETS	REPETITIONS
	DEADLIFT	6	1–5
	PUSHUP PROGRESSION	6	5–10

INTERVAL TRAINING	MOVEMENT	INTERVAL	DURATION
	ONE-KETTLEBELL SWING	60 SECONDS WORK, 90 SECONDS REST	7.5 MINUTES

Saturday—Medium

SUPERSET	MOVEMENT	SETS	REPETITIONS
	PULL-UP PROGRESSION	5	1–5
	LUNGE OR SPLIT-SQUAT PROGRESSION	5	5–10

INTERVAL TRAINING	MOVEMENT	INTERVAL	DURATION
	ONE-KETTLEBELL SWING	60 SECONDS WORK, 90 SECONDS REST	7.5 MINUTES

THE METABOLIC/ENDURANCE/STRENGTH PHASE

VOLUME PHASE WEEK FIVE

Sunday and/or Monday

| FOOD | JOURNAL REVIEW | PLANNING | PREPARATION | COOKING |

Tuesday—Hard

SUPERSET	MOVEMENT	SETS	REPETITIONS
	TWO-KETTLEBELL MILITARY PRESS	8	5–10
	TWO-KETTLEBELL SWING	8	10–20

Thursday—Hard

SUPERSET	MOVEMENT	SETS	REPETITIONS
	TWO-KETTLEBELL SQUAT	7	5–10
	TWO-KETTLEBELL BENT-OVER ROW	7	5–10

INTERVAL TRAINING	MOVEMENT	INTERVAL	DURATION
	ONE-KETTLEBELL SWING	60 SECONDS WORK, 90 SECONDS REST	10 MINUTES

Saturday—Medium

SUPERSET	MOVEMENT	SETS	REPETITIONS
	DEADLIFT	6	1–5
	PUSHUP PROGRESSION	6	5–10

INTERVAL TRAINING	MOVEMENT	INTERVAL	DURATION
	ONE-KETTLEBELL SWING	60 SECONDS WORK, 90 SECONDS REST	10 MINUTES

VOLUME PHASE WEEK SIX

Sunday and/or Monday

| FOOD | JOURNAL REVIEW | PLANNING | PREPARATION | COOKING |

Tuesday—Hard

SUPERSET	MOVEMENT	SETS	REPETITIONS
	PULL-UP PROGRESSION	8	1–5
	LUNGE OR SPLIT-SQUAT PROGRESSION	8	5–10

Thursday—Hard

SUPERSET	MOVEMENT	SETS	REPETITIONS
	TWO-KETTLEBELL MILITARY PRESS	7	5–10
	TWO-KETTLEBELL SWING	7	10–20

INTERVAL TRAINING	MOVEMENT	INTERVAL	DURATION
	ONE-KETTLEBELL SWING	60 SECONDS WORK, 90 SECONDS REST	12.5 MINUTES

Saturday—Medium

SUPERSET	MOVEMENT	SETS	REPETITIONS
	TWO-KETTLEBELL SQUAT	7	5–10
	TWO-KETTLEBELL BENT-OVER ROW	7	5–10

INTERVAL TRAINING	MOVEMENT	INTERVAL	DURATION
	ONE-KETTLEBELL SWING	60 SECONDS WORK, 90 SECONDS REST	12.5 MINUTES

THE METABOLIC/ENDURANCE/STRENGTH PHASE

WHAT ABOUT REST?

Between exercises in a superset, your rest is usually just the time spent switching exercises. If you're really feeling worked over, rest up to 30 seconds.

Rest between supersets varies depending on the rep range you're working in.

In the metabolic phase:
Rest 30–60 seconds between supersets.
In the endurance phase:
Rest 60 seconds between supersets.
In the strength phase:
Rest 60–120 seconds between supersets.

If you haven't done legitimate strength work before and you're used to go-go-go bootcamp workouts, it may seem very odd to have low reps and high rest. The trick is that *you need to go heavy enough that you need this much rest.*

Think heavier kettlebells and very challenging body-weight exercises in this phase.

For the volume phase, rest as long as you need to in order to get as many reps possible in each set. We don't need to watch the rest or compress the rest at all. What this is about is the *total number of reps done in that workout*.

The *Bring It!* phases follow these same rules. For the metabolic-endurance workouts in *Bring It!*, rest up to 30 seconds between exercises in the supersets. Then rest 60 seconds between supersets.

For the metabolic-strength workouts you'll find in *Bring It! Remix*, you'd rest up to 30 seconds between the exercises of each superset. And then you'd rest 60–120 between supersets.

JOSH

CHAPTER 25

ANSWERING THE NAGGING QUESTIONS

Giving you a range of 6–12 reps per set is a pretty wide open range. Normally workout programs will give you a range like 10–12, or even just 12 reps, and have you adjust the weight to hit it right every time. That's called single progression—here are the number of reps to hit, and you progress by adding weight. This works really well if you have access to a rack of dumbbells, or are working with a barbell and can accurately make small changes to how heavy it is over time.

The problem is, there are pretty big jumps between sizes of kettlebells. Going from an 8-kg kettlebell to a 12-kg is 50% more weight. A 50% jump is a ridiculous increase. In a perfect world we'd bring the weight up 2–5% per jump.

It's the same with bodyweight exercises—it can be a big jump to go from knee pushups to full pushups.

Enter the double progression. Having wide rep ranges makes it easy for you to find a way to make each rep range work within your abilities. You'll be able to find a progression of each exercise that works, and you should be able to work your way up using the kettlebells you own.

Here is how double progression works. The primary progression are the reps—*add a rep here, add a rep there*. When you max out the reps, go to the next bodyweight exercise progression, or the next kettlebell combination.

DOUBLE PROGRESSION

First, progress by adding reps per set.

Second, when you've maxed out the reps, progress by moving up a kettlebell or to the next bodyweight exercise.

This begs the question: *Where do I start?*

I'd rather have you start close to the top end of each rep range. This way you always get a chance to move up a bodyweight progression and a kettlebell combination at least once during each phase.

For example, in the metabolic phase, start with kettlebells you feel confident about doing at least 10 reps. The first week or two you can add a couple reps, get to 12, and *then* move up to the next heavier kettlebell combination.

If you aren't sure about being closer to the bottom of the rep range with a heavier kettlebell or closer to the top of the rep range with a lighter one, in this program I'd rather you be closer to the top end of the rep range with a lighter kettlebell.

The same goes for bodyweight exercises. I'd rather you start closer to the top of the rep range with an easier bodyweight progression.

WHAT IF I CAN'T HIT THE SAME NUMBER OF REPS EVERY SET?

I don't expect you to. If the plan was 12 reps per set and the first set you hit 12 reps, the second set you hit 10 reps, and the third set you hit 8 reps with good form, that's fine. Just don't progress the kettlebell weight or the bodyweight exercise until you can hit all 12 reps in all the sets.

Just work on adding a rep here, and a rep there. Keep your form solid. And only push it on the hardest workout of each week.

So continuing the example above, we're saying you did kettlebell military presses, you got one set of 12 reps, the second set you get 10 reps, and the third set you get 8 reps. And then the next workout with kettlebell military presses, you got 12 reps, 11 reps, and 10 reps the third set. You added a rep or two to the second and third sets, and that's great progress.

The next time you do kettlebell military presses, the program says to add a fourth set. When you add that set, maybe it looks like this: 12 reps, 12 reps, 11 reps, but then on that new fourth set you only get 7 reps. That's fine too.

And in that way, the program is going to force you to progress whether you like it or not—you'll be adding a set every week or every other week.

THE MONTHLY CYCLE OF EASY TO HARD

Now you have more in-depth knowledge of how cycles and phases work for fat loss than 99% of all personal trainers. Next let's jump into why each phase is set up the way it is.

The first week is relatively easy. Usually it's one workout where you do two or three sets, and then the other two workout days it's only one set. Everyone always says it seems really easy.

It *is* easy, and that's by design.

That first week you're doing a brand-new rep range. Just the novelty of that new rep range is enough to provide fat-loss results. Making the jump from sets of 12 to sets of 20, or from sets of 20 to sets of 6 is huge. It doesn't take a lot of volume to get what we're going for.

It's also a rest! Sometimes people call this a de-load week.

While each phase starts easy as a low number sets, it ends hard as a high number of sets. You'll get into a rhythm of each phase starting easy and ending hard, and then you've got another easy segment to recover. By the time you're recovered, it's getting hard again.

It all moves in a cycle.

The first time I saw this concept of waving the number of sets from week to week was in Pavel Tsatsouline's *Kettlebell Fast Tens* program. It was a six-week program where the number of sets started low, built up, then started low again, and built up again. I totally loved it and started experimenting with it with my fat-loss clients. It worked so well that I used almost the same template in 2007 when I wrote *Fighter Workouts for Fat Loss*, except that it had multiple six-week waving phases.

I originally wrote my *Platinum Coaching Club Workouts* in 2009 using a build-up in volume each week. That evolved into four-week programs. The coaching club members got great results, with two sets of everything the first week, three sets the second week, and then four sets of everything the third and fourth weeks. And that led me to write *System Six: Easy Fat Loss* the same way in 2011, except pushing the envelope with the absolute fewest sets and easiest possible workouts.

Then in 2013, I got to do a two-month internship at Results Fitness, where I saw them start everyone with one set the first week, two sets the second week, and three sets the third and fourth weeks. It was really cool to get to work with a few hundred clients, each working on their own monthly cycle of easy to hard. To be at one of the best fat-loss gyms in the world and see them doing the exact same thing was totally amazing.

What you now get in the *Pull Your Weight* program is the most refined, elegant, and effective evolution of this cycle.

THE WEEKLY CYCLE OF EASY TO HARD

You'll notice this whole program is cycles within cycles. The human body seems to respond really well to cycles.

I got hooked on the idea of weekly cycles through Pavel's book *Power to the People,* and then later, the program that more closely informs this one, *Enter the Kettlebell.* I really got hooked on the volume changing from a hard day to an easy day each week with *Enter the Kettlebell.*

Ever notice how every week, you feel great on Monday, and by Friday you're kinda tired? And then you have a weekend, rest up, and go do it all again?

That's also how the weeks of this workout program are arranged. Each week we start with the most important workout—food planning and preparation.

Right after that, you get the hard workout. That's immediately followed by a medium workout. And then, at the end of the week you get to recover with an easy workout.

The body responds really well to these kinds of cycles because it's the way we're designed, and it also matches how our lives are set up.

Years, seasons, months, weeks perfectly map to programs, cycles, phases, and weeks.

SHOULD I LIFT TO FAILURE?

The question of whether we should go 100% all-out on each set is as old as time. And, as usual, we find our answer somewhere in the middle of yes and no.

Some exercises you can get away with going to failure, and some exercises you usually shouldn't go anywhere near failure, at least not for fat loss.

On one end, we've got isolation movements—think of a machine biceps curl. This is an exercise where not only *can* we go to 100% failure, but it would be silly not to.

On the other end of the spectrum, we've got a barbell deadlift. For the average person, this is one of the more complex and, if done incorrectly, dangerous movements we have. For our purposes, you've got no business going anywhere near failure in the deadlift. We can get all the results without any of the risk, and still keep a couple reps in the bank.

And that's a key concept—that we can get all of the results we need for fat loss without compromising form on a big movement like a deadlift. The deadlift uses all of the biggest muscles in the body at the same time—the muscles in the legs and back. It's a powerful stimulus for fat loss just by itself. In fact, no amount of blasting your biceps at 100% with curls would come anywhere near the fat-loss stimulus of deadlifting at 80%.

Literally, all of the movements that are useless for fat loss are the same movements you can get away with doing all-out: curls, triceps, crunches, situps, leg extensions, machine leg curls, lateral raises, and so on.

The movements that are the most powerful for fat loss are generally exercises you don't need to push to 100% failure, or at least very rarely: deadlifts, squats, pull-ups, and standing military presses.

Then there are some exercises that fall in the middle. They're useful for fat loss, and you can push them pretty hard: lunging progressions, step-ups, bodyweight squatting progressions, and pushups.

Let me give a shout-out to Christian Thibadeau, as he was the first person I ever saw lay out a 'should I train to failure' continuum, with single-joint bodybuilding exercises on one side, and multi-joint barbell lifts on the other. He had a muscle-building context, and had Olympic lifts and other stuff in there as well so his version looked different than ours. I've massively modified ours for the kinds of movements we use for fat loss.

Now, let's take a look at the *Fat Loss Happens on Monday* version of the continuum.

Kettlebell swings show up in two columns because they can be very different, depending on your level of experience with them. If you're new to kettlebell swings, they fall in the third column—a little goes a long way, and you can get a great fat-loss response without pushing them very hard. This is cool, because in the beginning, you really need to think about getting your technique perfect.

Kettlebell swings fall into the second category if you're experienced with kettlebell swings. If you've been doing them for a couple years, you can definitely push them right up to the line, and that's what you want to do.

If we were listing combination exercises like thrusters and renegade rows, they would also fall into the third category: They're definitely great for fat loss. That being said, I wouldn't base a program on them the way we could with everything else in the third category, and even in the second category. Combination exercises are most effective when they're paired with movements from the second and third categories.

MOVEMENT CHOICE CONTINUUM		
WEAK FOR FAT LOSS	**GOOD FOR FAT LOSS**	**GREAT FOR FAT LOSS**
Biceps curls	One-kettlebell swings	Barbell deadlifts
Triceps press-downs	Pushup progressions	Two-kettlebell swings
Triceps kickbacks	Lunge progressions	Two-kettlebell front squats
Machine leg curls	Split-squat progressions	Two-kettlebell military presses
Leg extensions	Bent-over rows	Pull-ups
Crunches	Single-leg deadlifts	Barbell front squats
Situps		Barbell back squats
Hip adductor machine		Barbell military presses
Hip abductor machine		
These moves would have to be pushed to **100%** failure to be useful at all. More useful for extra volume on muscle gain and bodybuilding programs. Terrible use of time in fat-loss programs.	These moves can be pushed to **90–95%** most of the time. They're staple moves in any effective fat-loss program.	These moves produce a powerful fat-loss response when done in the **80–90%** range.
Not used in fat-loss programs. In any program, you'd leave **less than zero reps** in the bank. You'd go to failure, and then you'd push farther with drop sets and forced reps.	Leave **one rep** in the bank on easy and medium workout days. Leave **zero reps** in the bank on hard workout days.	Leave **two to three reps** in the bank on easy and medium workout days. Leave **one rep** in the bank on hard workout days.

HOW SHOULD I WARM UP?

If you're a beginner, use this short and simple warmup. You'll find descriptions and photos of these exercises beginning on page 235.

BEGINNER WARMUP CIRCUIT	
MOVEMENT	REPS
KNEE PUSHUPS WITH AB BRACING	10, 8, 6
PRISONER SPLIT-SQUAT	10, 8, 6
STICK HIP-HINGE DRILL	10, 8, 6

If you're intermediate, use this short and simple warmup.

INTERMEDIATE WARMUP CIRCUIT	
MOVEMENT	REPS
PUSHUP PLANK WITH AB BRACING	50S, 40S, 30S
PRISONER WALKING LUNGES	10, 8, 6
STICK HIP-HINGE DRILL	10, 8, 6

And if you're advanced, use this warmup.

ADVANCED WARMUP CIRCUIT	
MOVEMENT	REPS
PUSHUPS WITH AB BRACING	10, 8, 6
PRISONER REVERSE LUNGES	10, 8, 6
BODYWEIGHT SINGLE-LEG DEADLIFTS	10, 8, 6

Whichever your choice, this is about a 10-minute warmup.

If it takes longer than that, you're using a progression that's too hard. If you're short on time and need a shorter warmup, no problem—cut this warmup in half. If you need to go longer, keep adding descending sets.

I've trained clients outdoors and indoors and places that were indoors that felt like they were outdoors. When it's zero degrees and snowing outside in Colorado, we'd always do a longer warmup—more like 10-8-6-4-2. If it's the middle of summer and 100 degrees outside, we might warm up with one set of 10 of each and go.

Younger folks can get away with less warming up; older folks usually need more. None of this should be shocking, so feel free to adjust based on your individual situation and common sense.

PUSH, PULL, SQUAT, HIP HINGE

If you think of the workout as always being a push, a pull, a squat, and a hip hinge, the warmup is the same. The movement preparation for the push is the knee pushup, pushup plank, or pushups. The movement prep for the pull is the 'prisoner' part of prisoner lunges. The movement prep for the hip hinge is the stick hip-hinge drill or single-leg deadlifts. And the prep for the squat is the split-squats or lunges.

All of the warmup drills do two things.

The pushup, pushup plank, and pushup drill is both a specific warmup for pushups and kettlebell military presses, and it's also a core drill. You're going to squeeze the ground with your hands and brace your abs extra hard, like you were doing a crunch. You're going to exaggerate the core bracing of a normal pushup, and treat this like an extra core drill.

The prisoner lunges, walking lunges, and walking reverse lunges are another two-for-one. The lunge is a specific warmup for squats, lunges, or split-squats, while the 'prisoner' part is a warmup for rows and pull-ups. And that's why you can't be relaxed about having your hands behind your head—you need to pull your elbows back hard, and pull your shoulder blades back and down hard. It should be harder on the muscles between and below your shoulder blades than it is for your legs.

The stick hip-hinge drill is teaching an absolute perfect version of the movement you need for your swings, deadlifts, or single-leg deadlifts. That repetition of doing it perfectly over and over is going to transfer to doing it right when you add weight. Just make sure to keep your head, upper back, and tailbone against the stick the whole time. Then sit your butt backward and fold forward at your hips until you feel a little bit of stretch. The single-leg deadlifts without weight use the same idea, assuming you've already mastered the stick hip-hinge drill.

You could think of your warmup like this.

WARMUP TEMPLATE	
MOVEMENT	WARMUP
CORE	AB BRACING ON PUSHUPS
PUSH	KNEE PUSHUP, PUSHUP PLANK, PUSHUP
PULL	PRISONER SHOULDER & ELBOW PULLBACK
SQUAT	SPLIT-SQUAT, WALKING LUNGE, REVERSE LUNGE
HIP HINGE	HIP-HINGE STICK DRILL, SINGLE-LEG DEADLIFT

Do you need more specific warmups for the rest of the workout? Maybe. It would be a smart idea to do a set of goblet squats before you do heavy two-kettlebell squats. For people doing barbell deadlifts, I usually have them do a set at 50% of the work weight, and then another set at 75% of the work weight before doing the work sets listed in the program.

If you're advanced, do whatever you want. Have a kettlebell background? Do some Turkish getup practice. Have a yoga background? Do Sun Salutation A and B a few times each. If you're advanced, you can do what you know to get yourself ready—neural warmups from Z-Health, some Primal Move flows, a Results Fitness RAMP—whatever you already know that falls into what someone would call dynamic joint mobility.

I've had advanced clients do all of the above, or even rotate through any of those on a monthly basis so they don't get bored. I also like to have people progress the combinations into crawls and multiplanar lunges. The pushups progress to bear crawls—forward, backward, even sideways. Lunges can go forward, sideways, and rotational.

At any level, beginner, intermediate or advanced, any corrective exercise you've been given from a physical therapist or an FMS practitioner makes a great warmup. And putting corrective exercise in the warmup is smart. It means you actually do it at least three times per week.

DIRECT CORE WORK?

I'm so glad you asked.

Direct core work is one of those things where most people need some, but there's just never enough time. I have some clients I train for 30-minute sessions, and other clients I train for 60-minute sessions.

If we have extra time, direct core training is the first thing to add. If we're short on time, direct core training is the first thing we take out.

Core in the Warmup

In the warmup, I'd like you to treat the pushups like planks. Brace your abs, pull your ribs down, and tuck your tailbone under, like you're holding a mini-crunch position. Exaggerate the plank aspect of those pushups in the warmup.

The Four Directions of Core

Your core basically protects your spine in four directions. And if you think about that, all you need to do for core training is plank in those four directions, and you've got it made.

CORE TRAINING TEMPLATE	
DIRECTION	CORE EXERCISE
FORWARD	FRONT PLANK
SIDEWAYS	SIDE PLANK
BACKWARD	HIP BRIDGE, AKA BACK PLANK
ROTATION	SINGLE-LEG PLANK, SINGLE-LEG HIP BRIDGE, OPPOSITE ARM/LEG RAISE

Granted, you could take it a lot further than that. If you want to dive deeper into core training, like a whole book deeper, check out *The New Rules of Lifting for Abs*, by Lou Schouler and Alwyn Cosgrove. It has all kinds of more advanced progressions with toys like the stability balls, TRX®, and ValSlides®.

For our purposes, just stick with planks if you have extra time. If you don't have time, really focus on setting the core on all of your *Fat Loss Happens on Monday* exercises.

CORE TRAINING IN THE PULL YOUR WEIGHT PROGRAM

DIRECTION	CORE EXERCISE
FORWARD	PUSHUP PROGRESSIONS, PULL-UP PROGRESSIONS
BACKWARD	DEADLIFTS, KETTLEBELL SWINGS
ROTATION	SINGLE-LEG DEADLIFTS, SINGLE-LEG PUSHUPS, SPIDERMAN PUSHUPS, ONE-ARM SWINGS

HIGH INTENSITY INTERVAL TRAINING

What about high intensity interval training, HIIT? Whatever you want to call it—cardio, energy system work, metabolic training, interval training…what about that?

First off, the reason we like *high intensity* interval training is because it's fast. If you can get the same fat-loss results from 10 minutes of intervals as you would a half-hour of slow cardio, let's rock out some short, fast, effective intervals.

On Thursdays and Saturdays, you're going to do interval training with one-arm kettlebell swings. It's written into your workout program after your Thursday and Saturday workouts.

If you'd rather do shorter workouts five days per week, you can definitely do your intervals on separate days, like Wednesdays and Fridays. A case could be made for that being more effective, but most people are busy and have an easier time getting this done if they just do their intervals right after their workouts. As usual, *just getting it done* beats optimal timing.

The only rule is if you do interval training on the same day as your strength training workouts, always do the strength training first because *we always put the most important part first.*

The interval training is really simple.

Phase One: *20 seconds of kettlebell swings, followed by 40 seconds rest*

Phase Two: *30 seconds of kettlebell swings, followed by 60 seconds rest*

Phase Three: *30 seconds of kettlebell swings, followed by 30 seconds rest*

Phase Four: *60 seconds of kettlebell swings, followed by 120 seconds rest*

Phase Five: *30 seconds of kettlebell swings, followed by 30 seconds rest*

Phase Six: *60 seconds of kettlebell swings, followed by 90 seconds rest*

There's always as much rest as work, or even more rest than work. That's how we keep the intervals *high intensity*. It's about putting more work into the work interval; it's not about less rest between intervals.

It should be obvious, but just in case it's not—adjust which weight of kettlebell you're using based on the differing work-to-rest ratios. In general, err on the side of starting too light, and having to move up because it was too easy.

A couple notes on kettlebell swings for intervals: *First, every swing should be snappy.* Swings should be all butt and hamstrings. We definitely don't want you to feel swings in your shoulders, arms, or low back. If you start to feel it in any of those places, your intervals are done for the day.

Second: Swings should be fast. They should pop and be explosive, like a jump or a punch. If your swings slow down or lose explosiveness, you need to either drop to a lighter kettlebell or stop your intervals for the day.

If you're using a 16-kg kettlebell for swings, and your swing starts to lose form or lose explosiveness, you could drop down to the 12-kg kettlebell. And if that started to lose form or explosiveness, you could drop down to the 8-kg kettlebell. If the 8-kg kettlebell starts to feel heavy, you're done for the day.

Now, depending on what you have access to, you can switch out different tools for your interval training every other month. You could do swings one month and sprinting the next month. Then come back to swings again.

APPROVED MODES OF INTERVAL TRAINING

- TWO-ARM KETTLEBELL SWINGS
- ONE-ARM KETTLEBELL SWINGS
- TWO-KETTLEBELL SWINGS
- KETTLEBELL SNATCHES
- PUSHUPS
- ALTERNATING INTERVALS: KETTLEBELL SWINGS AND PUSHUPS
- LUNGES
- ALTERNATING INTERVALS: LUNGES AND KNEE PUSHUPS
- JUMP LUNGES
- ALTERNATING INTERVALS: JUMP LUNGES AND PUSHUPS
- BATTLING ROPES
- AIRDYNE BIKE
- SPIN BIKE
- OUTDOOR SPRINTS
- TREADMILL SPRINTS
- JUMP ROPE
- BURPEES
- BEAR CRAWLS
- WEIGHTED SLED PUSH
- WEIGHTED SLED PULL

As much as kettlebell swings and pushups are two of my favorite methods of doing energy system training, you've got other options. With energy system training, feel free to switch things up any time you get bored.

High intensity interval training is where *you can and should get the most variation.*

I don't even care if you change every workout: Do swings one workout, bike the next workout, and jump rope the next. That's all totally fine and will work really well with this program.

The most common variation, and my favorite, is to alternate swings and pushups, every other interval.

PAIN AND OTHER PROBLEMS IN THE WORKOUTS

Pain versus Pain versus Pain

Sometimes I think everyone has something that hurts or some past injury they're still nursing. Then again, I may be jaded about pain—I worked as the corrective exercise guy in a physical therapy office for three years. But in general, people have stuff that hurts. And most people don't really differentiate between good and bad pain.

We'll start by defining pain as a red flag—your body trying to warn you about something bad happening.

Let's get this sorted out really quickly, and then deal with what to do about it.

The muscle working or muscle soreness—This isn't pain the way we've defined it. This is just the muscle working or getting worked. You can tell because you feel it in the muscle, and it goes away.

Muscle stretching—This also isn't pain the way we've defined it. It's uncomfortable to stretch. But you know it's okay because you feel it in the muscle, not in the joint, and it goes away when you stop, or at most in a day or two.

Injury—This is the pain we're most concerned with. For our purposes we're going to make it really simple: *If it's pain* in the joint, it's bad. *Red flag. Stop.* If it doesn't go away in a few days to a week, go see a doctor or a physical therapist.

I recently saw somebody wearing a t-shirt that said *Pain isn't weakness leaving the body. Pain is injury looking for a hole to get in.*

Words to live by.

WHAT TO DO ABOUT THE WRONG KIND OF PAIN

Right now corrective exercise is booming—stabilize this and stretch that and balance things out. I think it's all great, and I'm a really big fan and a user of both the Functional Movement Screen (FMS) and the National Academy of Sports Medicine's Corrective Exercise Specialist (CES) systems.

Corrective exercises are great for people who don't move well and are potentially at risk of injury. In other words, they're good for avoiding future pain. They have little to do with pain you already have.

If you have pain now, there are two things you need to do.
Go see a medical professional—a D.O., P.T., or M.D.
Work around it.

The fast track to getting results is working around it.

You should definitely handle the problem. And, while you're handling it, you should work around it. Do every part of this program that doesn't hurt.

Look, we know that food makes up most of your fat-loss results anyway. If you have to cut or substitute a move to stay out of pain, *do it.*

For the first few years I was a personal trainer, I really sucked at corrective exercises. It seemed like nothing I did with corrective exercises made any difference. But all my clients still got amazing fat-loss results. We just did whatever we could.

If someone had pain squatting but not lunging, we did lots of lunges. If overhead pressing hurt, we just did dumbbell bench pressing or pushups instead.

It's actually a remarkably simple system we have here. You've got—

A push: *Pushups or Military Presses*

A pull: *Pull-ups or Bent-over Rows*

A squat: *Bodyweight or Kettlebell*

A hinge: *Deadlifts, Single-leg Deadlifts, or Kettlebell Swings*

If any of those hurt, the most obvious solution is to try to switch it out for one of the other options. For example, if kettlebell military presses don't work for you, do all pushups. Or conversely, if pushups don't work for you, do all military presses.

Easy.

The next option would be to alter a move based on equipment. The reason the program is wrapped around bodyweight and kettlebell work is so you can do it at home.

But if you have a gym membership you have other options. For example, if kettlebell military presses don't work, you could try seated incline dumbbell presses—and play with the highest incline you can get away with. Or if pushups don't work, you could do a dumbbell bench press. And you could most definitely use the assisted pull-up machine in lieu of the pull-up progression.

Last but not least, drop it completely. If there's no version of the exercise that works, just drop it. It'll give you more time to go find a physical therapist to help work that out.

And more time to focus on what really matters— your food.

IF PUSHUPS HURT YOUR WRISTS

It's super common for pushups to hurt at the wrist. First things first: *None of these exercises should hurt you. Don't hurt yourself.*

To reiterate the last two chapters: There's a difference between muscles working, muscle soreness, and getting tired, which are all normal, and pain in a joint. Pain in a joint is bad. If something hurts in the joint, you should go see a physical therapist.

That being said, pushups hurting wrists is common enough that it's worth addressing separately. And we can almost always work around it.

Options to work around wrist pain—

> *Pushup handles*—You can get these for under $20 at any sporting goods store and it's usually the best solution.
>
> *Doorway pull-up bar*—If you have a doorway pull-up bar for your pull-ups, you can use it just like pushup handles.
>
> *Yoga Wedge*—Yoga supply companies make a special wedge to alleviate wrist pain in yoga postures. This works great for some people's wrists.
>
> *Pushup Board*—This is basically a 2x4 on a stand. You can make it yourself; it'd be a lot cheaper than the $50 to buy it. That being said, if you're really into pushups or if you're an SFG or RKC trainee, you'll like having something you can try to 'break in half' to create extra tension and lock your shoulders into place in that great hardstyle way. It could be worth it to you.
>
> *The handles of Hex dumbbells*—Hex dumbbells work just as well as pushup handles in a pinch.
>
> *Heavy Kettlebell Handles*—You can do pushups on the handles of your two heaviest kettlebells. You don't want to use light kettlebells for this, as you run the risk of a kettlebell getting unsteady and rolling.

Any of these are easy ways to make pushups not hurt your wrists.

IF KETTLEBELL MILITARY PRESSES DON'T WORK FOR YOUR SHOULDERS

If you work out in a gym, or if your home gym has an adjustable bench, the easiest way to fix a problem with the military press is to set a bench to the highest incline that still works for your shoulders. So instead of a military press, we do an incline press. It doesn't matter if it's with kettlebells or dumbbells—both work fine.

A great bodyweight option, from Eric Cressey, is a combination of a pushup and the yoga downward dog movement. At the top of every pushup, do a downward dog, that's one repetition. It can be made easier by doing the pushup on your knees and made harder by elevating the feet. It's a great way to start working toward overhead movements and get the shoulders moving a little better overhead at the same time. For lack of a better name, we'll call these pushup-to-down-dogs.

Pushup-to-down-dogs are described on page 290.

Long-term, if military presses don't work, you're going to want to look into putting some serious time into posture work, thoracic spine mobility, 360° diaphragmatic breathing, and shoulder mobility. Basically you need to get to the point where your shoulders move well enough that you can do military presses.

For a lot people, this really just amounts to doing some stretching. Others are going to hit a wall and need to see an FMS-certified instructor who can point them in the right direction of some more advanced corrective exercises. And for a few, you may even need to see a physical therapist.

In the meantime, do either incline presses if you have the equipment available, or pushup-to-down-dogs. Go ahead and get all the results you can out of your workouts while you're doing the correctives.

WORKING IN CORRECTIVE EXERCISES

By the time I left the physical therapy office where I worked, I felt like everyone over 35 had probably injured something at some point. If you've already hurt something and your physical therapist has treated and cleared you for exercise, but told you to keep doing the corrective exercises, you should do that.

One thing I learned from Gray Cook is to have people superset the correctives with the strength exercises. It would look like the following.

Monday—Medium

SUPERSET ONE	MOVEMENT	SETS	REPETITIONS
	DEADLIFT	3	6–12
	PUSHUP PROGRESSION	3	6–12
	CORRECTIVE EXERCISE #1	3	12

SUPERSET TWO	MOVEMENT	SETS	REPETITIONS
	PULL-UP PROGRESSION	3	6–12
	LUNGE OR SPLIT-SQUAT PROGRESSION	3	6–12
	CORRECTIVE EXERCISE #2	3	12

It really works to have corrective exercises in the program like this. It gives you a little more rest between sets—meaning you're going to be stronger in each set—and you get to use your rest time productively.

On top of that, some corrective exercises are fairly metabolic themselves, so one way or the other you're getting a better workout, and you're getting your corrective exercises in also.

Let's say you've been told to keep up with thoracic mobility and pec stretching. You'd do this—

SUPERSET ONE	MOVEMENT	SETS	REPETITIONS
	DEADLIFT	3	6–12
	PUSHUP PROGRESSION	3	6–12
	QUADRUPED THORACIC ROTATION	3	10

SUPERSET TWO	MOVEMENT	SETS	REPETITIONS
	PULL-UP PROGRESSION	3	6–12
	LUNGE OR SPLIT-SQUAT PROGRESSION	3	6–12
	DOORWAY PEC STRETCH	3	30 SECONDS

Now if you were really messed up—welcome to the club—and the physical therapist told you to keep up with six corrective exercises, use the first four as your warmup, and then put the two most important into the workout.

WARMUP

MOVEMENT	SETS	REPETITIONS
FOAM ROLL THORACIC SPINE EXTENSION	1	1 MINUTE
FOAM ROLL PEC STRETCH	1	1 MINUTE
BAND EXTERNAL ROTATION	1	10
Ts, Ys, AND Ws	1	20

SUPERSET ONE

MOVEMENT	SETS	REPETITIONS
DEADLIFT	3	6–12
PUSHUP PROGRESSION	3	6–12
QUADRUPED THORACIC ROTATION	3	10

SUPERSET TWO

MOVEMENT	SETS	REPETITIONS
PULL-UP PROGRESSION	3	6–12
LUNGE OR SPLIT-SQUAT PROGRESSION	3	6–12
DOORWAY PEC STRETCH	3	30 SECONDS

Ultimately, if you had to see a physical therapist earlier, it's like you get to have your physical therapist build your warmup for you. It'll be a warmup specific to you, and sets you up to get more out of the rest of your workout.

If you haven't been hurt—you're the exception—but feel like you might have a posture issue or a mobility issue that's holding you back, go see an FMS-certified kettlebell instructor.

This is really the best, simplest way to keep up with your corrective exercises—keep them in your program. If you have a posture issue from working at a desk, you may have to keep doing those exercises until you retire.

Or if you had a big injury, you may have corrective exercises you need to do for the rest of your life. You may as well put them in your program.

Whatever it is, the best way to do corrective exercises is to do a little bit every time you work out. Consistency and frequency is the whole deal. Putting it in as a five-minute warmup, or as one-minute breaks between sets is a genius way to fit it in to the workouts you're doing anyway.

Again, big ups to Gray Cook for that idea.

IF YOU'RE HAVING PROBLEMS WITH BARBELL DEADLIFTS

Usually the issues people have with deadlifts mostly come from not knowing how to fold at and create power from the hips. This can usually get sorted out from the progression plan and the warmup—spending a lot of time with the stick hip-hinge drill and Romanian deadlifts.

Some people just get beat up with barbell deadlifts. The trap-bar deadlift is an easy substitution that agrees with almost everyone. Lots of people who struggle with the deadlift can get it after spending a few months trap-bar deadlifting. Some people love the trap bar, and just stick with that.

The trap-bar deadlift is a great way to get strong, using a really easy, really forgiving movement. Not every gym has one, but it's an awesome investment for your home gym.

If you keep working toward the barbell deadlift and the stick hip-hinge drill and Romanian deadlifting don't sort you out, I recommend getting someone to help—like an SFG or RKC kettlebell instructor, or an FMS-certified trainer. Ideally you'd try to find someone who is both kettlebell and FMS-certified.

TIME CONSTRAINTS

I think everyone was blown away the first time they read Alwyn Cosgrove's *Hierarchy of Fat Loss* and saw how simply he laid out the best use of time in a fat-loss program. I've been playing with the concept of putting what's important first, and ruthlessly cutting out less-effective workout options ever since reading that article five years ago.

Here is how prioritization works with *Fat Loss Happens on Monday*.

If you have *unlimited* time—

- **Food Journal Review, Food Planning/Preparing/Cooking**
- **The Warmup**
- **Kettlebell/Bodyweight Workouts (three times per week)**
- **Interval Training (two times per week)**
- **Direct Core Training**
- **Corrective Exercise**
- **Slow Cardio/Yoga/Hiking/Running/Tennis/whatever else you enjoy**

If you only have time for this program, cut out everything else.

- **Food Journal Review, Food Planning/Preparing/Cooking**
- **The Warmup**
- **Kettlebell/Bodyweight Workouts (three times per week)**
- **Interval Training (two times per week)**

If you're shorter on time than that, cut out the warmup and the energy system work, and just do the parts that have the most impact on how your body looks.

- **Food Journal Review, Food Planning/Preparing/Cooking**
- **Kettlebell/Bodyweight Workouts (three times per week)**

Many people will be shocked that interval training doesn't make the cut. Remember, it's good for burning some calories, but it doesn't *change your shape the way the kettlebell and bodyweight training will.*

If you cut the warmup, you'll use the first set of your bodyweight and kettlebell training as your warmup. In other words, you'll start off easier or lighter and build up each set. Since your first sets in the workout are becoming warmup sets, this means you're going to get fewer hard workout sets in. But that's the game when we're short on time—a short workout is 10 times better than no workout.

You'll also notice that food planning, preparing, and cooking are still the number one priority.

If you're really, really short on time, and only have time for one thing, you can cut to the most essential and only do kettlebell and bodyweight workouts two times per week.

- **Food Journal Review, Food Planning/Preparing/Cooking**
- **Kettlebell/Bodyweight Workouts (two times per week)**

If you do the two-times-per-week model, just roll with the workouts, in order, exactly how it's written. Your four-week phases will take six weeks, and six-week phases will take nine weeks. That's totally fine, you're still getting the same number of exposures to each rep range—the same number of workouts.

Or, if you're really short on time, here's the deal: Only do what's going to make the absolute biggest impact.

By now you should know that isn't the workouts.

- **Food Journal Review, Food Planning/Preparing/Cooking**

Miss a workout if you need to, for sure, but never miss your journal review, food planning, preparing, and cooking.

WHAT DO I DO WHEN I FEEL LIKE CRAP?

Let's say you only got two hours sleep and your dog ate your homework and your boss yelled at you and you missed lunch. Should you still go for that four sets of 12 because that's what the plan says?

This may shock you… *wait for it…*

No.

When you feel like crap and can't believe you're even staring at kettlebells and bodyweight exercises at all, the standard recommendation is to do *one set* of everything, and then go rest and take care of yourself.

This whole program is an attempt to cycle the workload from easy to hard on a regular schedule. But in reality, life will force its own schedule on you.

Don't worry about it. Don't try to make up that workout later and don't back up a week on the plan either. Just do one set of everything, and move on.

We're putting the nutrition first, right? Don't stress about one lost workout.

I repeat, *we're putting the nutrition first.* Just focus on your one nutrition habit for the week, and the one meal you're applying it to. That's it.

And usually we can keep the weight of the kettlebells and which bodyweight progressions we're on the same—just dial back the number of sets.

I could say the same thing about an entire phase: If you're having a really stressful month at work, and when you get to three sets of 12 you just can't get any farther, you don't need to push to four sets of 12, do or die. Just finish out the phase with three sets of 12.

It's not the end of the world.

Why?

Because we're putting the nutrition habits first!

PULL YOUR WEIGHT REVIEW

Food planning and shopping is your first and most important workout of the week.

Food preparation and cooking is your second most important workout of the week.

You can do less working out if you get the food right.

It doesn't matter how your workout feels; what matters is that you progress to heavier kettlebell combinations, and harder bodyweight progressions.

Women should be slowly working toward doing three chin-ups and deadlifting their bodyweight for three reps.

Men should be slowly working toward doing 10 pull-ups and deadlifting one-and-a-half times their bodyweight for three reps.

Bodyweight exercises can be made easier or harder, just like using lighter or heavier kettlebells, by working with a progression of easier to harder versions of that exercise.

A good fat-loss program has multiple seasons and months.

A cycle is like a season of workouts.

A phase is like a month of workouts.

Everything moves in predictable, repeating, preplanned cycles from easy to hard.

BRING IT!

JOSH

CHAPTER 26

THE *BRING IT!* PROGRAM

In a perfect world, this program would be used for a twice-per-year challenge. Things are humming along nicely already, but this is an opportunity to take it to the next level. And that's exactly where it can fit inside of the previous program—whenever you want to amp things up, maybe New Years or summertime or whenever.

Other times, you'll use the *Bring It!* program because you're a little behind the timeline.

Sometimes you have a hard deadline or goal, and you need immediate results. This is kind of like back in school: It would have been great if you'd studied all semester, but you didn't, and now you need to cram for the final. That's the most common use of the *Bring It!* program.

It doesn't matter if it's a birthday, reunion, vacation, whatever. You need results, and you need them now.

What we're going to do here is use the emotional leverage of that hard goal, and implement everything from *One Change* all at the same time. At the same time we do that, we're going to amp up the principles from the *Pull Your Weight* program and squeeze all the results out of the workout program we can in this short time frame.

In short, when you need results yesterday, you're going to *Bring It!*

THE *BRING IT!* PROGRAM IS DIFFERENT

In the *Pull Your Weight* program, we're doing smart fat-loss workouts and we're angling toward increasing strength over time. Most of the focus is actually on making small changes in diet—one meal and one habit each week. It's a long-term program, thinking long-term results.

But twice a year when it's time to *Bring It!* we have to do things a little differently. You want to lock things down, making your body a priority, and kicking ass in both workouts and diet.

For the workouts, we're going to use target density circuits. If there's a most effective way for short-term fat-loss workouts, it's circuits. We're going to massively jack up the intensity of the circuits by compressing the rest in a density window, and then we're going to perfect the weight you're using by giving you a target.

Intensity is a power tool. It's very effective for fat loss when judiciously used.

Circuit training is a great way to increase intensity for fat loss, when it's done correctly. And it's almost never done correctly. Usually the work-to-rest ratio is so small that it just turns into a more interesting version of cardio.

Essentially, circuit training then loses everything about it that makes it more effective for fat loss.

It's a fine line. How do you compress the rest just enough to get the intensity we want? Compress the rest too much, and you trade intensity for cardio. Have too much rest, and it just turns into normal strength training.

JUST RIGHT FOR FAT LOSS: TARGET DENSITY CIRCUITS

I started this journey long ago just doing circuits. Do a set amount of work, and do it as fast as you can. It's kind of like CrossFit, except with proper exercise form the whole time.

But I found that for fat loss, we really wanted the circuit to last about 20 minutes. Shorter than 20 minutes and we wouldn't get everything we could out of it. Longer than 20 minutes, it just started to get less intense and become a dressed-up version of aerobics.

So I flipped the script on work versus time, and made it time versus work: It's a 20-minute window, and we see how much work we can pack into it. This is like Charles Staley's escalating density training, except we're doing it for fat loss.

Now we've got circuits, and we've got a 20-minute density training window. The next thing to add is a target number of rounds. Most people get this part terribly wrong. If it's too heavy, it becomes a strength set. If it's too light, again it might as well just be a group exercise class.

Here are the targets: **Five rounds is the starting place, and nine rounds is the ending place.**

If you get fewer than five rounds, you know the kettlebell weight or the bodyweight progression you're using is too hard. If you get more than nine rounds, you know the weight is too light or the bodyweight progression is too easy.

And, try to set up the kettlebell weights and bodyweight progression in each circuit so that all of the movements are about the same level of difficulty.

BRING IT! NUTRITION

We're kicking up the workout intensity in this program, so guess what? We're also kicking up the nutrition intensity.

The funny thing is, we aren't actually going to do anything different than we do in the *One Change* program. We're doing the same Eleven Habits. The difference here is we're going to do them all at the same time.

The genius of adding them one at a time, slowly, and working on one meal at a time, is that you're building each one into your lifestyle…forever.

But in the *Bring It!* phase, we don't have that kind of time. We're going to do all 11 at once.

Habit 1: *Plan your meals for the week, either on Sunday or Monday. Grid your free meals ahead of time.*

Habit 2: *Go shopping for the food on your plan, either on Sunday or Monday.*

Habit 3: *Prepare, cook, and portion the food on your plan on Sunday or Monday.*

Habit 4: *Keep a daily food journal. Review your food journal weekly, either on Sunday or Monday.*

Habit 5: *Make sure you're getting protein at every meal. Shoot for three-quarters of a gram of protein per pound of target bodyweight, per day.*

Habit 6: *Review your food journal for total calories consumed. Compare your total calories to your weekly weight change.*

Habit 7: *Eat slowly. A meal should take at least 15 minutes.*

Habit 8: *Stop eating when you're 80% full.*

Habit 9: *Make sure you're getting good fats at most meals. Add good fat to meals you normally feel hungry after and see if that helps you feel full.*

Habit 10: *Check the quality of your carbohydrates. Are you getting most of your carbohydrates from brown rice, quinoa, brown rice pasta, sprouted-grain bread, fruit, and vegetables?*

Habit 11: *Keep a gratitude journal—every day, write down one thing you like about your body, are proud of about your body, or are grateful for about your body.*

In normal life, it's hard to work in new habits. But if you have a hard deadline, like a wedding or a vacation or an important birthday or a class reunion, the leverage you get from that deadline can propel you to do everything at the same time. Lean on the emotional leverage of the deadline.

I'm mostly a positive motivator. But in the short term, the negative motivation of looking bad at an event or other deadline is really powerful. I've had clients where we struggled with implementing the habits one at a time for a couple months, but magically two months from a hard deadline, they implement them all at the same time.

Let's get real, these *won't* stick as long-term habits, but sometimes we don't care. We want to look awesome for that deadline. After that, we'll go back to the *One Change* program and start building real habits for life.

In the *Bring It!* program, these three habits have to immediately be on point.

Habit 1: Plan your meals every day, ahead of time, or every week, ahead of time.

Habit 2: Go shopping.

Habit 3: Prepare, cook, and portion your food every Monday.

Before you even look at the workouts, review your food journal, go to the store, and get the food you need.

I'm going to keep things extra simple for you in this phase.

Food is protein: *seafood, meat, poultry, pork.*

Good fats will help you feel full and give you energy: *Avocado, nuts, oils.*

Allowed carbohydrates are *vegetables, fruit, brown rice, quinoa, sweet potatoes, and yams.*

If it's not on the list above, you can't eat it in this phase—not until your free day.

On your free day, pretty much anything is fair game, but don't go too crazy. In the *Bring It!* program, think of your free day as a time to eat whatever quality you want, but not to go crazy binging on massive amounts of quantity.

One other thing about free days in the *Bring It!* program—limit the week's alcohol to two drinks on your free day. That's it for the week. If you can't do that, you can't *Bring It!*

If you remember quantity of food equals scale weight, and quality of food equals leanness, you'll see we're playing the same game as in the *One Change* program. We're just playing the game much faster.

We use the emotional leverage of a hard deadline to massively accelerate the implementation of the food habits and food quality, and we massively accelerate the results. It's that simple.

TO CARBOHYDRATE CYCLE, OR NOT TO CARBOHYDRATE CYCLE?

It's pretty simple: *Don't do it if you don't have to or don't want to.*

I know a lot of great trainers who when under the gun will immediately go to carbohydrate cycling. And I get it—research shows it's more effective for fat loss than caloric restriction alone.

That being said, I'll never forget when I first interviewed celebrity trainer Valerie Waters about nutrition. She said she doesn't use anything near that complicated, and she gets literally the hottest celebrities on earth in perfect shape for movies and for the red carpet!

Clearly, it's not a requirement. For my first seven years as a trainer, I never used any nutrient timing at all…ever. It was just a matter of the same three principles.

Quantity
Protein
Quality: Carbs and Fat

It's always that simple.

That being said, a lot of my clients really enjoy carbohydrate cycling. It's a fun game to play. And if you've already

EACH WORKOUT IN THE *BRING IT!* PROGRAM

The *Bring It!* program has two phases.
Target Density Circuits
Metabolic Strength

First let's take a look at the workouts in the target density training phase.

FIVE BY FIVE OR THREE BY FIVE

This is the only workout in the target density circuit phase that will be slow. Sets of five is a classic strength program. The biggest benefit of the five sets of five reps days is that the stronger you get, the harder you can push it on the other bootcamp-style days.

Five by five just means five sets of five reps. Three by five means three sets of five reps.

In the five by five workout, you'll have a pushup progression, a pull-up progression, and deadlifts. Go as heavy as you can, and do five sets of five reps. You can rest as much as you want, and you can lift at any tempo you choose. Five reps isn't very many, so you should be able to go heavier than normal.

People always ask, "What weight should I use?"

You should use the heaviest weight where you can maintain good form. If you haven't worked on low-rep strength before, it's sometimes hard for people to know how hard to go. It doesn't feel hard in the same way high reps feel hard—exhaustion, soreness, and heart pounding. It's hard in a totally different feel, being on the edge of how much you can lift with good form. Really work on getting tight, squeezing the bar—or the ground on the pushups—and lifting heavy.

The strength days in the target density circuit phase are low reps, sets of five. You're going to really want to work on tightening up, bracing your core, and squeezing the bar, because you're going heavy and getting strong this time.

Most people really aren't strong enough to get the bodies they want. This is our time to fix that. This is a great time to work on harder movements in the pull-up progression, and adding weight to your deadlifts.

THE FIRST 20-MINUTE WORKOUT

20-MINUTE TARGET DENSITY CIRCUIT	MOVEMENT	REPETITIONS
	THRUSTER	10
	PULL-UP PROGRESSION	5

This is a favorite workout. The first time I saw anyone combine thrusters and pull-ups was in a CrossFit workout called Fran. CrossFit did it a little differently; they do a set amount of work, and time how long it takes. They have a specific weight they always use, and they use a barbell for the thrusters. And they do kipping pull-ups…so, actually what they do is completely different.

For us, with fat loss as our goal, we set the time in a density window and have a fat-loss targeted number of rounds.

HOW THE TARGET DENSITY CIRCUIT WORKS

Do 10 thrusters (see the exercise section for the description), then five pull-ups, and repeat that as many times as you can in 20 minutes. Rest whenever you need to, even in the middle of sets.

Now, here is how that will look in real life: You crank through the first set of 10 thrusters and five of whatever pull-up progression you're doing (three-second pull-up hangs, partial pull-ups, whatever), then rest for 30 seconds.

The next set, you do eight thrusters, rest 10 seconds, and then do the other two. Then do the same thing with the pull-ups—you can do about four, then rest 10 seconds, and do another.

On the third round, you can only do four thrusters, then you rest, do two more, then do two more, then do another one…and another.

Now go right into the pull-ups, but it's about the same—you can get through two pull-ups, rest, do one more, and then do one more, and then do the last one.

Partial pull-ups work great for this workout, as do pull-up negatives. The three-second pull-up hangs work fine, too. Just don't rush them.

And remember: Set the five reps of the pull-up progression and the 10 reps of the thrusters to be about the same difficulty. Try to set up the superset of the two of them so you can get through five to nine rounds in 20 minutes.

THE SECOND 20-MINUTE WORKOUT

20-MINUTE TARGET DENSITY CIRCUIT	MOVEMENT	REPETITIONS
	ONE-KETTLEBELL SWING	25
	RENEGADE ROW	5
	WALKING LUNGE	50 FEET

Do 25 swings, then do five renegade rows with each arm, and then walking lunges for 50 feet. That's round one. For a lot of people, it may initially be hard to get five rounds in 20 minutes. Enjoy!

THE THIRD 20-MINUTE WORKOUT

20-MINUTE TARGET DENSITY CIRCUIT	MOVEMENT	REPETITIONS
	ONE-KETTLEBELL BENT-OVER ROW	10
	PUSHUP PROGRESSION	10
	TWO-KETTLEBELL SQUAT	10

This is probably the most straightforward of the target density circuits. Just set up the bent-over rows, the pushup progression, and the kettlebell squats all at about the same difficulty, and let 'er rip!

Rest as needed, and keep perfect form.

Again, try to set up this tri-set so you can complete five to nine rounds in 20 minutes.

THE DIFFERENCE BETWEEN THE *PULL YOUR WEIGHT* PROGRAM AND THE *BRING IT!* PROGRAM

Now that you know how the target density phase works, the next question is how does the metabolic strength phase in the *Bring It!* program work?

The strength phase in *Bring It!* is different in three big ways.

1. Instead of being given a large rep range to work through, say between 6–12, in *Bring It!* you're given a very small range of reps to hit, like 10–12. You'll adjust the bodyweight progression and the kettlebells however you need to in order to land in that rep range. Feel free to adjust the progression and kettlebells as needed—each workout or even each set, depending on what you're capable of that day.

2. In *Bring It!* the first two weeks will be sets of 10–12 repetitions, and the last two weeks are sets of 12–15. It's going to jump up on you pretty hard those last two weeks. Again, adjust the bodyweight progressions and the kettlebell weights you're using as needed. Go to lower weights or easier progressions as needed to be able to hit those rep ranges.

3. Instead of two supersets of two exercise combinations, the *Bring It!* program is a giant set of four exercises all done one after another, and you don't rest until you've completed all four.

RULES FOR TARGET DENSITY CIRCUITS

If you complete fewer than five rounds in 20 minutes, you used weights that were too heavy.

If you complete more than nine rounds in 20 minutes, you used weights that were too light.

Unlike traditional timed workouts or density workouts, target density circuits are designed to be *self-regulating*. You always know how to adjust the weights to get *the best fat-loss workout possible*.

THE *BRING IT!* PROGRAM

BRING IT! WEEK ONE
Sunday and/or Monday

FOOD	JOURNAL REVIEW	PLANNING	PREPARATION	COOKING

Tuesday: Strength

STRENGTH SUPERSET	MOVEMENT	SETS	REPETITIONS
	DEADLIFT	5	4–5
	PUSHUP PROGRESSION	5	4–5

STRENGTH	MOVEMENT	SETS	REPETITIONS
	WALKING LUNGE	2	50 FEET

STRENGTH	MOVEMENT	SETS	REPETITIONS
	PULL-UP PROGRESSION	5	4–5

INTERVAL TRAINING	MOVEMENT	INTERVAL	DURATION
	ONE-KETTLEBELL SWING	30 SECONDS WORK, 30 SECONDS REST	6 MINUTES

Thursday: Target Density Circuit: 20 Minutes

20-MINUTE TARGET DENSITY CIRCUIT	MOVEMENT	REPETITIONS
	THRUSTER	10
	PULL-UP PROGRESSION	5

STRENGTH AND CORE SUPERSET	MOVEMENT	SETS	REPETITIONS
	SINGLE-LEG DEADLIFT	1	4–5
	PLANK PROGRESSION	1	30–60 SECONDS

Saturday: Strength

STRENGTH SUPERSET	MOVEMENT	SETS	REPETITIONS
	REAR-FOOT-ELEVATED SPLIT-SQUAT	5	4–5
	PULL-UP PROGRESSION	5	4–5

STRENGTH	MOVEMENT	SETS	REPETITIONS
	WALKING LUNGE	2	50 FEET

STRENGTH	MOVEMENT	SETS	REPETITIONS
	PUSHUP PROGRESSION	5	4–5

INTERVAL TRAINING	MOVEMENT	INTERVAL	DURATION
	ONE-KETTLEBELL SWING	30 SECONDS WORK, 30 SECONDS REST	8 MINUTES

BRING IT! WEEK TWO

Sunday and/or Monday

| FOOD | JOURNAL REVIEW | PLANNING | PREPARATION | COOKING |

Tuesday: Target Density Circuits, 20 Minutes

20-MINUTE TARGET DENSITY CIRCUIT	MOVEMENT	REPETITIONS
	ONE-KETTLEBELL BENT-OVER ROW	10
	PUSHUP PROGRESSION	10
	TWO-KETTLEBELL SQUAT	10

STRENGTH AND CORE SUPERSET	MOVEMENT	SETS	REPETITIONS
	SINGLE-LEG DEADLIFT	2	4–5
	PLANK PROGRESSION	2	30–60 SECONDS

Thursday: Strength

STRENGTH SUPERSET	MOVEMENT	SETS	REPETITIONS
	DEADLIFT	5	4–5
	PUSHUP PROGRESSION	5	4–5

STRENGTH	MOVEMENT	SETS	REPETITIONS
	WALKING LUNGE	2	50 FEET

STRENGTH	MOVEMENT	SETS	REPETITIONS
	PULL-UP PROGRESSION	5	4–5

INTERVAL TRAINING	MOVEMENT	INTERVAL	DURATION
	ONE-KETTLEBELL SWING	30 SECONDS WORK, 30 SECONDS REST	10 MINUTES

Saturday: Target Density Circuits, 20 Minutes

20-MINUTE TARGET DENSITY CIRCUIT	MOVEMENT	REPETITIONS
	ONE-KETTLEBELL SWING	25
	RENEGADE ROW	5
	WALKING LUNGE	50 FEET

STRENGTH AND CORE SUPERSET	MOVEMENT	SETS	REPETITIONS
	TWO-KETTLEBELL MILITARY PRESS	2	4–5
	HIP BRIDGE AND SIDE PLANK PROGRESSION	2	30–60 SECONDS

BRING IT! WEEK THREE

Sunday and/or Monday

FOOD	JOURNAL REVIEW	PLANNING	PREPARATION	COOKING

Tuesday: Strength

STRENGTH SUPERSET	MOVEMENT	SETS	REPETITIONS
	DEADLIFT	5	4–5
	PUSHUP PROGRESSION	5	4–5

STRENGTH	MOVEMENT	SETS	REPETITIONS
	WALKING LUNGE	2	50 FEET

STRENGTH	MOVEMENT	SETS	REPETITIONS
	PULL-UP PROGRESSION	5	4–5

INTERVAL TRAINING	MOVEMENT	INTERVAL	DURATION
	ONE-KETTLEBELL SWING	30 SECONDS WORK, 30 SECONDS REST	12 MINUTES

Thursday: Target Density Circuits, 20 Minutes

20-MINUTE TARGET DENSITY CIRCUIT	MOVEMENT	REPETITIONS
	ONE-KETTLEBELL SWING	25
	RENEGADE ROW	5
	WALKING LUNGE	50 FEET

STRENGTH AND CORE SUPERSET	MOVEMENT	SETS	REPETITIONS
	TWO-KETTLEBELL MILITARY PRESS	3	4–5
	HIP BRIDGE AND SIDE PLANK PROGRESSION	3	30–60 SECONDS

Saturday: Target Density Circuits, 20 Minutes

20-MINUTE TARGET DENSITY CIRCUIT	MOVEMENT	REPETITIONS
	THRUSTER	10
	PULL-UP PROGRESSION	5

STRENGTH AND CORE SUPERSET	MOVEMENT	SETS	REPETITIONS
	SINGLE-LEG DEADLIFT	3	4–5
	PLANK PROGRESSION	3	30–60 SECONDS

BRING IT! WEEK FOUR

Sunday and/or Monday

FOOD	JOURNAL REVIEW	PLANNING	PREPARATION	COOKING

Tuesday: Target Density Circuits, 20 Minutes

20-MINUTE TARGET DENSITY CIRCUIT	MOVEMENT	REPETITIONS
	ONE-KETTLEBELL BENT-OVER ROW	10
	PUSHUP PROGRESSION	10
	TWO-KETTLEBELL SQUAT	10

STRENGTH AND CORE SUPERSET	MOVEMENT	SETS	REPETITIONS
	SINGLE-LEG DEADLIFT	3	4–5
	PLANK PROGRESSION	3	30–60 SECONDS

Thursday: Target Density Circuits, 20 Minutes

20-MINUTE TARGET DENSITY CIRCUIT	MOVEMENT	REPETITIONS
	ONE-KETTLEBELL SWING	25
	RENEGADE ROW	5
	WALKING LUNGE	50 FEET

STRENGTH AND CORE SUPERSET	MOVEMENT	SETS	REPETITIONS
	TWO-KETTLEBELL MILITARY PRESS	3	4–5
	HIP BRIDGE AND SIDE PLANK PROGRESSION	3	30–60 SECONDS

Saturday: Target Density Circuits, 20 Minutes

20-MINUTE TARGET DENSITY CIRCUIT	MOVEMENT	REPETITIONS
	THRUSTER	10
	PULL-UP PROGRESSION	5

STRENGTH AND CORE SUPERSET	MOVEMENT	SETS	REPETITIONS
	SINGLE-LEG DEADLIFT	3	4–5
	PLANK PROGRESSION	3	30–60 SECONDS

BRING IT! WEEK FIVE

Sunday and/or Monday

FOOD	JOURNAL REVIEW	PLANNING	PREPARATION	COOKING

Tuesday: Metabolic Endurance

CORE	MOVEMENT	SETS	REPETITIONS
	HIP BRIDGE OR SIDE PLANK PROGRESSION	2	15–45 SECONDS
	PLANK PROGRESSION	2	15–45 SECONDS

CIRCUIT	MOVEMENT	SETS	REPETITIONS
	TWO-KETTLEBELL MILITARY PRESS	2	10–12
	TWO-KETTLEBELL SQUAT	2	10–12
	PULL-UP PROGRESSION	2	10–12
	SINGLE-LEG DEADLIFT	2	10–12

INTERVAL TRAINING	MOVEMENT	INTERVAL	DURATION
	ONE-KETTLEBELL SWING	30 SECONDS WORK, 60 SECONDS REST	3 MINUTES

Thursday: Metabolic Endurance

CORE	MOVEMENT	SETS	REPETITIONS
	HIP BRIDGE OR SIDE PLANK PROGRESSION	2	15–45 SECONDS
	PLANK PROGRESSION	2	15–45 SECONDS

CIRCUIT	MOVEMENT	SETS	REPETITIONS
	PUSHUP PROGRESSION	2	10–12
	SINGLE-LEG DEADLIFT	2	10–12
	PULL-UP PROGRESSION	2	10–12
	WALKING LUNGE	2	50 FEET

INTERVAL TRAINING	MOVEMENT	INTERVAL	DURATION
	ONE-KETTLEBELL SWING	30 SECONDS WORK, 60 SECONDS REST	4.5 MINUTES

Saturday: Metabolic Endurance

CORE	MOVEMENT	SETS	REPETITIONS
	HIP BRIDGE OR SIDE PLANK PROGRESSION	2	15–45 SECONDS
	PLANK PROGRESSION	2	15–45 SECONDS

THE BRING IT! PROGRAM

CIRCUIT	MOVEMENT	SETS	REPETITIONS
	TWO-KETTLEBELL MILITARY PRESS	2	10–12
	TWO-KETTLEBELL SQUAT	2	10–12
	PULL-UP PROGRESSION	2	10–12
	REAR-FOOT-ELEVATED SPLIT-SQUAT	2	10–12

INTERVAL TRAINING	MOVEMENT	INTERVAL	DURATION
	ONE-KETTLEBELL SWING	30 SECONDS WORK, 60 SECONDS REST	6 MINUTES

BRING IT! WEEK SIX

Sunday and/or Monday

FOOD	JOURNAL REVIEW	PLANNING	PREPARATION	COOKING

Tuesday: Metabolic Endurance

CORE	MOVEMENT	SETS	REPETITIONS
	HIP BRIDGE OR SIDE PLANK PROGRESSION	2	30–60 SECONDS
	PLANK PROGRESSION	2	30–60 SECONDS

CIRCUIT	MOVEMENT	SETS	REPETITIONS
	PUSHUP PROGRESSION	3	10–12
	TWO-KETTLEBELL SQUAT	3	10–12
	TRIPOD ROW	3	10–12
	SINGLE-LEG DEADLIFT	3	10–12

INTERVAL TRAINING	MOVEMENT	INTERVAL	DURATION
	ONE-KETTLEBELL SWING	30 SECONDS WORK, 60 SECONDS REST	7.5 MINUTES

Thursday: Metabolic Endurance

CORE	MOVEMENT	SETS	REPETITIONS
	HIP BRIDGE OR SIDE PLANK PROGRESSION	2	30–60 SECONDS
	PLANK PROGRESSION	2	30–60 SECONDS

CIRCUIT	MOVEMENT	SETS	REPETITIONS
	TWO-KETTLEBELL MILITARY PRESS	3	10–12
	SINGLE-LEG DEADLIFT	3	10–12
	PULL-UP PROGRESSION	3	10–12
	LUNGE OR SPLIT-SQUAT PROGRESSION	3	10–12

INTERVAL TRAINING	MOVEMENT	INTERVAL	DURATION
	ONE-KETTLEBELL SWING	30 SECONDS WORK, 60 SECONDS REST	9 MINUTES

Saturday: Metabolic Endurance

CORE	MOVEMENT	SETS	REPETITIONS
	HIP BRIDGE OR SIDE PLANK PROGRESSION	2	30–60 SECONDS
	PLANK PROGRESSION	2	30–60 SECONDS

CIRCUIT	MOVEMENT	SETS	REPETITIONS
	RENEGADE ROW	3	4–6
	THRUSTER	3	10–12
	SINGLE-LEG DEADLIFT	3	10–12

INTERVAL TRAINING	MOVEMENT	INTERVAL	DURATION
	ONE-KETTLEBELL SWING	30 SECONDS WORK, 60 SECONDS REST	11.5 MINUTES

BRING IT! WEEK SEVEN

Sunday and/or Monday

| FOOD | JOURNAL REVIEW | PLANNING | PREPARATION | COOKING |

Tuesday: Metabolic Endurance

CORE	MOVEMENT	SETS	REPETITIONS
	HIP BRIDGE OR SIDE PLANK PROGRESSION	2	30–60 SECONDS
	PLANK PROGRESSION	2	30–60 SECONDS

CIRCUIT	MOVEMENT	SETS	REPETITIONS
	TWO-KETTLEBELL MILITARY PRESS	3	12–15
	TWO-KETTLEBELL SQUAT	3	12–15
	PULL-UP PROGRESSION	3	12–15
	SINGLE-LEG DEADLIFT	3	12–15

INTERVAL TRAINING	MOVEMENT	INTERVAL	DURATION
	ONE-KETTLEBELL SWING	30 SECONDS WORK, 60 SECONDS REST	13 MINUTES

Thursday: Metabolic Endurance

CORE	MOVEMENT	SETS	REPETITIONS
	HIP BRIDGE OR SIDE PLANK PROGRESSION	2	30–60 SECONDS
	PLANK PROGRESSION	2	30–60 SECONDS

CIRCUIT	MOVEMENT	SETS	REPETITIONS
	PUSHUP PROGRESSION	3	12–15
	SINGLE-LEG DEADLIFT	3	12–15
	TRIPOD ROW	3	12–15
	WALKING LUNGE	3	50 FEET

INTERVAL TRAINING	MOVEMENT	INTERVAL	DURATION
	ONE-KETTLEBELL SWING	30 SECONDS WORK, 60 SECONDS REST	14.5 MINUTES

Saturday: Metabolic Endurance

CORE	MOVEMENT	SETS	REPETITIONS
	HIP BRIDGE OR SIDE PLANK PROGRESSION	2	30–60 SECONDS
	PLANK PROGRESSION	2	30–60 SECONDS

CIRCUIT	MOVEMENT	SETS	REPETITIONS
	TWO-KETTLEBELL MILITARY PRESS	3	12–15
	TWO-KETTLEBELL SQUAT	3	12–15
	PULL-UP PROGRESSION	3	12–15
	LUNGE OR SPLIT-SQUAT PROGRESSION	3	12–15

INTERVAL TRAINING	MOVEMENT	INTERVAL	DURATION
	ONE-KETTLEBELL SWING	30 SECONDS WORK, 60 SECONDS REST	14.5 MINUTES

BRING IT! WEEK EIGHT

Sunday and/or Monday

FOOD	JOURNAL REVIEW	PLANNING	PREPARATION	COOKING

Tuesday: Metabolic Endurance

CORE	MOVEMENT	SETS	REPETITIONS
	HIP BRIDGE OR SIDE PLANK PROGRESSION	2	60–90 SECONDS
	PLANK PROGRESSION	2	60–90 SECONDS

CIRCUIT	MOVEMENT	SETS	REPETITIONS
	PUSHUP PROGRESSION	3	12–15
	TWO-KETTLEBELL SQUAT	3	12–15
	TRIPOD ROW	3	12–15
	SINGLE-LEG DEADLIFT	3	12–15

INTERVAL TRAINING	MOVEMENT	INTERVAL	DURATION
	ONE-KETTLEBELL SWING	30 SECONDS WORK, 60 SECONDS REST	14.5 MINUTES

Thursday: Metabolic Endurance

CORE

MOVEMENT	SETS	REPETITIONS
HIP BRIDGE OR SIDE PLANK PROGRESSION	2	60–90 SECONDS
PLANK PROGRESSION	2	60–90 SECONDS

CIRCUIT

MOVEMENT	SETS	REPETITIONS
TWO-KETTLEBELL MILITARY PRESS	3	12–15
SINGLE-LEG DEADLIFT	3	12–15
PULL-UP PROGRESSION	3	12–15
LUNGE OR SPLIT-SQUAT PROGRESSION	3	12–15

INTERVAL TRAINING

MOVEMENT	INTERVAL	DURATION
ONE-KETTLEBELL SWING	30 SECONDS WORK, 60 SECONDS REST	14.5 MINUTES

Saturday: Metabolic Endurance

CORE

MOVEMENT	SETS	REPETITIONS
HIP BRIDGE OR SIDE PLANK PROGRESSION	2	60–90 SECONDS
PLANK PROGRESSION	2	60–90 SECONDS

CIRCUIT

MOVEMENT	SETS	REPETITIONS
RENEGADE ROW	3	6–8
THRUSTER	3	12–15
SINGLE-LEG DEADLIFT	3	12–15

INTERVAL TRAINING

MOVEMENT	INTERVAL	DURATION
ONE-KETTLEBELL SWING	30 SECONDS WORK, 60 SECONDS REST	14.5 MINUTES

JOSH

CHAPTER 27

BRING IT! REMIX

You're going to *Bring It!* twice a year.

And if you had to, you could even *Bring It!* for 16 weeks straight. While this isn't the preferable way to go, sometimes it's necessary. I've had clients do these longer *Bring It!* programs for really big events—weddings, divorces, high school reunions, decade birthdays, or decade anniversaries.

Again, the preferred way to do it is to use the *Pull Your Weight* program most of the time, and slowly work your way to your goal, or even within striking distance of your goal, and then *Bring It!* when you need an eight-week boost or a challenge.

But like I said, things don't always go according to plan. At your discretion, you can use this second *Bring It!* program, the *Remix,* as your second go-round each year, or even run them both back to back.

This *Bring It!* program works off of the original principles, but has a few small changes.

1. The target density circuit phase in *Bring It! Remix* has two 10-minute density windows instead of one 20-minute density window. You'll do the first circuit for 10 minutes, rest three minutes, and then do the second 10-minute circuit.

2. Shoot for two to four rounds in each 10-minute target density circuit.

3. The strength days in the target density circuit phase are even heavier—sets of three heavy reps. You're going to really want to work on tightening up, bracing your core, and squeezing the bar, because you're going heavy and getting strong this time. Most people really aren't strong enough to get the bodies they want. This is our time to fix that. This is a great time to work on harder movements of the pull-up progression, and for adding weight to your deadlifts.

4. In the *Bring It! Remix* metabolic strength phase, the first two weeks are sets of 8–10 reps, and the last two weeks are sets of 6–8. With the reps per set decreasing, you're going to be working on getting freaky strong.

THE *BRING IT! REMIX* PROGRAM

BRING IT! REMIX WEEK ONE

Sunday and/or Monday

| FOOD | JOURNAL REVIEW | PLANNING | PREPARATION | COOKING |

Tuesday: Strength

STRENGTH SUPERSET	MOVEMENT	SETS	REPETITIONS
	DEADLIFT	5	2–3
	PUSHUP PROGRESSION	5	2–3

STRENGTH	MOVEMENT	SETS	REPETITIONS
	WALKING LUNGE	2	50 FEET

STRENGTH	MOVEMENT	SETS	REPETITIONS
	PULL-UP PROGRESSION	5	2–3

INTERVAL TRAINING	MOVEMENT	INTERVAL	DURATION
	ONE-KETTLEBELL SWING	30 SECONDS WORK, 30 SECONDS REST	6 MINUTES

Thursday: Target Density, Two 10-Minute Circuits

10-MINUTE TARGET DENSITY CIRCUIT	MOVEMENT	REPETITIONS
	TWO-KETTLEBELL SQUAT	5
	TWO-KETTLEBELL SWING	10

10-MINUTE TARGET DENSITY CIRCUIT	MOVEMENT	REPETITIONS
	PULL-UP PROGRESSION	5
	PUSHUP PROGRESSION	10

STRENGTH AND CORE SUPERSET	MOVEMENT	SETS	REPETITIONS
	HIP BRIDGE OR SIDE PLANK PROGRESSION	3	30–60 SECONDS
	PLANK PROGRESSION	3	30–60 SECONDS

Saturday: Strength

STRENGTH SUPERSET	MOVEMENT	SETS	REPETITIONS
	TWO-KETTLEBELL SQUAT	5	2–3
	PULL-UP PROGRESSION	5	3

STRENGTH	MOVEMENT	SETS	REPETITIONS
	WALKING LUNGE	2	50 FEET

STRENGTH	MOVEMENT	SETS	REPETITIONS
	PUSHUP PROGRESSION	5	2–3

INTERVAL TRAINING	MOVEMENT	INTERVAL	DURATION
	ONE-KETTLEBELL SWING	30 SECONDS WORK, 30 SECONDS REST	8 MINUTES

BRING IT! REMIX WEEK TWO

Sunday and/or Monday

FOOD	JOURNAL REVIEW	PLANNING	PREPARATION	COOKING

Tuesday: Target Density, Two 10-Minute Circuits

10-MINUTE TARGET DENSITY CIRCUIT	MOVEMENT	REPETITIONS
	THRUSTER	10
	RENEGADE ROW	5

10-MINUTE TARGET DENSITY CIRCUIT	MOVEMENT	REPETITIONS
	THRUSTER	10
	TWO-KETTLEBELL SWING	10

STRENGTH AND CORE SUPERSET	MOVEMENT	SETS	REPETITIONS
	PULL-UP PROGRESSION	3	2–3
	HIP BRIDGE AND SIDE PLANK PROGRESSION	3	30–60 SECONDS

Thursday: Strength

STRENGTH SUPERSET	MOVEMENT	SETS	REPETITIONS
	DEADLIFT	5	2–3
	PUSHUP PROGRESSION	5	2–3

STRENGTH	MOVEMENT	SETS	REPETITIONS
	WALKING LUNGE	2	50 FEET

STRENGTH	MOVEMENT	SETS	REPETITIONS
	PULL-UP PROGRESSION	5	2–3

INTERVAL TRAINING	MOVEMENT	INTERVAL	DURATION
	ONE-KETTLEBELL SWING	30 SECONDS WORK, 30 SECONDS REST	10 MINUTES

Saturday: Target Density, Two 10-Minute Circuits

10-MINUTE TARGET DENSITY CIRCUIT	MOVEMENT	REPETITIONS
	RENEGADE ROW	5
	TWO-KETTLEBELL SWING	10

10-MINUTE TARGET DENSITY CIRCUIT	MOVEMENT	REPETITIONS
	PUSHUP PROGRESSION	10
	TWO-KETTLEBELL SWING	10

STRENGTH AND CORE SUPERSET	MOVEMENT	SETS	REPETITIONS
	PULL-UP PROGRESSION	3	2–3
	PLANK PROGRESSION	3	30–60 SECONDS

BRING IT! REMIX WEEK THREE

Sunday and/or Monday

FOOD	JOURNAL REVIEW	PLANNING	PREPARATION	COOKING

Tuesday: Strength

STRENGTH SUPERSET	MOVEMENT	SETS	REPETITIONS
	TWO-KETTLEBELL SQUAT	5	2–3
	PULL-UP PROGRESSION	5	2–3

STRENGTH	MOVEMENT	SETS	REPETITIONS
	WALKING LUNGE	2	50 FEET

STRENGTH	MOVEMENT	SETS	REPETITIONS
	PUSHUP PROGRESSION	5	2–3

INTERVAL TRAINING	MOVEMENT	INTERVAL	DURATION
	ONE-KETTLEBELL SWING	30 SECONDS WORK, 30 SECONDS REST	12 MINUTES

Thursday: Target Density, Two 10-Minute Circuits

10-MINUTE TARGET DENSITY CIRCUIT	MOVEMENT	REPETITIONS
	THRUSTER	10
	PULL-UP PROGRESSION	5

10-MINUTE TARGET DENSITY CIRCUIT	MOVEMENT	REPETITIONS
	PUSHUP PROGRESSION	10
	PULL-UP PROGRESSION	5

STRENGTH AND CORE SUPERSET	MOVEMENT	SETS	REPETITIONS
	SINGLE-LEG DEADLIFT	3	2–3
	PLANK PROGRESSION	3	30–60 SECONDS

Saturday: Target Density, Two 10-Minute Circuits

10-MINUTE TARGET DENSITY CIRCUIT	MOVEMENT	REPETITIONS
	TWO-KETTLEBELL SQUAT	5
	TWO-KETTLEBELL SWING	10

10-MINUTE TARGET DENSITY CIRCUIT	MOVEMENT	REPETITIONS
	PULL-UP PROGRESSION	5
	PUSHUP PROGRESSION	10

STRENGTH AND CORE SUPERSET	MOVEMENT	SETS	REPETITIONS
	HIP BRIDGE OR SIDE-PLANK PROGRESSION	3	2–3
	PLANK PROGRESSION	3	30–60 SECONDS

BRING IT! REMIX WEEK FOUR

Sunday and/or Monday

FOOD	JOURNAL REVIEW	PLANNING	PREPARATION	COOKING

Tuesday: Target Density, Two 10-Minute Circuits

10-MINUTE TARGET DENSITY CIRCUIT	MOVEMENT	REPETITIONS
	THRUSTER	10
	RENEGADE ROW	5

10-MINUTE TARGET DENSITY CIRCUIT	MOVEMENT	REPETITIONS
	THRUSTER	10
	TWO-KETTLEBELL SWING	10

STRENGTH AND CORE SUPERSET	MOVEMENT	SETS	REPETITIONS
	PULL-UP PROGRESSION	3	2–3
	HIP BRIDGE AND SIDE PLANK PROGRESSION	3	30–60 SECONDS

Thursday: Target Density, Two 10-Minute Circuits

10-MINUTE TARGET DENSITY CIRCUIT	MOVEMENT	REPETITIONS
	RENEGADE ROW	5
	TWO-KETTLEBELL SWING	10

10-MINUTE TARGET DENSITY CIRCUIT	MOVEMENT	REPETITIONS
	PUSHUP PROGRESSION	10
	PULL-UP PROGRESSION	5

STRENGTH AND CORE SUPERSET	MOVEMENT	SETS	REPETITIONS
	PULL-UP PROGRESSION	3	2–3
	HIP BRIDGE AND SIDE PLANK PROGRESSION	3	30–60 SECONDS

Saturday: Target Density, Two 10-Minute Circuits

10-MINUTE TARGET DENSITY CIRCUIT	MOVEMENT	REPETITIONS
	THRUSTER	10
	PULL-UP PROGRESSION	5

10-MINUTE TARGET DENSITY CIRCUIT	MOVEMENT	REPETITIONS
	PUSHUP PROGRESSION	10
	PULL-UP PROGRESSION	5

STRENGTH AND CORE SUPERSET	MOVEMENT	SETS	REPETITIONS
	SINGLE-LEG DEADLIFT	3	2–3
	PLANK PROGRESSION	3	30–60 SECONDS

BRING IT! REMIX WEEK FIVE

Sunday and/or Monday

| FOOD | JOURNAL REVIEW | PLANNING | PREPARATION | COOKING |

Tuesday: Metabolic Strength

CORE	MOVEMENT	SETS	REPETITIONS
	HIP BRIDGE OR SIDE PLANK PROGRESSION	2	15–45 SECONDS
	PLANK PROGRESSION	2	15–45 SECONDS

CIRCUIT	MOVEMENT	SETS	REPETITIONS
	TWO-KETTLEBELL MILITARY PRESS	2	8–10
	TWO-KETTLEBELL SQUAT	2	8–10
	PULL-UP PROGRESSION	2	8–10
	SINGLE-LEG DEADLIFT	2	8–10

INTERVAL TRAINING	MOVEMENT	INTERVAL	DURATION
	ONE-KETTLEBELL SWING	30 SECONDS WORK, 60 SECONDS REST	4.5 MINUTES

Thursday: Metabolic Strength

CORE	MOVEMENT	SETS	REPETITIONS
	HIP BRIDGE OR SIDE PLANK PROGRESSION	2	15–45 SECONDS
	PLANK PROGRESSION	2	15–45 SECONDS

CIRCUIT	MOVEMENT	SETS	REPETITIONS
	PUSHUP PROGRESSION	2	8–10
	SINGLE-LEG DEADLIFT	2	8–10
	TRIPOD ROW	2	8–10
	WALKING LUNGE	2	50 FEET

INTERVAL TRAINING	MOVEMENT	INTERVAL	DURATION
	ONE-KETTLEBELL SWING	30 SECONDS WORK, 60 SECONDS REST	4.5 MINUTES

Saturday: Metabolic Strength

CORE	MOVEMENT	SETS	REPETITIONS
	HIP BRIDGE OR SIDE PLANK PROGRESSION	2	15–45 SECONDS
	PLANK PROGRESSION	2	15–45 SECONDS

CIRCUIT	MOVEMENT	SETS	REPETITIONS
	TWO-KETTLEBELL MILITARY PRESS	2	8–10
	TWO-KETTLEBELL SQUAT	2	8–10
	PULL-UP PROGRESSION	2	8–10
	LUNGE OR SPLIT-SQUAT PROGRESSION	2	8–10

INTERVAL TRAINING	MOVEMENT	INTERVAL	DURATION
	ONE-KETTLEBELL SWING	30 SECONDS WORK, 60 SECONDS REST	6 MINUTES

BRING IT! REMIX WEEK SIX

Sunday and/or Monday

FOOD	JOURNAL REVIEW	PLANNING	PREPARATION	COOKING

Tuesday: Metabolic Strength

CORE	MOVEMENT	SETS	REPETITIONS
	HIP BRIDGE OR SIDE PLANK PROGRESSION	2	30–60 SECONDS
	PLANK PROGRESSION	2	30–60 SECONDS

CIRCUIT	MOVEMENT	SETS	REPETITIONS
	PUSHUP PROGRESSION	3	8–10
	TWO-KETTLEBELL SQUAT	3	8–10
	TRIPOD ROW	3	8–10
	SINGLE-LEG DEADLIFT	3	50 FEET

INTERVAL TRAINING	MOVEMENT	INTERVAL	DURATION
	ONE-KETTLEBELL SWING	30 SECONDS WORK, 60 SECONDS REST	7.5 MINUTES

Thursday: Metabolic Strength

CORE	MOVEMENT	SETS	REPETITIONS
	HIP BRIDGE OR SIDE PLANK PROGRESSION	2	30–60 SECONDS
	PLANK PROGRESSION	2	30–60 SECONDS

CIRCUIT	MOVEMENT	SETS	REPETITIONS
	TWO-KETTLEBELL MILITARY PRESS	3	8–10
	SINGLE-LEG DEADLIFT	3	8–10
	PULL-UP PROGRESSION	3	8–10
	WALKING LUNGE	3	50 FEET

INTERVAL TRAINING	MOVEMENT	INTERVAL	DURATION
	ONE-KETTLEBELL SWING	30 SECONDS WORK, 60 SECONDS REST	9 MINUTES

Saturday: Metabolic Strength

CORE	MOVEMENT	SETS	REPETITIONS
	HIP BRIDGE OR SIDE PLANK PROGRESSION	2	30–60 SECONDS
	PLANK PROGRESSION	2	30–60 SECONDS

CIRCUIT	MOVEMENT	SETS	REPETITIONS
	RENEGADE ROW	3	8–10
	THRUSTER	3	8–10
	SINGLE-LEG DEADLIFT	3	8–10

INTERVAL TRAINING	MOVEMENT	INTERVAL	DURATION
	ONE-KETTLEBELL SWING	30 SECONDS WORK, 60 SECONDS REST	11.5 MINUTES

BRING IT! REMIX WEEK SEVEN

Sunday and/or Monday

| FOOD | JOURNAL REVIEW | PLANNING | PREPARATION | COOKING |

Tuesday: Metabolic Strength

CORE	MOVEMENT	SETS	REPETITIONS
	HIP BRIDGE OR SIDE PLANK PROGRESSION	2	30–60 SECONDS
	PLANK PROGRESSION	2	30–60 SECONDS

CIRCUIT	MOVEMENT	SETS	REPETITIONS
	TWO-KETTLEBELL MILITARY PRESS	3	6–8
	TWO-KETTLEBELL SQUAT	3	6–8
	PULL-UP PROGRESSION	3	6–8
	SINGLE-LEG DEADLIFT	3	6–8

INTERVAL TRAINING	MOVEMENT	INTERVAL	DURATION
	ONE-KETTLEBELL SWING	30 SECONDS WORK, 60 SECONDS REST	13 MINUTES

Thursday: Metabolic Strength

CORE	MOVEMENT	SETS	REPETITIONS
	HIP BRIDGE OR SIDE PLANK PROGRESSION	2	30–60 SECONDS
	PLANK PROGRESSION	2	30–60 SECONDS

CIRCUIT	MOVEMENT	SETS	REPETITIONS
	PUSHUP PROGRESSION	3	6–8
	SINGLE-LEG DEADLIFT	3	6–8
	TRIPOD ROW	3	6–8
	WALKING LUNGE	3	50 FEET

INTERVAL TRAINING	MOVEMENT	INTERVAL	DURATION
	ONE-KETTLEBELL SWING	30 SECONDS WORK, 60 SECONDS REST	14.5 MINUTES

Saturday: Metabolic Strength

CORE	MOVEMENT	SETS	REPETITIONS
	HIP BRIDGE OR SIDE PLANK PROGRESSION	2	30–60 SECONDS
	PLANK PROGRESSION	2	30–60 SECONDS

CIRCUIT	MOVEMENT	SETS	REPETITIONS
	TWO-KETTLEBELL MILITARY PRESS	3	6–8
	TWO-KETTLEBELL SQUAT	3	6–8
	PULL-UP PROGRESSION	3	6–8
	LUNGE OR SPLIT-SQUAT PROGRESSION	3	6–8

INTERVAL TRAINING	MOVEMENT	INTERVAL	DURATION
	ONE-KETTLEBELL SWING	30 SECONDS WORK, 60 SECONDS REST	14.5 MINUTES

BRING IT! REMIX WEEK EIGHT

Sunday and/or Monday

| FOOD | JOURNAL REVIEW | PLANNING | PREPARATION | COOKING |

Tuesday: Metabolic Strength

CORE	MOVEMENT	SETS	REPETITIONS
	HIP BRIDGE OR SIDE PLANK PROGRESSION	2	60–90 SECONDS
	PLANK PROGRESSION	2	60–90 SECONDS

CIRCUIT	MOVEMENT	SETS	REPETITIONS
	PUSHUP PROGRESSION	4	6–8
	TWO-KETTLEBELL SQUAT	4	6–8
	TRIPOD ROW	4	6–8
	SINGLE-LEG DEADLIFT	4	6–8

INTERVAL TRAINING	MOVEMENT	INTERVAL	DURATION
	ONE-KETTLEBELL SWING	30 SECONDS WORK, 60 SECONDS REST	14.5 MINUTES

Thursday: Metabolic Strength

CORE	MOVEMENT	SETS	REPETITIONS
	HIP BRIDGE OR SIDE PLANK PROGRESSION	1	60–90 SECONDS
	PLANK PROGRESSION	1	60–90 SECONDS

CIRCUIT	MOVEMENT	SETS	REPETITIONS
	TWO-KETTLEBELL MILITARY PRESS	4	6–8
	SINGLE-LEG DEADLIFT	4	6–8
	TRIPOD ROW	4	6–8
	WALKING LUNGE	4	50 FEET

INTERVAL TRAINING	MOVEMENT	INTERVAL	DURATION
	ONE-KETTLEBELL SWING	30 SECONDS WORK, 60 SECONDS REST	14.5 MINUTES

Saturday: Metabolic Strength

CORE	MOVEMENT	SETS	REPETITIONS
	HIP BRIDGE OR SIDE PLANK PROGRESSION	2	60–90 SECONDS
	PLANK PROGRESSION	2	60–90 SECONDS

CIRCUIT	MOVEMENT	SETS	REPETITIONS
	RENEGADE ROW	4	6–8
	THRUSTER	4	6–8
	SINGLE-LEG DEADLIFT	4	6–8

INTERVAL TRAINING	MOVEMENT	INTERVAL	DURATION
	ONE-KETTLEBELL SWING	30 SECONDS WORK, 60 SECONDS REST	14.5 MINUTES

BRING IT! REVIEW

Twice a year, it's time to kick ass.

As always, food preparation is your first and most important workout of the week.

When you're doing a *Bring It!* phase, use the emotional leverage of your approaching goal date to do all of the nutrition habits…*now.*

Don't leave fat-loss circuits to chance. Use a target density circuit—20 minutes, five to nine rounds in *Bring It!* or two 10-minute, two to four rounds of *Bring It! Remix.*

EXERCISE INSTRUCTIONS

JOSH

CHAPTER 28

THE EXERCISE INSTRUCTIONS

For each exercise, we're going to list four things.

Ready: *What you need for that exercise*
Set: *The right starting position*
Go: *How to properly execute the movement*
Josh Says: *This is exactly what I would say to you, as you're doing the movement…in real life.*

The *Josh Says* cues are going to be completely different from what you're used to—they're external cues. They'll be about moving something outside of your body toward a goal.

This is super fun. There's been some amazing new research on the kinds of coaching cues that are most effective for teaching movement. Long story short: External cues have been proven to be 100% more effective than internal cues.

I got to do an amazing workshop with Nick Winkelman, director of education and performance systems at Athletes Performance in Arizona. I would say Nick is the leading guy at synthesizing all of the research on external cuing, including that of Gabrielle Wulf, and applying it with the pro athletes he trains. It completely changed the way I coach every movement, and you're going to get coached that way now.

Another major point Nick has is that any time you can't use an external cue, use an unusual and weird analogy. There are a couple times we'll do that here, too.

I'd like to give a major shout-out to Craig Rasmussen, Mike Wunsch, and Ash Thomas, with whom I had long conversations about external cueing during my internship at Results Fitness.

An external cue is moving something outside of yourself toward a goal. An internal cue is any cue that's about moving your body. It turns out people just don't respond to internal cues, and internal cues are the slowest and hardest way to learn a new movement.

And almost every fitness book in the world only has internal cues.

The *Josh Says* cues may sound kinda silly—things like 'reach your back pockets toward the back wall.' But there's now 10 years of research showing conclusively that it's 100% more effective than if you think about 'sitting back with your hips.'

If external cues are more effective, both for learning and for retention, why do we use internal cues in the *Ready*, *Set*, and *Go* parts? The external cues are a little bit silly, and they don't necessarily make sense without having the basic cues to set things up. Think about the *Ready*, *Set*, and *Go* parts while you're setting up for the movement. But while you're doing the movement, only think about the external *Josh Says* cues.

For more in-depth instructions, consider the following books or DVDs.

KETTLEBELL EXERCISES

Enter the Kettlebell, **by Pavel**—This DVD has all of the drills that most of us originally used to learn the kettlebell swing, and also has a great primer on the military press.

Return of the Kettlebell, **by Pavel**—The best book or DVD for learning double-kettlebell swings, squats, and military presses.

Simple and Sinister, **by Pavel**—This book has some newer cues for learning the swing that are really great, as well as some new drills for refining the swing. If you're totally new to the swing, you'd be better off with the *Enter the Kettlebell* DVD, but if you've been doing swings and want to go a little deeper with your practice, get *Simple and Sinister*.

BODYWEIGHT EXERCISES

Pushing the Limits, **by Al Kavadlo**—This is a great book that goes in depth on pushup and squat progressions and variations. It covers every variation of the squat and pushup we use in *Fat Loss Happens on Monday*, and then goes into more advanced progressions.

Naked Warrior, **by Pavel**—If you want to progress to one-arm pushups and pistols, this is the book to get. The tension techniques taught in this book will make you significantly stronger on every lift in the strength phase and strength days of *Fat Loss Happens on Monday*.

CORE EXERCISES

The New Rules of Lifting for Abs, **by Lou Schuler and Alwyn Cosgrove**—If you want to go farther than the plank progressions in *Fat Loss Happens on Monday*, this book will take you as far as you want to go. This is *the* book on how to get a strong functional midsection that will make you stronger in your workouts. And lest you think you can core workout your way to ripped abs, Lou and Alwyn break it down: *New Rule #16: All that said, calories still matter more than anything else.*

CORRECTIVE EXERCISES

RAMP: The 21st Century Warmup, **by Results Fitness**—This DVD is about warmups, but these warmup programs are assembled from corrective exercises that almost everyone needs. It outlines different correctives by body part, and then outlines some sets of correctives together. The only really great videos I've found for corrective exercises are designed for trainers. While the *RAMP* DVD is also designed for trainers, it's totally accessible to the enduser. Besides being a great resource for corrective exercises, it's also provides six amazing corrective-based warmup programs.

DEADLIFT PROGRESSION, BARBELL

1: Stick Deadlift Drill

2: Deadlift, Romanian

3: Deadlift, Barbell

DEADLIFT, BARBELL ALTERNATIVE

Deadlift, Trap Bar

1: STICK DEADLIFT DRILL

Ready
- You need a dowel rod or broomstick.

Set
- Hold the stick so it's touching the back of your head, the top of your back, and your tailbone.

Go
- Sit your hips backward and fold your upper body forward.
- Keep the stick in contact with your head, upper back, and tailbone the entire time.
- Flex your butt and drive your hips forward.

Josh Says
- *To start:* Reach the bottom of the stick to the back wall.
- *And:* Reach the top of the stick to the front wall.
- *To finish:* Drive your belt buckle to the wall in front of you.

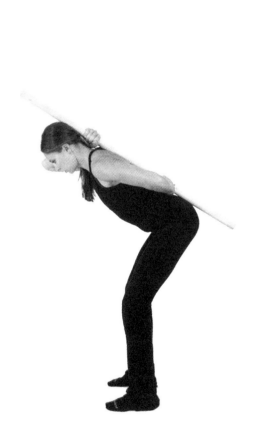
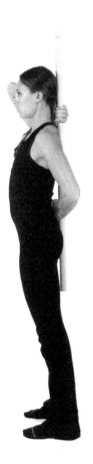

2: DEADLIFT, ROMANIAN

Ready

- You need two kettlebells.

Set

- Pick the kettlebell up just like the stick deadlift drill on the previous page.

Go

- Sit your hips back using the same body angle as the stick drill.
- Flex your butt and drive your hips forward.
- Repeat sitting your hips back every repetition.
- Keep your back totally straight as in the stick drill throughout the entire movement.
- Set the kettlebell down using the same body angle as the stick drill.

Josh Says

- *To start:* Reach your back pockets to the back wall.
- *And:* Reach your hat to the wall in front of you.
- Remember the *Stick Deadlift Drill*. Keep the stick on your back straight.
- *To finish:* Drive your belt buckle to the wall in front of you.
- *And:* Push the heels of your shoes down hard into the floor.

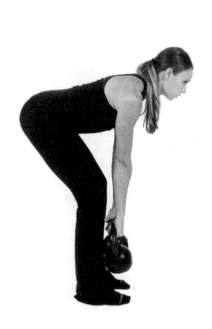
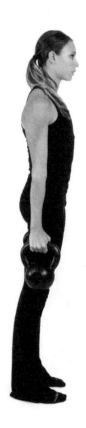

3: DEADLIFT, BARBELL

Ready
- You'll need a barbell, loaded with the appropriate amount of weight for your current strength level and the day's opening rep range.

Set
- Stand with the barbell right underneath you, with your shins touching the bar.
- Sit your hips back as in the stick drill, and grab the barbell with your hands outside your legs.

Go
- Sit your hips back—like the stick drill.
- Let your knees bend a little bit as you're sitting your hips back.
- Squeeze the barbell, flex your butt, and brace your abs, all before you break the barbell off the ground.
- Drive through your heels.
- Flex your butt and drive your hips forward.
- Repeat sitting your hips back every repetition.
- Keep your back totally straight as in the stick drill through the entire movement.

Josh Says
- *To start:* Reach your back pockets to the wall behind you.
- *And:* Remember the hinge stick drill. Keep the stick on your back straight.
- *And:* Keep the barbell touching your pants the whole time.
- *To finish:* Push the ground away.
- *Or:* Drive the heels of your shoes down hard into the floor.
- *And:* Drive your belt buckle to the wall in front of you.

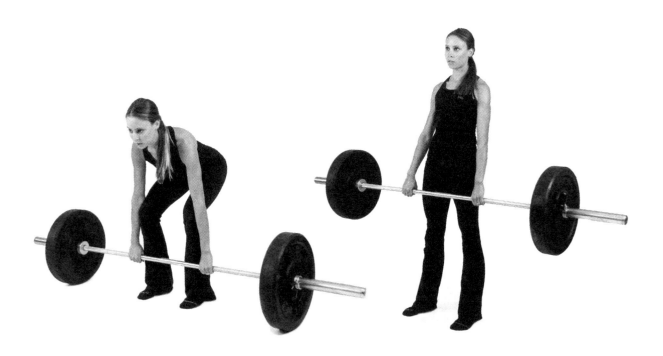

DEADLIFT, TRAP BAR (BARBELL DEADLIFT ALTERNATIVE)

Barbell Deadlift Alternative

- Not everyone's back initially agrees with deadlifts.
- Many people find that trap-bar deadlifts feel great, even if barbell deadlifts don't.
- This is a great way to work on serious strength in a more forgiving version of the deadlift.

It's Still a Deadlift

- One of the advantages and disadvantages of the trap bar is that you can deadlift with it, squat with it, or do a combination deadlift-squat.
- Remember to replicate the stick deadlift drill.
- If your trap-bar deadlift looks more like a squat, work on keeping your hips higher, like a deadlift, and don't add weight until your form looks like these pictures.

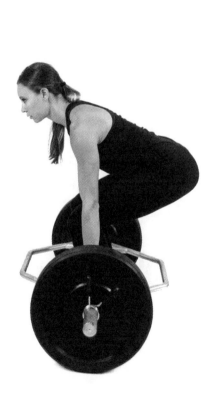
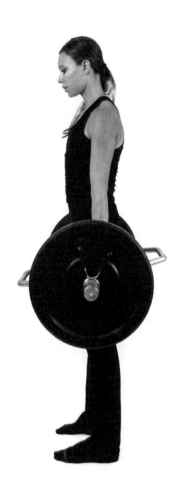

DEADLIFT PROGRESSION, SINGLE-LEG

1: Stick Deadlift Drill
   (See page 238)

2: Deadlift, Single-Leg Assisted

3: Deadlift, Single-Leg, Opposite-Hand

4: Deadlift, Single-Leg, Two Kettlebells

2: DEADLIFT, SINGLE-LEG ASSISTED

Ready

- You need one kettlebell, set a foot out in front of you, and something to hold on to: A stick, the wall, a chair, or a railing.

Set

- If you're standing on your left leg, you'll hold the kettlebell in your right hand. The kettlebell will always be in the opposite hand from the leg you're standing on.
- Your free hand holds onto the stick or the wall to help with balance.
- Do all of the reps on your less-awesome leg first, and then do your awesome leg.

Go

- Hinge at your hips, while gravity pulls the kettlebell toward the ground.
- Then flex your butt and drive your hips forward.
- Keep your back totally straight as in the stick drill throughout the entire movement.

Josh Says

- *To start:* Reach your back pockets towards the wall behind you.
- *And:* Reach your hat to the wall in front of you.
- *To finish:* Drive your belt buckle to the wall in front of you.

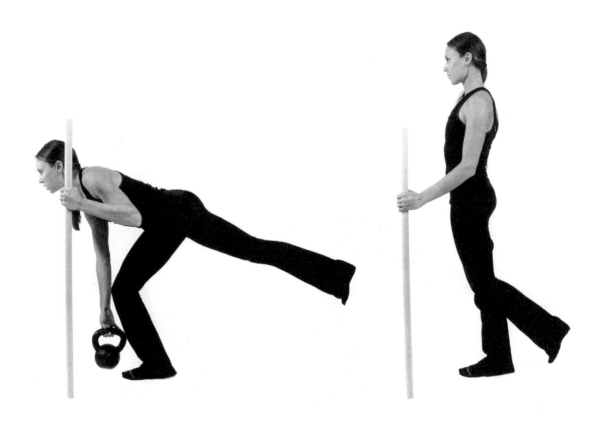

3: DEADLIFT, SINGLE-LEG, OPPOSITE-HAND

Ready

- You need one kettlebell, set a foot out in front of you.

Set

- If you're standing on your left leg, you'll hold the kettlebell in your right hand. The kettlebell will always be in the opposite hand from the leg you're standing on.

Go

- Hinge at your hips, while gravity pulls the kettlebell toward the ground.
- Then flex your butt and drive your hips forward.
- Always keep your shoulders and hips square.

Josh Says

- *To start:* Reach your back pockets toward the wall behind you.
- *And:* Reach your hat to the wall in front of you.
- *And:* Remember the hinge stick drill. Keep the stick on your back straight.
- *To finish:* Drive your belt buckle to the wall in front of you.

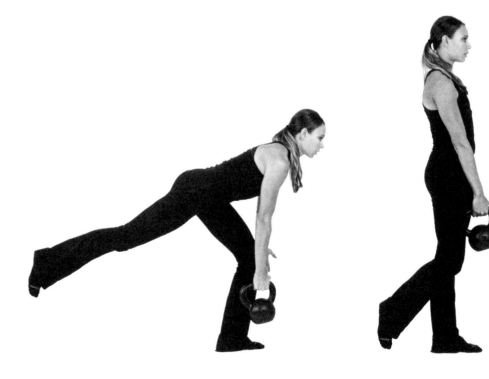

4: DEADLIFT, SINGLE-LEG, TWO KETTLEBELLS

Ready
- You'll need two kettlebells, either of the same or different weights.

Set
- If you're standing on your left leg, you'll hold the heavier kettlebell in your right hand. The heavier kettlebell will always be in the opposite hand from the leg you're standing on.
- Hold the lighter kettlebell on the same side as the leg you're standing on.
- Do all of the reps on your less-awesome leg first, and then do your awesome leg.

Go
- Hinge at your hips, while gravity pulls the kettlebells toward the ground.
- Then flex your butt and drive your hips forward.

Josh Says
- *To start:* Reach your back pockets toward the wall behind you.
- *And:* Reach your hat to the wall in front of you.
- *And:* Remember the hinge stick drill. Keep the stick on your back straight.
- *To finish:* Drive your belt buckle to the wall in front of you.

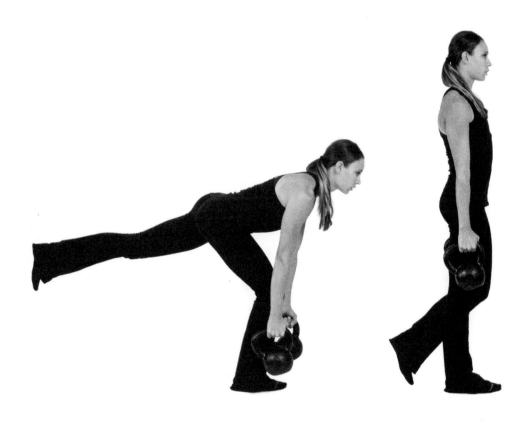

LUNGE/SPLIT-SQUAT PROGRESSION

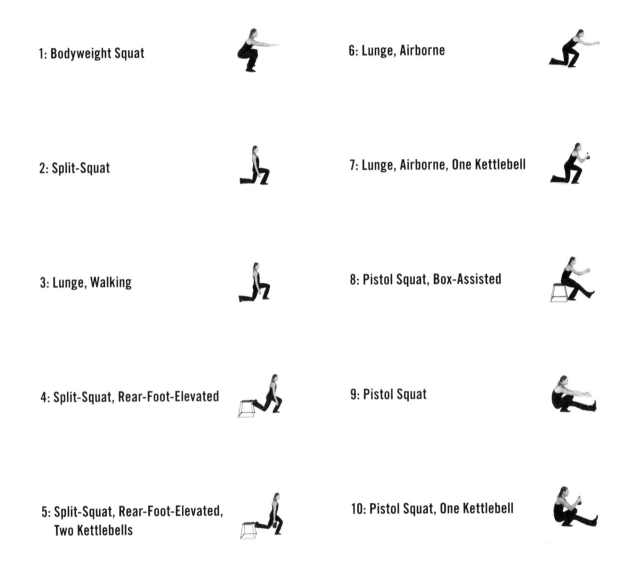

1: Bodyweight Squat

2: Split-Squat

3: Lunge, Walking

4: Split-Squat, Rear-Foot-Elevated

5: Split-Squat, Rear-Foot-Elevated, Two Kettlebells

6: Lunge, Airborne

7: Lunge, Airborne, One Kettlebell

8: Pistol Squat, Box-Assisted

9: Pistol Squat

10: Pistol Squat, One Kettlebell

1: BODYWEIGHT SQUAT

Ready
- No equipment is required for this exercise.

Set
- Put your arms straight out in front for counterbalance.

Go
- Sit your butt straight down.
- Keep most of the weight through your heels, but also keep your big toe down.
- Push your knees out so they stay in line with your feet.
- Arch your low back hard and keep your chest up.

Josh Says
- *To start:* Pull your back pockets back and down toward the floor.
- *In the middle:* The seams on the side of your pants—push those out to the side walls.
- *And:* Keep the logo on the front of your shirt up.
- *To finish:* Push the floor away.
- *Or:* Drive the heels of your shoes down into the floor.

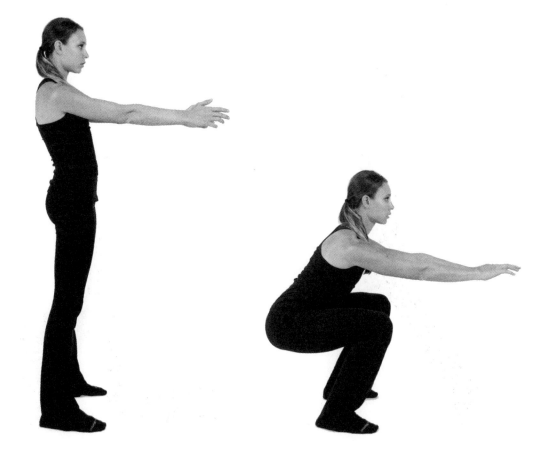

2: SPLIT-SQUAT

Ready
- No equipment is required for this exercise.

Set
- With your feet hip width apart, take a step backward.

Go
- Bend both knees and bring your back knee toward the floor.
- Keep most of the weight through the heel of your front foot—do most of the work with the front leg.
- Keep your front knee in line with your front foot.
- Stay as tall as possible—don't bend forward.
- Drive through your heel and come back up.
- Do all of the reps with your less-awesome leg, and then do all of the reps with your awesome leg.

Josh Says
- *To start:* Drop your back knee straight to the floor.
- *In the middle:* At the bottom, keep pulling your hat up to the ceiling.
- *And:* Push the seam of your front pant leg out to the side wall.
- *To finish:* Push the floor away.
- *And:* Drive the heel of your front shoe down into the floor.

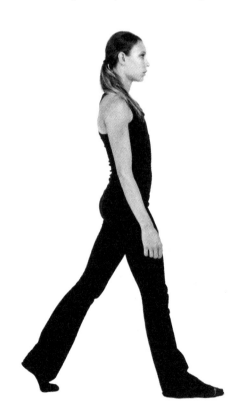
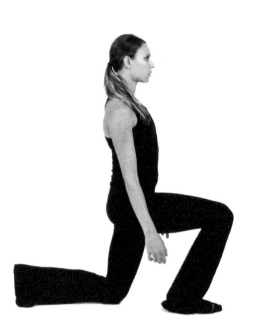

3: LUNGE, WALKING

Ready
- No equipment is required for this exercise.

Set
- Take a normal stance with your feet hip width apart and under you.

Go
- Take a step forward.
- Bend both knees and bring your back knee toward the floor.
- Keep most of the weight through the heel of your front foot—do most of the work with the front leg.
- Keep your front knee in line with your front foot.
- Stay as tall as possible—don't bend forward.
- Drive through your heel and come back up.
- Alternate legs each rep.

Josh Says
- *To start:* Drop your back knee straight to the floor.
- *In the middle:* At the bottom, keep pulling your hat up to the ceiling.
- *And:* Push the seam of your front pant leg out to the side wall.
- *To finish:* Push the floor away.
- *Or:* Drive the heel of your front shoe down into the floor.

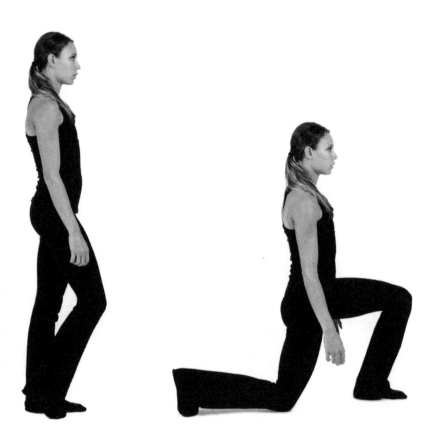

4: SPLIT-SQUAT, REAR-FOOT-ELEVATED

Ready
- You'll need a chair, box, or bench to put your back foot on.

Set
- Your back foot goes on the box.
- If necessary, hop your front foot forward so it's the same distance from the back foot as it would be in a normal split-squat.

Go
- Bend both knees and bring your back knee toward the floor.
- Keep most of the weight through the heel of your front foot—do most of the work with the front leg.
- Keep your front knee in line with your front foot.
- Stay as tall as possible—don't bend forward.
- Drive through your heel and come back up.
- Do all of the reps with your less-awesome leg, and then do all of the reps with your awesome leg.

Josh Says
- *To start:* Drop your back knee down toward the floor.
- *In the middle:* Push the seam of your front pant leg out to the side wall.
- *To finish:* Push the floor away.
- *Or:* Drive the heel of your front shoe down into the floor.

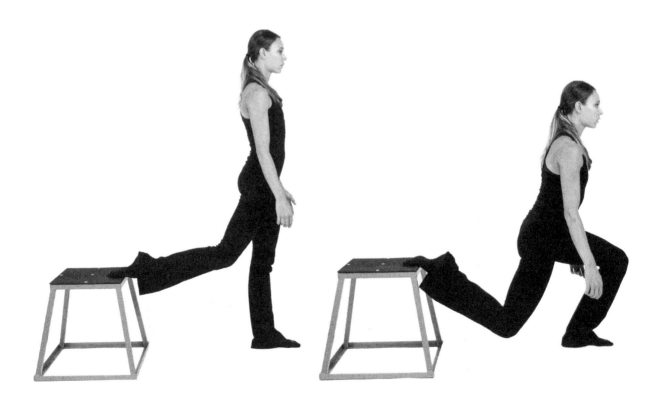

5: SPLIT-SQUAT, REAR-FOOT-ELEVATED, TWO KETTLEBELLS

Ready

- You'll need a chair, box, or bench to put your back foot on.
- You'll also need two kettlebells.

Set

- Hold two kettlebells in the suitcase position.
- Your back foot goes on the box.
- If necessary, hop your front foot forward so it's the same distance from the back foot as in a split-squat that's not rear-foot-elevated.

Go

- Bend both knees and bring your back knee down toward the floor.
- Keep most of the weight through the heel of your front foot—do most of the work with the front leg.
- Keep your front knee in line with your front foot.
- Stay as tall as possible—don't bend forward.
- Drive through your heel, and come back up.
- Do all of the reps with your less-awesome leg, and then do all of the reps with your awesome leg.

Josh Says

- *To start:* Drop your back knee straight to the floor.
- *In the middle:* Push the seam of your front pant leg out to the side wall.
- *To finish:* Push the floor away.
- *And:* Drive the heel of your front shoe down into the floor.

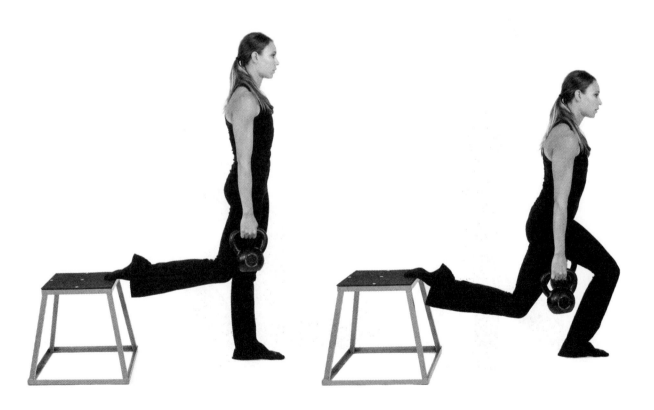

6: LUNGE, AIRBORNE

Ready
- No equipment is required, but you may want to use a light kettlebell as a counterbalance.

Set
- Stand on one leg.
- Bend the knee of the unweighted leg.
- Imagine you're doing a rear-foot-elevated split-squat with an invisible box.

Go
- Bend your other knee and squat with the leg you're standing on.
- Fold at your hips so your head and chest come forward as far as possible, and reach forward with your hands.
- Sit your butt way back.
- Drive through your heel and come back up.
- Do all of the reps with your less-awesome leg, and then do all of the reps with your awesome leg.

Josh Says
- *To start:* Pull your back pockets to the back wall.
- *And:* Reach for the wall in front of you.
- *To finish:* Push the floor away.
- *And:* Bring your belt buckle to the wall in front of you.

Bonus Tip
- Using a light kettlebell as a counterbalance will make it easier for most people.

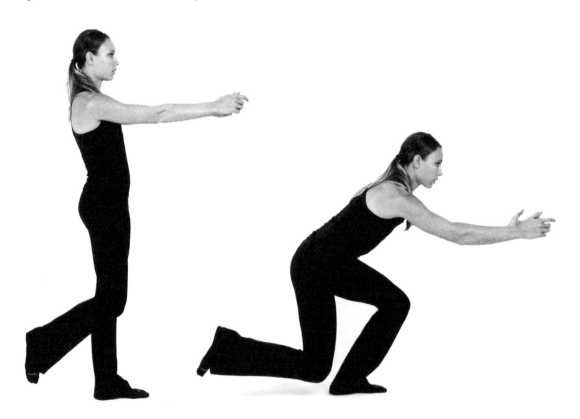

7: LUNGE, AIRBORNE, ONE KETTLEBELL

Ready
- You will need one kettlebell.

Set
- Stand on one leg.
- Bend the knee of the unweighted leg.
- Imagine you're doing a rear-foot-elevated split-squat with an invisible box.
- Hold the kettlebell in the goblet position.

Go
- Bend your other knee and squat with the leg you're standing on.
- Fold at your hips so your head and chest come forward as far as possible.
- Sit your butt way back.
- Drive through your heel and come back up.
- Do all of the reps with your less-awesome leg, and then do all of the reps with your awesome leg.

Josh Says
- *To start:* Pull your back pockets to the back wall.
- *And:* Reach for the wall in front of you with your hat.
- *To finish:* Push the floor away.
- *And:* Bring your belt buckle to the wall in front of you.

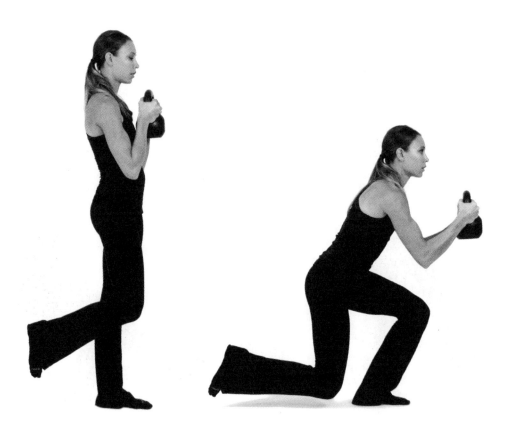

8: PISTOL SQUAT, BOX-ASSISTED

Ready
- You'll need a box or chair to squat down to—higher boxes are easier; lower boxes are harder.
- You may want to use a light kettlebell as a counterbalance.

Set
- Back your heels right up to the chair or box.
- Stand on one leg.

Go
- Bend your knee and squat with the leg you're standing on.
- Sit your butt way back.
- Fold at your hips so your head and chest come forward as far as possible.
- Sit your butt backward until it just barely touches the chair or box.
- Drive through your heel and come back up.
- Do all of the reps with your less-awesome leg, and then do all of the reps with your awesome leg.

Josh Says
- *To start:* Pull your back pockets to the back wall.
- *And:* Reach for the wall in front of you.
- *To finish:* Push the floor away.
- *And:* Reach your hat toward the ceiling.

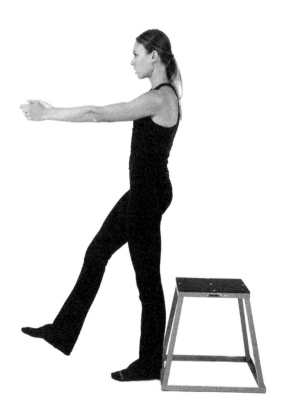
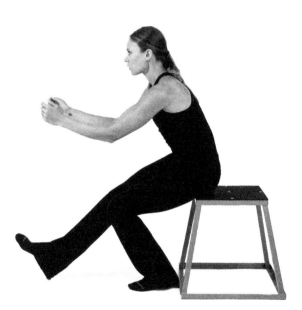

9: PISTOL SQUAT

Ready
- No equipment is required for this exercise.
- You may want to use a light kettlebell as a counterbalance.

Set
- Stand on one leg.

Go
- Bend your knee and squat with the leg you're standing on.
- Sit your butt way back.
- Fold at your hips so your head and chest come forward as far as possible.
- Sit your butt backwards until your butt hits your ankle.
- Drive through your heel and come back up.
- Do all of the reps with your less-awesome leg, and then do all of the reps with your awesome leg.

Josh Says
- *To start:* Pull your back pockets to the back wall.
- *Or:* Pull your back pockets to your shoe.
- *In the middle:* Reach for the wall in front of you.
- *To finish:* Push the floor away.
- *And:* Reach your hat toward the ceiling.

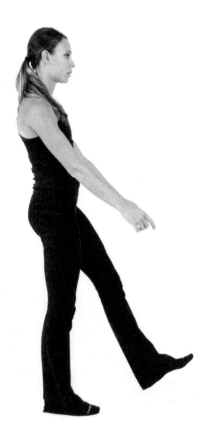
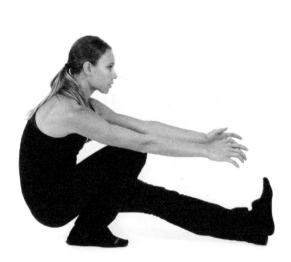

10: PISTOL SQUAT, ONE KETTLEBELL

Ready
- You will need one kettlebell.

Set
- Stand on one leg.
- Hold a kettlebell in the goblet position.

Go
- Bend your knee and squat with the leg you're standing on.
- Sit your butt way back.
- Fold at your hips so your head and chest come forward as far as possible.
- Sit your butt backward until your butt hits your ankle.
- Drive through your heel and come back up.
- Do all of the reps with your less-awesome leg, and then do all of the reps with your awesome leg.

Josh Says
- *To start:* Pull your back pockets to the back wall.
- *Or:* Pull your back pockets to your shoe.
- *In the middle:* Reach for the wall in front of you.
- *To finish:* Push the floor away.
- *And:* Reach your hat toward the ceiling.

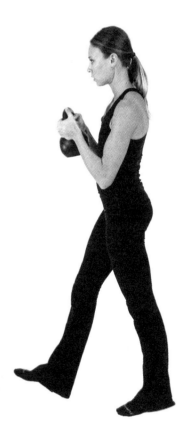
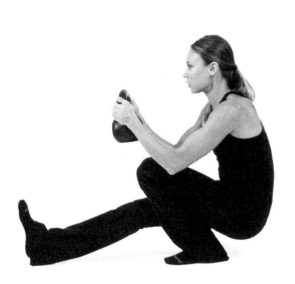

PULL-UP PROGRESSION

Door-Frame Pull-Up Bar

Band Assistance for Pull-Ups

1: Pull-Up Hang, Three Seconds

2: Pull-Up Hang, Active Shoulders, Three Seconds

3: Chin-Up, Top Hold, One Second

4: Chin-Up Negative, Three Seconds

5: Chin-Up, 1/4

6: Chin-Up, 1/2

7: Chin-Up, 3/4

8: Chin-Up

9: Pull-Up

10: Pull-Up, Tactical

DOOR FRAME PULL-UP BAR

- If you're working out at home, the easiest way to do pull-ups is to use a pull-up bar that snaps into place on a door frame.

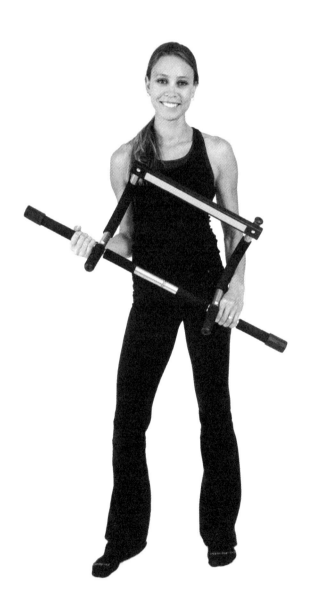

BAND ASSISTANCE FOR PULL-UPS

The Easiest and Cheapest Way to Make Pull-Ups Easier
- You can get any strength of light to heavy looped bands from either EliteFTS, Jumpstretch, or Iron Woody.
- Loop the band over a pull-up bar, then thread it through. Put only one foot into the band; you'll need the other foot free to step down to the floor when you are done.

Any Step in the Progression
- Can be used to make the pull-up hangs easier.
- Can be used to make the ¼, ½, and ¾ chin-ups easier.
- Can be used to make chin-ups, pull-ups, and tactical pull-ups easier.

Totally Helpful, But Not Necessary
- The pull-up progression was designed to be done without a band, so band assistance is not necessary.
- If you're new to working out or a little overweight, the band can help with the initial pull-up hangs.
- If you're advanced, the band can be used if you get stuck on a step in the progression.

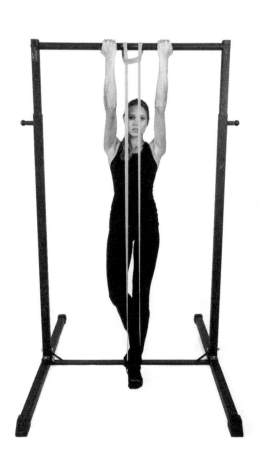
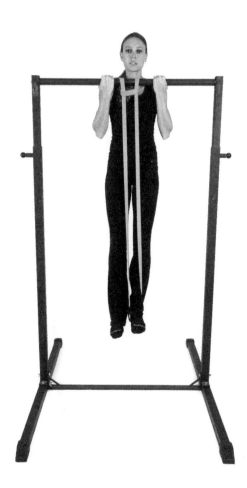

1: PULL-UP HANG, THREE SECONDS

Ready
- You'll need a pull-up bar or doorframe pull-up bar.

Set
- Grab the bar, with your palms facing forward and hands just outside of shoulder width.
- Wrap your thumbs around the bar opposite the fingers.
- Brace your abs hard, like you're doing a mini-crunch.
- Pull your ribs down and tuck your butt under.

Go
- Pull your shoulders down and back, hard, while you brace your abs hard for three seconds. Then relax.

Josh Says
- *To start:* Brace your abs like I was going to punch you in the stomach.
- *Or:* Imagine you're wearing a button-up shirt. Bring the bottom three buttons together.
- *And:* Point your belt buckle toward the ceiling.
- *And:* Squeeze the bar.

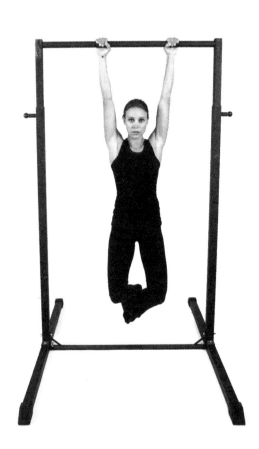

2: PULL-UP HANG, ACTIVE SHOULDERS, THREE SECONDS

Ready
- You'll need a pull-up bar or doorframe pull-up bar.

Set
- Grab the bar, palms facing forward with your hands just outside of shoulder width.
- Wrap your thumbs around the bar opposite the fingers.
- Pull your shoulders down and back, hard.
- Brace your abs hard, like you're doing a mini-crunch.
- Pull your ribs down and tuck your butt under.

Go
- Pull your shoulders down and back, lifting your body.
- Keep your elbows totally straight the whole time.

Josh Says
- *To start:* Imagine your ears are super hot and you have to keep your shoulders away from them to not get burned!
- *Or:* Get lots of air between your ears and your shoulders.
- *And:* Pull your shirt sleeves down toward the floor.

Bonus Tip
- It can be helpful to practice this in front of a mirror—without a pull-up bar—if you're having trouble getting the shoulder movement.

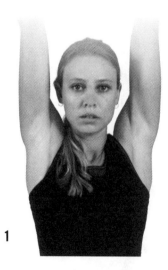

Shoulders are relaxed and up by the ears. The body hangs down.

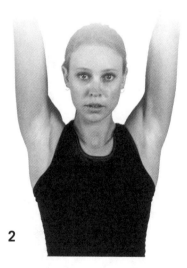

Pull the shoulders back and down, away from the ears. Pulling the shoulders down pulls the body up.

3: CHIN-UP, TOP HOLD, ONE SECOND

Ready
- You'll need a pull-up bar or doorframe pull-up bar.
- You'll also need a box, step, or chair that helps you get your chin over the pull-up bar.

Set
- From a box, step, or chair, grab the pull-up bar with your palms facing you and hands just inside of shoulder width.
- Wrap your thumbs around the bar, opposite the fingers.
- Pull your ribs down and tuck your butt under.

Go
- Step or jump off the box, step, or chair to bring yourself to the top of the pull-up bar.
- Squeezing the pull-up bar hard with your hands, pull your shoulders down and back, hard.
- Brace your abs hard for one second.
- Try to keep your chin higher than the bar the entire hold at the top.

Josh Says
- *To start:* Pull the bar to your shirt.
- *And:* Imagine your ears are super hot and you have to keep your shoulders away from them to not get burned!
- *And:* Get lots of air between your ears and your shoulders.
- *And:* Brace your abs like I was going to punch you in the stomach.
- *And:* Point your belt buckle toward the ceiling.

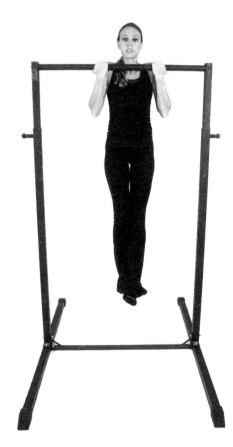

THE EXERCISE INSTRUCTIONS

4: CHIN-UP NEGATIVE, THREE SECONDS

Ready
- You'll need a pull-up bar or doorframe pull-up bar.
- You'll also need a box, step, or chair to help get your chin over the pull-up bar.

Set
- From a box, step, or chair, grab the pull-up bar with your palms facing you and your hands just inside of shoulder width.
- Wrap your thumbs around the bar.
- Pull your ribs down and tuck your butt under.

Go
- Step or jump off the box, step, or chair to bring yourself to the top of the pull-up bar.
- Squeezing the pull-up bar hard with your hands, pull your shoulders down and back, hard.
- Try to lower yourself slowly and smoothly for all three seconds.

Josh Says
- *To start:* Jump up to the bar.
- *And:* Get lots of air between your ears and your shoulders.
- *And:* Brace your abs like I was going to punch you in the stomach.
- *And:* Lower down three… slow… seconds.

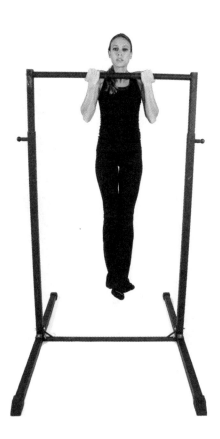
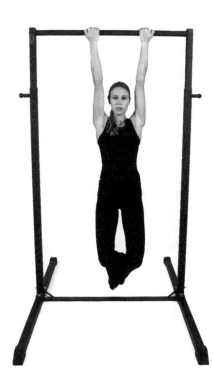

5: CHIN-UP, ¼

Ready
- You'll need a pull-up bar or doorframe pull-up bar.
- You'll also need a box, step, or chair to help get your chin over the pull-up bar.

Set
- From a box, step, or chair, grab the pull-up bar with your palms facing you and your hands just inside of shoulder width.
- Wrap your thumbs around the bar.
- Pull your ribs down and tuck your butt under.

Go
- Step or jump off the box, step, or chair to bring yourself to the top of the pull-up bar.
- Pull your shoulders down back and hard.
- Brace your abs hard, like you're doing a mini-crunch.
- Lower yourself down a quarter of the way down, and then immediately pull yourself back up.
- Reset your shoulders, and then repeat.

Josh Says
- *To start:* Pull the bar to your shirt.
- *And:* Get lots of air between your ears and your shoulders.
- *Then:* Lower down a quarter of the way, then explode back up to the bar!
- *And:* Brace your abs like I was going to punch you in the stomach.
- *And:* Point your belt buckle toward the ceiling.

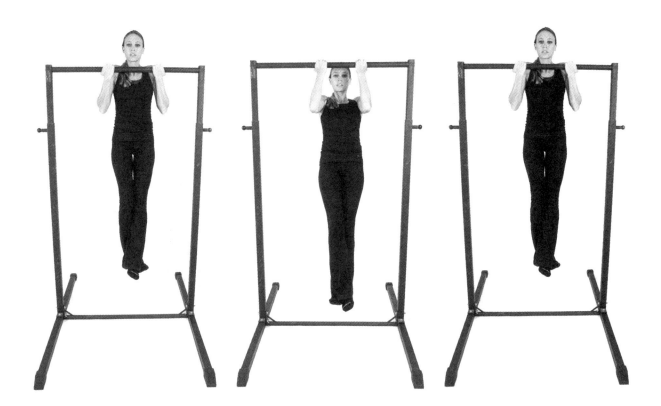

6: CHIN-UP, ½

Ready
- You'll need a pull-up bar or doorframe pull-up bar.
- You'll also need a box, step, or chair to help get your chin over the pull-up bar.

Set
- From a box, step, or chair, grab the pull-up bar with your palms facing you and your hands just inside of shoulder width.
- Wrap your thumbs around the bar.
- Pull your ribs down and tuck your butt under.

Go
- Step or jump off the box, step, or chair to bring yourself to the top of the pull-up bar.
- Pull your shoulders down back and hard.
- Brace your abs hard, like you're doing a mini-crunch.
- Lower yourself half of the way down, and then immediately pull yourself back up.
- Reset your shoulders, and then repeat.

Josh Says
- *To start:* Pull the bar to your shirt.
- *And:* Get lots of air between your ears and your shoulders.
- *Then:* Lower down half of the way, then explode back up to the bar!
- *And:* Brace your abs like I was going to punch you in the stomach.
- *And:* Point your belt buckle toward the ceiling.

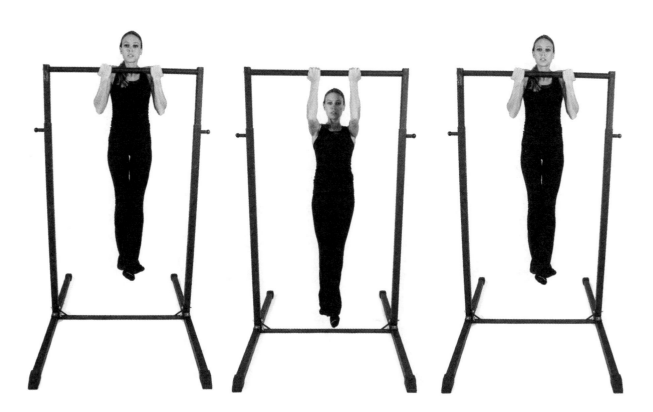

7: CHIN-UP, ¾

Ready
- You'll need a pull-up bar or doorframe pull-up bar.
- You'll also need a box, step, or chair to help get your chin over the pull-up bar.

Set
- From a box, step, or chair, grab the pull-up bar with your palms facing you and your hands just inside of shoulder width.
- Wrap your thumbs around the bar.
- Pull your ribs down and tuck your butt under.

Go
- Pull your shoulders down, back, and hard.
- Brace your abs hard, like you're doing a mini-crunch.
- Lower yourself three-quarters of the way down, and then immediately pull yourself back up.
- Reset your shoulders, and then repeat.

Josh Says
- *To start:* Pull the bar to your shirt.
- *And:* Get lots of air between your ears and your shoulders.
- *Then:* Lower down three-quarters of the way, then explode back up to the bar!
- *And:* Brace your abs like I was going to punch you in the stomach.
- *And:* Point your belt buckle toward the ceiling.

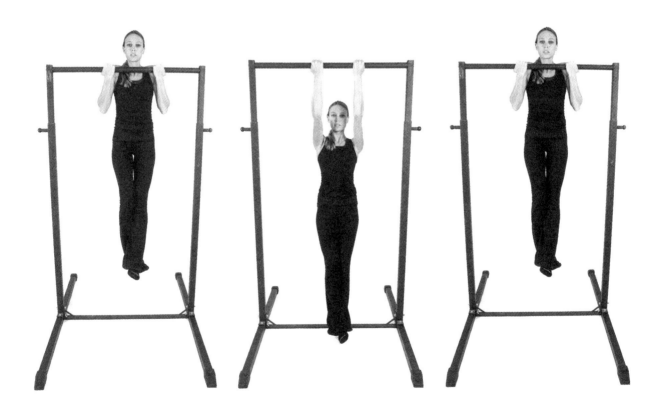

8: CHIN-UP

Ready
- You'll need a pull-up bar or doorframe pull-up bar.

Set
- From a standing position on the floor or from a box, grab the pull-up bar with your palms facing you, hands just inside of shoulder width.
- Wrap your thumbs around the bar, opposite the fingers.
- Pull your shoulders down, back, and hard.
- Brace your abs hard, like you're doing a mini-crunch.
- Pull your ribs down and tuck your butt under.

Go
- Pull yourself up until your chin is over the bar.
- Lower yourself down until your arms are straight, and then immediately pull yourself back up.

Josh Says
- *To start:* Pull the bar to your shirt.
- *And:* Get lots of air between your ears and your shoulders.
- *And:* Brace your abs like I was going to punch you in the stomach.
- *And:* Point your belt buckle toward the ceiling.
- *Or:* Explode up to the bar.

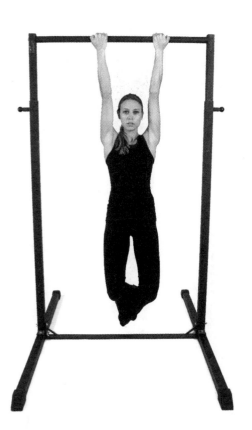
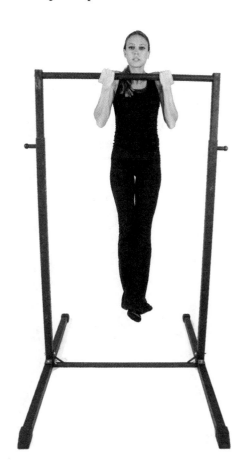

9: PULL-UP

Ready
- You'll need a pull-up bar or doorframe pull-up bar.

Set
- From a standing position on the floor or from a box, grab the pull-up bar with your palms facing forward, and your hands just wider than shoulder width.
- Wrap your thumbs around the bar, opposite the fingers.
- Pull your shoulders down and back, hard.
- Brace your abs hard, like you're doing a mini-crunch.
- Pull your ribs down and tuck your butt under.

Go
- Pull yourself up until your chin is over the bar.
- Lower yourself down until your arms are straight, and then immediately pull yourself back up.

Josh Says
- *To start:* Pull the bar to your shirt.
- *And:* Get lots of air between your ears and your shoulders.
- *And:* Brace your abs like I was going to punch you in the stomach.
- *And:* Point your belt buckle toward the ceiling.
- *Or:* Explode up to the bar.

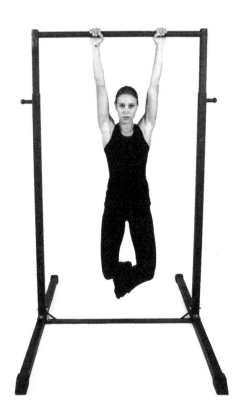
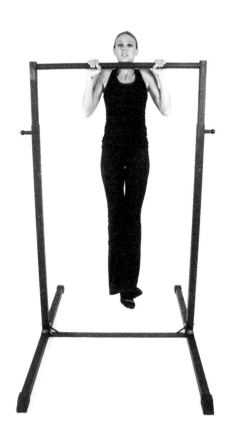

10: PULL-UP, TACTICAL

Ready
- You'll need a pull-up bar or doorframe pull-up bar.

Set
- From a standing position on the floor or from a box, grab the pull-up bar with your palms facing forward, and your hands just wider than shoulder width.
- Your thumbs will be on the same side as your fingers.
- Pull your shoulders down and back, hard.
- Brace your abs hard, like you're doing a mini-crunch.
- Pull your ribs down and tuck your butt under.

Go
- Pull yourself up until your neck or chest touches the bar.
- Lower yourself down slowly until your arms are straight.
- Wait for one count, then pull yourself back up.

Josh Says
- *To start:* Pull the bar to your shirt.
- *And:* Get lots of air between your ears and your shoulders.
- *And:* Brace your abs like I was going to punch you in the stomach.
- *And:* Point your belt buckle toward the ceiling.
- *Or:* Explode up to the bar.

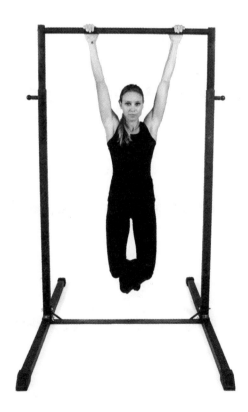
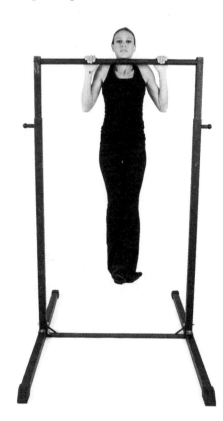

PUSHUP PROGRESSION

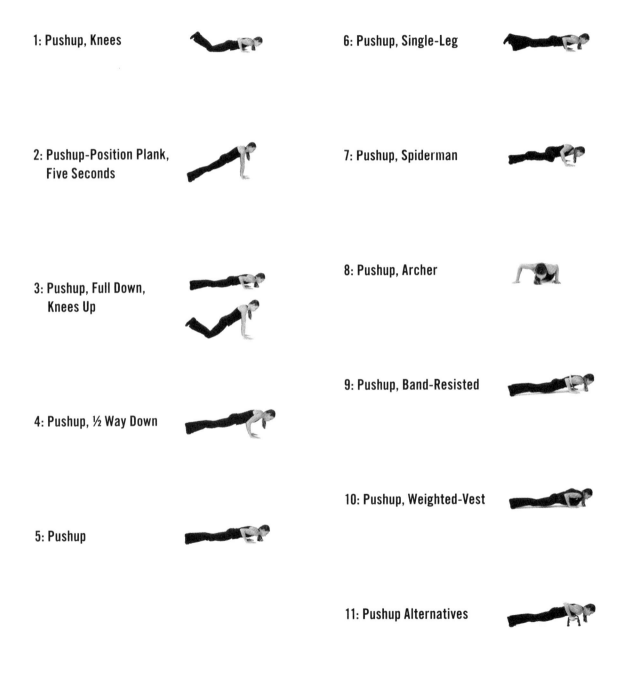

1: Pushup, Knees

2: Pushup-Position Plank, Five Seconds

3: Pushup, Full Down, Knees Up

4: Pushup, ½ Way Down

5: Pushup

6: Pushup, Single-Leg

7: Pushup, Spiderman

8: Pushup, Archer

9: Pushup, Band-Resisted

10: Pushup, Weighted-Vest

11: Pushup Alternatives

1: PUSHUP, KNEES

Ready
- Find a soft or padded surface for your knees: carpet, double- or triple-folded yoga mat, double- or triple-folded beach towel, or an airex pad.

Set
- On your hands and knees, move your knees back until your knees, hips, and shoulders all make a straight line.
- Lengthen your spine, get tall, and replicate what perfect posture would look like standing up.
- Brace your abs hard, like you're doing a mini-crunch.
- Pull your ribs down and tuck your butt under.

Go
- Do a pushup.

Josh Says
- *To start*: Brace your abs like I was going to punch you in the stomach.
- *Or*: Bring the logo on the front of your shirt and belt buckle together.
- *And*: Reach your hat to the front wall.
- *Then*: Push the ground away.

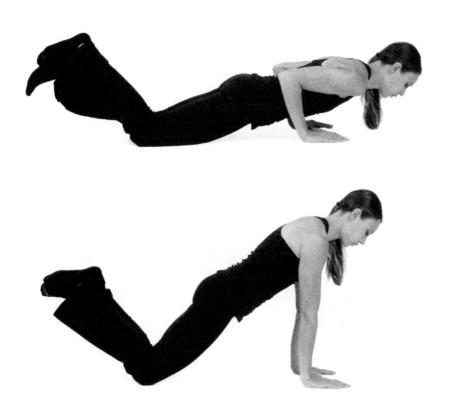

2: PUSHUP-POSITION PLANK, FIVE SECONDS

Ready
- No equipment is required for this exercise.

Set
- From your hands and knees, move your feet back until your feet, hips, and shoulders all make a straight line.
- Lengthen your spine, get tall, and replicate what perfect posture would look like standing up.
- Brace your abs hard, like you're doing a mini-crunch.
- Pull your ribs down and tuck your butt under.

Go
- Brace hard for five seconds. Then relax.

Josh Says
- *To start:* Brace your abs like I was going to punch you in the stomach.
- *Or:* Bring the logo on the front of your shirt and your belt buckle together.
- *And:* Reach your hat to the front wall.
- *To finish:* Squeeze the ground.
- *And:* Push the ground away.

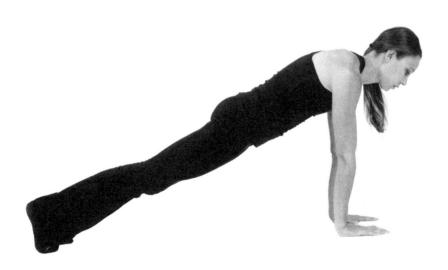

3: PUSHUP, FULL DOWN, KNEES UP

Ready
- Find a soft or padded surface for your knees: carpet, double- or triple-folded yoga mat, double- or triple-folded beach towel, or an airex pad.

Set
- From your hands and knees, move your feet back until your feet, hips, and shoulders all make a straight line.
- Lengthen your spine, get tall, and replicate what perfect posture would look like standing up.
- Brace your abs hard, like you're doing a mini-crunch.
- Pull your ribs down and tuck your butt under.

Go
- Lower yourself down in a full pushup from your toes.
- Put your knees down and push up from your knees.
- At the top of the knee pushup, straighten your legs back into a full pushup position.

Josh Says
- *To start:* Brace your abs like I was going to punch you in the stomach.
- *Or:* Bring the logo on the front of your shirt and your belt buckle together.
- *And:* Reach your hat to the front wall.
- *To finish:* Squeeze the ground.
- *And:* Push the ground away.

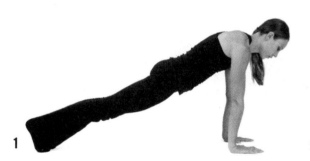
1

2

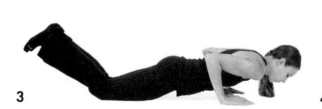
3

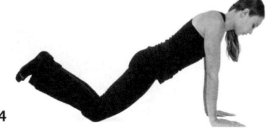
4

4: PUSHUP, ½ WAY DOWN

Ready
- No equipment is required for this exercise.

Set
- From your hands and knees, move your feet back until your feet, hips, and shoulders all make a straight line.
- Lengthen your spine, get tall, and replicate what perfect posture would look like standing up.
- Brace your abs hard, like you're doing a mini-crunch.
- Pull your ribs down and tuck your butt under.

Go
- Lower yourself half of the way down into a pushup, then press back up.

Josh Says
- *To start:* Brace your abs like I was going to punch you in the stomach.
- *Or:* Bring the logo on the front of your shirt and your belt buckle together.
- *And:* Reach your hat to the front wall.
- *To finish:* Squeeze the ground.
- *And:* Push the ground away.

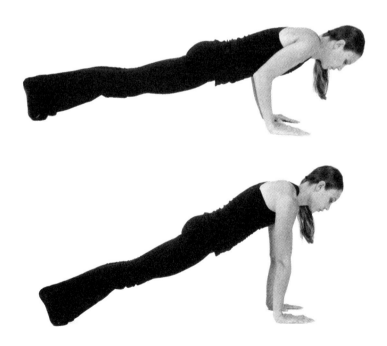

5: PUSHUP

Ready
- No equipment is required for this exercise.

Set
- From your hands and knees, move your feet back until your feet, hips, and shoulders all make a straight line.
- Lengthen your spine, get tall, and replicate what perfect posture would look like standing up.
- Brace your abs hard, like you're doing a mini-crunch.
- Pull your ribs down and tuck your butt under.

Go
- Do a pushup.

Josh Says
- *To start:* Brace your abs like I was going to punch you in the stomach.
- *Or:* Bring the logo on the front of your shirt and your belt buckle together.
- *And:* Reach your hat to the front wall.
- *To finish:* Squeeze the ground.
- *And:* Push the ground away.

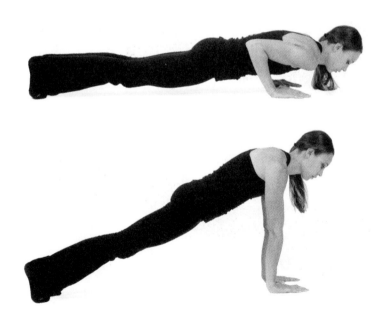

6: PUSHUP, SINGLE-LEG

Ready
- No equipment is required for this exercise.

Set
- From your hands and knees, move your feet back until your feet, hips, and shoulders all make a straight line.
- Lengthen your spine, get tall, and replicate what perfect posture would look like standing up.
- Brace your abs hard, like you're doing a mini-crunch.
- Pull your ribs down and tuck your butt under.
- Lift one foot an inch off of the ground.

Go
- Do half of the pushups on one leg, then switch and finish on the other leg.

Josh Says
- *To start:* Brace your abs like I was going to punch you in the stomach.
- *Or:* Bring the logo on the front of your shirt and your belt buckle together.
- *And:* Keep your pants pockets level.
- *To finish:* Squeeze the ground.
- *And:* Push the ground away.

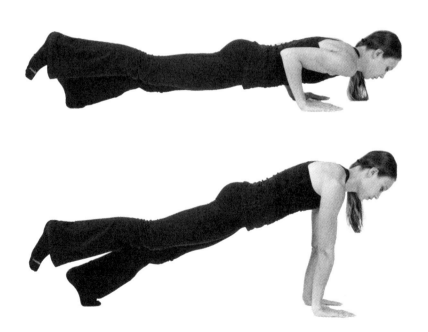

7: PUSHUP, SPIDERMAN

Ready

- No equipment is required for this exercise.

Set

- From your hands and knees, move your feet back until your feet, hips, and houlders all make a straight line.
- Lengthen your spine, get tall, and replicate what perfect posture would look like standing up.
- Brace your abs hard, like you're doing a mini-crunch.
- Pull your ribs down and tuck your butt under.

Go

- As you do the pushup, bring one knee as close to your elbow on the same side as you can.
- Switch legs every rep.

Josh Says

- *To start:* Brace your abs like I was going to punch you in the stomach.
- *Or:* Bring the logo on the front of your shirt and your belt buckle together.
- *And:* Pull your knee to your elbow.
- *To finish:* Squeeze the ground.
- *And:* Push the ground away.

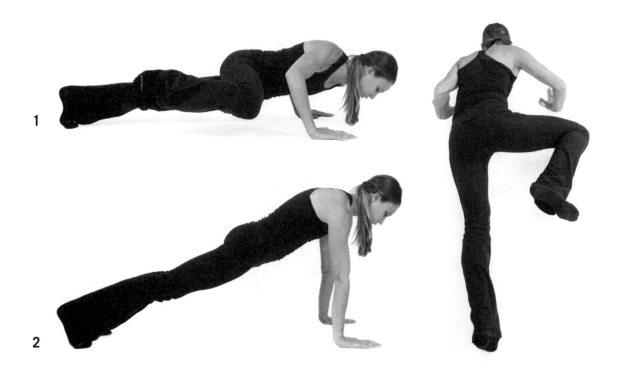

8: PUSHUP, ARCHER

Ready

- No equipment is required for this exercise.

Set

- Set one hand as close to your body as possible.
- Tuck that elbow in to your body.
- Set the other hand as far out as possible—the farther that hand is away, the harder the archer pushup will be.
- Move your feet back until your feet, hips, and shoulders all make a straight line.
- Lengthen your spine, get tall, and replicate what perfect posture would look like standing up.
- Brace your abs hard, like you're doing a mini-crunch.
- Pull your ribs down and tuck your butt under.

Go

- Do the number of reps for each set on *both arms*.

Josh Says

- *To start:* Brace your abs like I was going to punch you in the stomach.
- *Or:* Bring the logo on the front of your shirt and your belt buckle together.
- *To finish:* Squeeze the ground.
- *And:* Push the ground away.

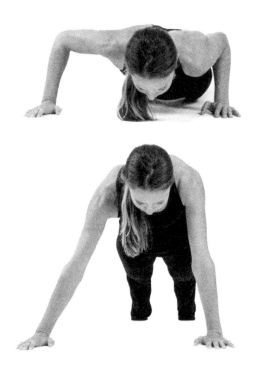

9: PUSHUP, BAND-RESISTED

The Easiest and Cheapest Way to Make Pushups Harder

- You can get any strength of light to heavy looped bands from either EliteFTS, Jumpstretch, or Iron Woody.
- Loop the band around the palm of your hand, then either over or under your arm, and around your back.

Add Weight to the Basic Pushups

- Works best for pushups and single-leg pushups.
- Start with a lighter band, and work your way up to heavier bands.
- If you're really strong, there's a point where you'll need to move up to a weighted vest instead of heavier and heavier bands.

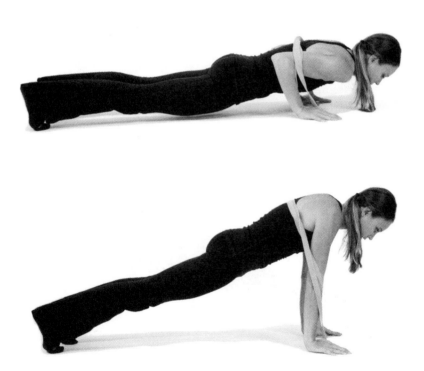

10: PUSHUP, WEIGHTED-VEST

The Best Way to Make Pushups Harder

- You can get weight vests anywhere from 10–80 pounds.
- You can use the weighted vest for any of the pushups in the pushup progression.

Add Weight to the Progression

- You can use the weighted vest for any of the pushups in the pushup progression.
- Standard protocol is to add 10 pounds, then work your way back through pushups, single-leg pushups, Spiderman pushups, and then archer pushups.
- Then add another 10 pounds and do it all again.

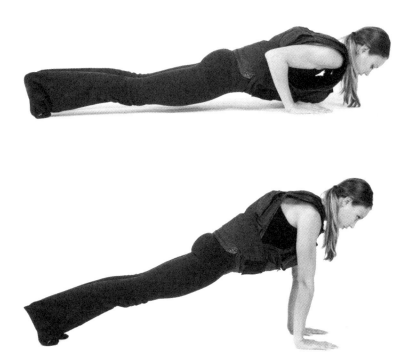

11: PUSHUP ALTERNATIVES

- Not everyone's wrists like pushups on the floor.
- Any of these options could make pushups agree with tender wrists.
- These alternatives work with every pushup in the progression.

Pushup Handles

- The easiest to find and cheapest alternative.
- The neutral wrist position works well for most people.

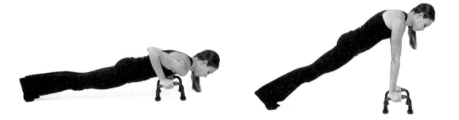

Yoga Wedge

- Many people who's wrists are tight from typing find that the yoga wedge feels good and is a good stretch.
- Can be a good half-step for getting back to floor pushups.

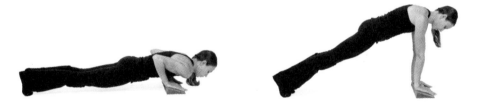

Pushup Board

- Can generate extra tension and strength by trying to 'break the board in half' like the barbell in a bench press.
- As a bonus, 'breaking the board in half' can also screw the shoulders into that shoulder-friendly externally rotated position.

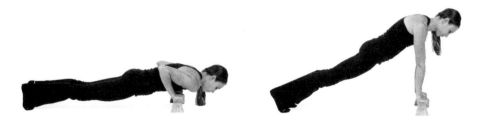

TWO-KETTLEBELL SWING PROGRESSION

Kettlebell Swing Safety

1: **Stick Deadlift Drill**
   (See page 238)

2: **Deadlift, Romanian**
   (See page 239)

3: **Kettlebell Swing, One Kettlebell**

4: **Kettlebell Swing, Two Kettlebells**

KETTLEBELL SWING SAFETY: PICKING IT UP AND PUTTING IT DOWN

Ready
- Set the kettlebell or 'bells far enough in front of you that you have to tip the handle to grab it.

Picking Kettlebells Up with a Swing
- Hike the kettlebell or 'bells back hard to the back wall.
- Then go explode up—right into your first swing.

Setting Kettlebells Down with a Swing
- Hike the kettlebell or 'bells back to the back wall.
- Let them swing out and set them down in exactly the reverse of how you picked it up.

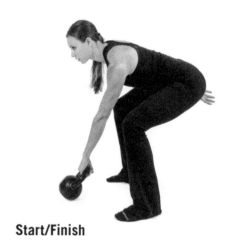

Start/Finish

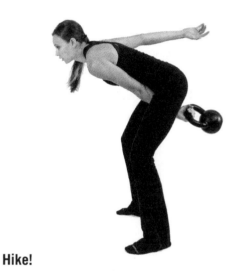

Hike!

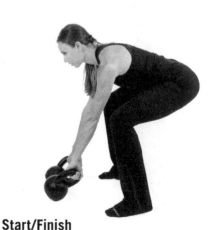

Start/Finish

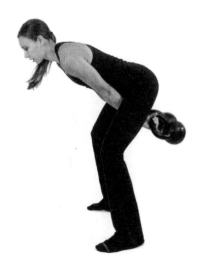

Hike!

3: KETTLEBELL SWING, ONE KETTLEBELL

Ready
- You need one kettlebell, set out in front of you.

Set
- Sit your hips back as in the *Stick Deadlift Drill* and grab the kettlebell.

Go
- Hike the kettlebell back behind your butt.
- Flex your butt and snap your hips forward.
- Engage your lats and stop the kettlebell from going above shoulder height.
- Repeat hiking the kettlebell back behind you each rep.
- Keep your back totally straight as in the *Stick Deadlift Drill* throughout the entire movement.

Josh Says
- *To start:* Hike the kettlebell to the back wall.
- *To finish:* Explode up!
- *And:* Drive your belt buckle to the wall in front of you!
- *Also:* Drive the heels of your shoes down hard into the floor.

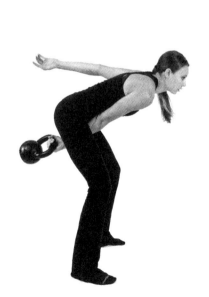
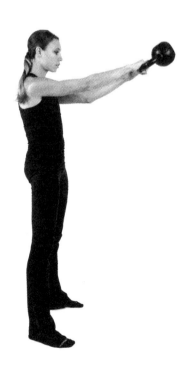

4: KETTLEBELL SWING, TWO KETTLEBELLS

Ready
- You need two kettlebells, set a foot out in front of you.
- Set your feet wide enough that you can get two kettlebells between your legs.

Set
- Sit your hips back as in the *Stick Deadlift Drill* and grab the kettlebells.

Go
- Hike the kettlebells back behind your butt.
- Flex your butt and snap your hips forward.
- Engage your lats and stop the kettlebell from going above shoulder height.
- Repeat hiking the kettlebell back behind you each rep.
- Keep your back totally straight as in the stick drill throughout the entire movement.

Josh Says
- *To start:* Hike the kettlebells to the back wall.
- *To finish:* Explode up!
- *And:* Drive your belt buckle to the wall in front of you!
- *Also to finish:* Drive the heels of your shoes down hard into the floor.
- *And:* Keep the kettlebells even.

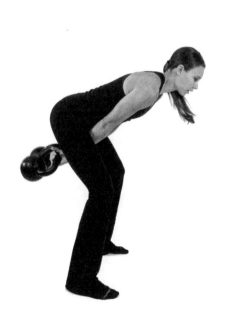
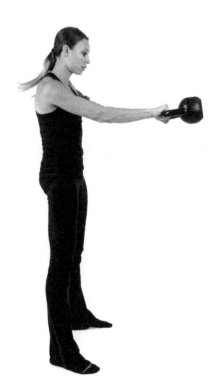

KETTLEBELL MILITARY PRESS PROGRESSION

1: Push Press, One Kettlebell

2: Military Press, One Kettlebell

3: Military Press, Two Kettlebells

MILITARY PRESS ALTERNATIVE

Downward Dog Pushup

1: PUSH PRESS, ONE KETTLEBELL

Ready
- You will need one kettlebell.

Set
- Clean the kettlebell to your chest in front of your shoulders in the rack position.

Go
- Sit your butt into a quarter-squat.
- Explode up into a standing military press in one fast, continuous movement.

Josh Says
- *To start:* Do a mini-squat.
- *To finish:* Explode the kettlebell up to the ceiling.
- *Or:* Jump the kettlebell up to the ceiling.

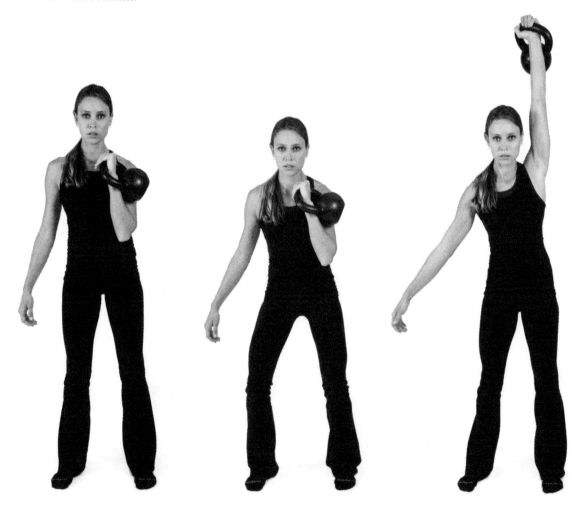

2: MILITARY PRESS, ONE KETTLEBELL

Ready
- You'll need one kettlebell, set a foot out in front of you.

Set
- Clean the kettlebell to your shoulder.
- Brace your butt and your abs.
- Pull your shoulder blade back and down.

Go
- Squeeze the kettlebell handle, and press it up over your head.

Josh Says
- *To start:* Punch the kettlebell up to the ceiling.
- *And:* Imagine your ears are super hot and you have to keep your shoulders away from them to not get burned!
- *Or:* Keep some air between your shoulder and your ear.
- *And:* Push your shoes down into the floor.

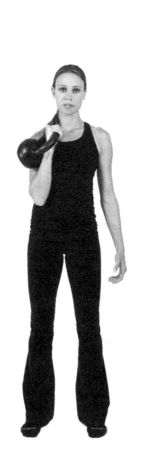
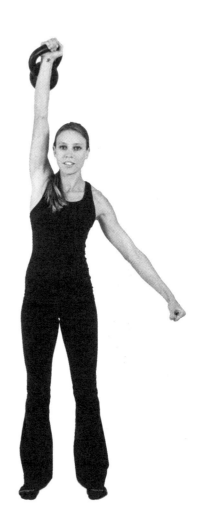

3: MILITARY PRESS, TWO KETTLEBELLS

Ready
- You'll need two kettlebells, set a foot out in front of you.

Set
- Clean both kettlebells to your shoulders.
- Brace your butt and your abs.
- Pull your shoulder blades back and down.

Go
- Squeeze the kettlebell handles, and press both kettlebells up over your head.

Josh Says
- *To start:* Punch the kettlebells up to the ceiling.
- *And:* Keep some air between your shoulders and your ears.
- *And:* Push your shoes down into the floor.
- *And:* Keep both kettlebells even as they go up.

Bonus Tip
- If your shoulders are really tight and cause you to struggle with two-kettlebell military presses, you may need to stick with single-kettlebell military presses while you're working on your shoulder flexibility and t-spine mobility.

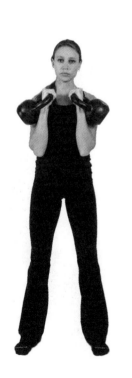
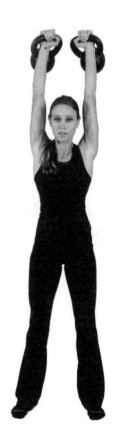

DOWNWARD DOG PUSHUPS (MILITARY PRESS ALTERNATIVE)

Military Press Alternative
- Not everyone's shoulders agree with military presses.
- Many people find that downward dog pushups feel great, even if military presses don't.
- This is a great way to work on a little overhead strength while simultaneously teaching your shoulder complex how to move better.

It's Just about Shoulders
- Unlike a true yoga downward dog, we don't care if your back rounds or your knees bend. We just want you to push your hands as far overhead as is comfortable.

To Make It Easier
- Do the pushup on your knees, then downward dog on your toes.

To Make It Harder
- Elevate your feet on a box, chair, or bench. The higher your feet, the harder it will be.

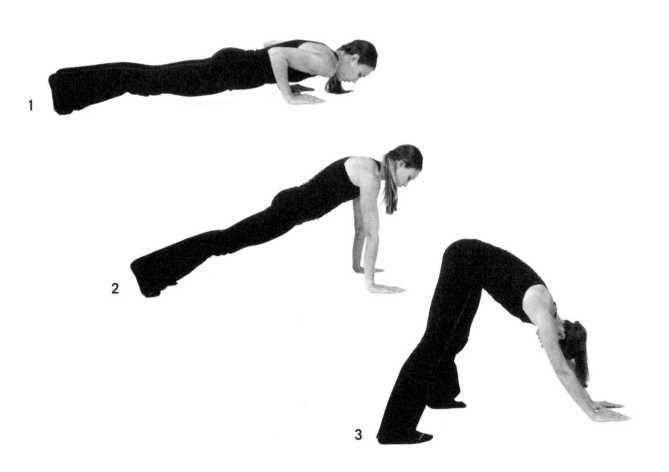

KETTLEBELL SQUAT PROGRESSION

1: Goblet Squat

2: Squat, One Kettlebell

3: Squat, Two Kettlebells

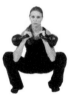

1: GOBLET SQUAT

Ready
- You'll need one kettlebell for this exercise.

Set
- Pick the kettlebell up with both hands, or clean it to chest height.
- Tuck your elbows in toward your body and hold the kettlebell a few inches away from your chest.

Go
- Sit your butt straight down. You're squatting between your legs, not back.
- Keep most of the weight through your heels, but also keep your big toe down.
- Push your knees out so they're on the same line as your feet.
- Arch your low back hard and keep your chest up.
- Return to the standing position.

Josh Says
- *To start:* Pull your back pockets back and down toward the floor.
- *In the middle:* Push the seams of your pants out toward the walls.
- *And:* Keep the logo on the front of your shirt up.
- *To finish:* Push the floor away from you.
- *Or:* Push the ground away.
- *Or:* Push the kettlebell up to the ceiling.

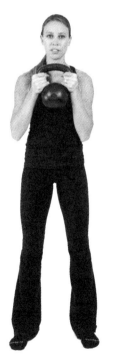
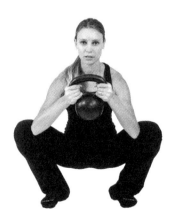

2: SQUAT, ONE KETTLEBELL

Ready
- You'll need one kettlebell, set a foot out in front of you.

Set
- Clean the kettlebell to your shoulder.

Go
- Sit your butt back and down.
- Keep most of the weight through your heels, but also keep your big toe down.
- Push your knees out so they're on the same line as your feet.
- Arch your low back hard and keep your chest up.
- Keep your shoulders and hips square the whole time.
- Return to the standing position.
- Switch sides every set.

Josh Says
- *To start:* Pull your back pockets back and down toward the floor.
- *In the middle:* Push the seams of your pants out toward the walls.
- *And:* Keep the logo on the front of your shirt up.
- *To finish:* Push the floor away from you.
- *Or:* Push the kettlebell up to the ceiling.

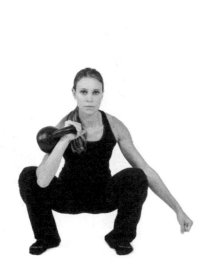
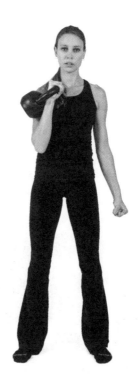

3: SQUAT, TWO KETTLEBELLS

Ready
- You'll need two kettlebells, the same weight or different weights, set a foot out in front of you.

Set
- Clean the kettlebells to your shoulders.

Go
- Sit your butt straight down.
- Keep most of the weight through your heels, but also keep your big toe down.
- Push your knees out so they're on the same line as your feet.
- Arch your low back hard and keep your chest up.
- Return to the sanding position.
- If the kettlebells are different weights, switch sides every set.

Josh Says
- *To start:* Pull your back pockets back and down toward the floor.
- *In the middle:* Push the seams of your pants out toward the side walls.
- *And:* Keep the logo on the front of your shirt up.
- *To finish:* Push the floor away from you.
- *Or:* Push the kettlebells up to the ceiling.

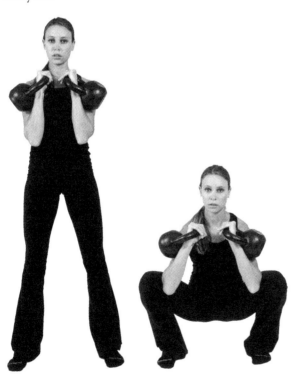
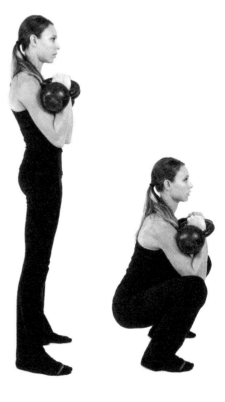

NON-PROGRESSION EXERCISES

WARMUP

Prisoner Lunge

PULL YOUR WEIGHT

Bent-Over Row

BRING IT!

Tripod Row

Thruster

Renegade Row

PRISONER LUNGE

Ready

- No equipment is required for this exercise.

Set

- Get in a normal standing stance with your feet hip width and under you.
- Lace your fingers behind your head in the 'getting arrested' pose.
- Pull your elbows back hard.
- Pull your shoulder blades down hard.

Go

- Take a step forward.
- Bend both knees and bring your back knee toward the floor.
- Keep most of the weight through the heel of your front foot—do most of the work with the front leg.
- Keep your front knee in line with your toes.
- Stay as tall as possible—don't bend forward.
- Drive through the heel of your front foot and come up, bringing your back foot forward.
- Alternate legs each rep. Start with your less-awesome side stepping forward.

Josh Says

- *Most important:* It's all about pulling your shirt sleeves to the wall behind you the whole time.
- *And:* Imagine your ears are super hot and you have to keep your shoulders away from them to not get burned!
- *Or:* Keep some air between your ears and your shoulders.
- *And:* At the bottom, keep pulling your hat up to the ceiling.

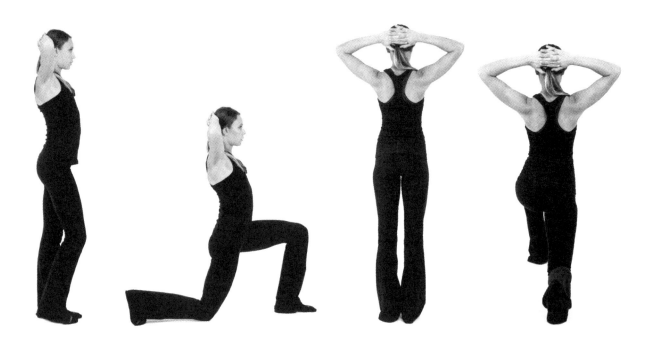

BENT-OVER ROW

Ready
- You'll need a kettlebell for this exercise.

Set
- Take a wide stance with the kettlebell slightly in front of you.
- Fold forward at your hips, until you can rest your elbow on your thigh just above your knee.
- Grab the kettlebell.

Go
- Pull the kettlebell back so your elbow is just behind your body.
- Do all of the reps on your less-awesome arm first, and then do your awesome arm.

Josh Says
- *To start:* Imagine a piece of tape on your elbow—pull that tape to the ceiling.
- *And:* Imagine your ears are super hot and you have to keep your shoulders away from them to not get burned!
- *And:* Remember the hinge stick drill. Keep the stick on your back straight.

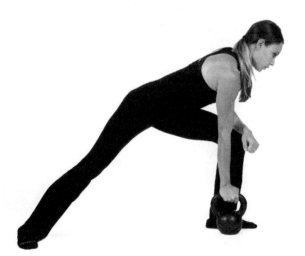 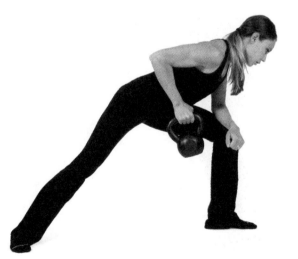

TRIPOD ROW

Ready
- You'll need a kettlebell and a box, bench, or chair for this exercise.

Set
- Take a wide stance with the kettlebell slightly in front of you.
- Fold forward at your hips, until you can rest your hand on the box, bench, or chair.
- Grab the kettlebell.

Go
- Pull the kettlebell back so your elbow is just behind your body.
- Do all of the reps on your less-awesome arm first, and then do your awesome arm.

Josh Says
- *To start:* Imagine a piece of tape on your elbow—pull that tape to the ceiling.
- *And:* Imagine your ears are super hot and you have to keep your shoulders away from them to not get burned!
- *And:* Remember the hinge stick drill. Keep the stick on your back straight.

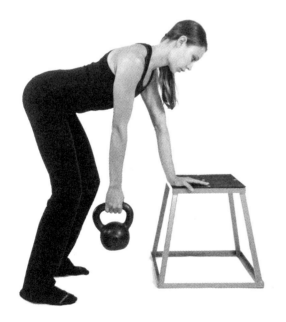
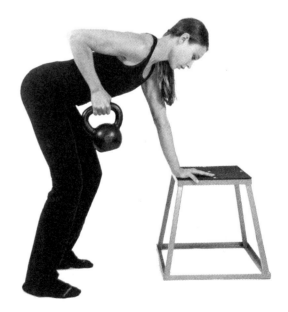

THRUSTER

Ready
- You'll need two kettlebells, the same weight or different weights.

Set
- Clean the kettlebells to your chest in front of your shoulders, in the rack position.

Go
- Sit your butt back and down.
- Keep most of the weight through your heels, but also keep your big toe down.
- Push your knees out.
- Arch your low back hard and keep your chest up.
- When you get to the bottom of the squat, explode up into a standing military press in one fast, continuous movement.
- If the kettlebells are different weights, switch sides every set.

Josh Says
- *To start:* Squat.
- *To finish:* Explode the kettlebells up to the ceiling.

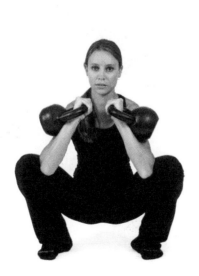
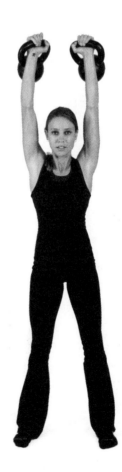

RENEGADE ROW

Ready

- You will need two heavy-ish kettlebells that are the same weight. The heavier the kettlebells are, the safer you are from having the kettlebell tip over while you're balancing on it.
- Or you could use two hex dumbbells that are the same weight. With these, you'll have less chance of them tipping over.

Set

- Get into a pushup position, with your hands on the kettlebell handles instead of on the floor.
- Lengthen your spine, get tall, and replicate what perfect posture would look like standing up.
- Brace your abs hard, like you're doing a mini-crunch.
- Pull your ribs down and tuck your butt under.

Go

- Put all of your weight on one hand, then pull the other kettlebell toward you in a rowing motion.
- Set that kettlebell down, put all of your weight on it, and then row the other kettlebell.

Josh Says

- *To start:* Brace your abs like I was going to punch you in the stomach.
- *And then:* Imagine a piece of tape on your elbow—pull the piece of tape to the ceiling.
- *And:* Keep both of your pants pockets level the whole time.

Bonus Tip:

- If you don't have the core strength for renegade rows, work on the *Front-Plank Progression* instead.

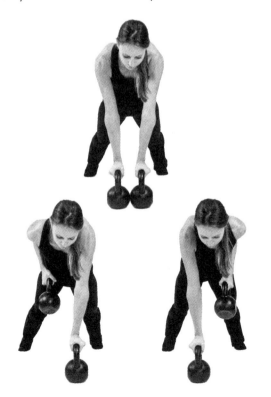
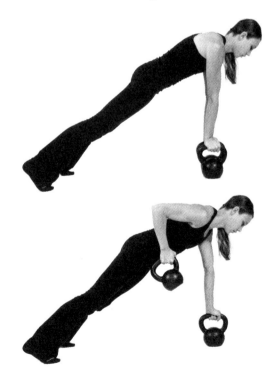

CORE: FRONT-PLANK PROGRESSION

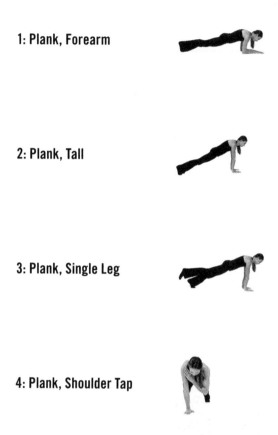

1: Plank, Forearm

2: Plank, Tall

3: Plank, Single Leg

4: Plank, Shoulder Tap

*If you need core progressions beyond the shoulder-tap plank, get *The New Rules of Lifting for Abs,* by Lou Schuler and Alwyn Cosgrove. Alternate between the advanced steps in their *Front-Plank Progression* and either ValSlide body saws, Swiss ball rollouts, or TRX fallouts.

1: PLANK, FOREARM

Ready
- No equipment is required for this exercise.

Set
- Starting from your elbows and knees, move your feet back until your feet, hips, and shoulders all make a straight line.
- Lengthen your spine, get tall, and replicate what perfect posture would look like standing up.
- Brace your abs hard, like you're doing a mini-crunch.
- Pull your ribs down and tuck your butt under.

Go
- Brace hard while you get tall.

Josh Says
- *To start:* Brace your abs like I was going to punch you in the stomach.
- *Or:* Imagine a logo on the front of your shirt. Pull the logo down toward your belt buckle, and pull your belt buckle toward the logo.
- *And:* Reach your hat to the wall in front of you.

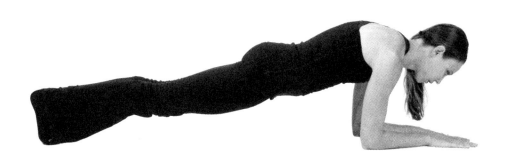

2: PLANK, TALL

Ready
- No equipment is required for this exercise.

Set
- Starting from your hands and knees, move your feet back until your feet, hips, and shoulders all make a straight line.
- Lengthen your spine, get tall, and replicate what perfect posture would look like standing up.
- Brace your abs hard, like you're doing a mini-crunch.
- Pull your ribs down and tuck your butt under.

Go
- Brace hard while you get tall.

Josh Says
- *To start:* Brace your abs like I was going to punch you in the stomach.
- *Or:* Imagine a logo on the front of your shirt. Pull the logo down toward your belt buckle, and pull your belt buckle toward the logo.
- *And:* Reach your hat to the wall in front of you.

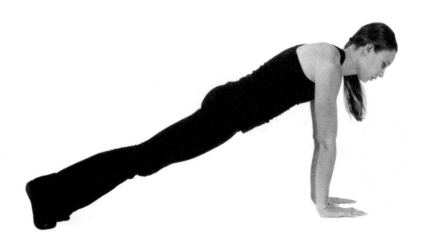

3: PLANK, SINGLE LEG

Ready
- No equipment is required for this exercise.

Set
- From your hands and knees, move your feet back until your feet, hips, and shoulders all make a straight line.
- Lengthen your spine, get tall, and replicate what perfect posture would look like standing up.
- Brace your abs hard, like you're doing a mini-crunch.
- Pull your ribs down and tuck your butt under.
- Lift one foot an inch off of the ground.

Go
- Brace hard while you get tall and keep your hips square.
- Switch feet each set.

Josh Says
- *To start:* Brace your abs like I was going to punch you in the stomach.
- *Or:* Imagine a logo on the front of your shirt. Pull the logo down toward your belt buckle, and pull your belt buckle toward the logo.
- *And:* Keep your pants side pockets level.

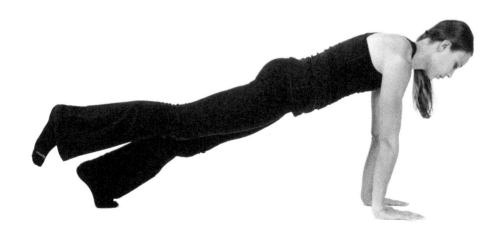

4: PLANK, SHOULDER TAP

Ready
- No equipment is required for this exercise.

Set
- From your hands and knees, move your feet back until your feet, hips, and shoulders all make a straight line.
- Lengthen your spine, get tall, and replicate what perfect posture would look like standing up.
- Brace your abs hard, like you're doing a mini-crunch.
- Pull your ribs down and tuck your butt under.
- Lift one foot an inch off of the ground.

Go
- Put all of your weight on one hand, then touch your shoulder with the other hand.
- Alternate one hand and then the other for the duration of the plank time.

Josh Says
- *To start:* Brace your abs like I was going to punch you in the stomach.
- *Or:* Imagine a logo on the front of your shirt. Pull the logo down toward your belt buckle, and pull your belt buckle toward the logo.
- *And:* Keep your pants side pockets level.
- *And:* Keep your shoulders level.

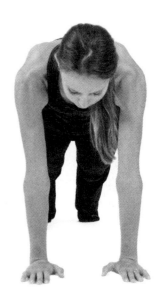
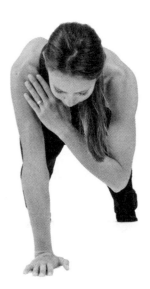

CORE: SIDE-PLANK PROGRESSION

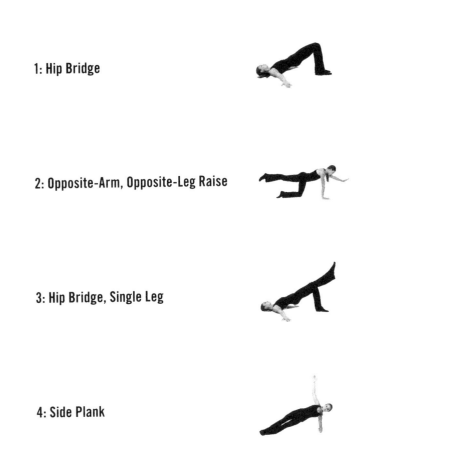

1: Hip Bridge

2: Opposite-Arm, Opposite-Leg Raise

3: Hip Bridge, Single Leg

4: Side Plank

*If you need core progressions beyond the side plank, get *The New Rules of Lifting for Abs*, by Lou Schuler and Alwyn Cosgrove. Alternate between their *ValSlide Pushaway Progression* and the advanced steps in their *Side-Plank Progression*.

THE EXERCISE INSTRUCTIONS 307

1: HIP BRIDGE

Ready
- No equipment is required for this exercise.

Set
- Lie on your back, feet flat on the floor with your knees bent to a 90° angle.
- Brace your abs hard, like you're doing a mini-crunch.
- Pull your ribs down and tuck your butt under.

Go
- Flex your butt and drive your hips up.

Josh Says
- *To start:* Brace your abs like I was going to punch you in the stomach.
- *And:* Flex your butt like I was going to kick you in the butt.
- *And then:* Drive your belt buckle to the ceiling.

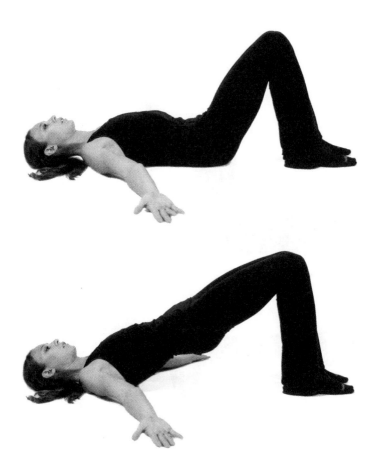

2: OPPOSITE-ARM, OPPOSITE-LEG RAISE

Ready

- No equipment is required for this exercise.

Set

- Get in a quadruped position, on your hands and knees.
- Lengthen your spine from your head to your tailbone—get tall.
- Brace your abs hard, like you're doing a mini-crunch.
- Flex your butt.

Go

- Extend one leg back and the opposite arm out.
- Keep your hips square to the floor—don't rotate.
- Switch sides and redo the motion.

Josh Says

- *To start:* Brace your abs like I was going to punch you in the stomach.
- *And:* Flex your butt like I was going to kick you in the butt.
- *And:* Reach your hat to the wall in front of you.
- *Then:* Lift your opposite arm and leg.
- *And:* Keep your pants pockets level.

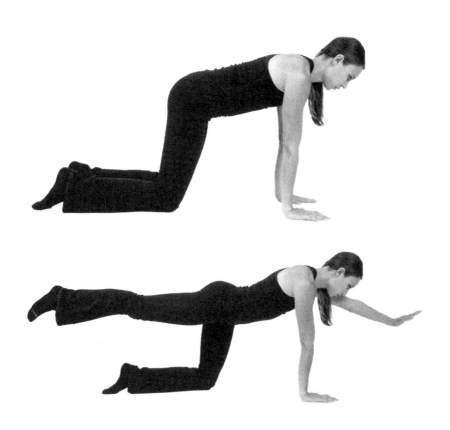

3: HIP-BRIDGE, SINGLE LEG

Ready
- No equipment is required for this exercise.

Set
- Lie on your back with your feet flat on the floor and your knees bent to a 90° angle.
- Brace your abs hard, like you're doing a mini-crunch.
- Pull your ribs down and tuck your butt under.

Go
- Flex your butt and drive your hips up.
- Straighten one leg.
- Brace your butt and abs hard enough that your hips stay level throughout the movement. Don't drop the hip on the side with the extended leg.

Josh Says
- *To start:* Brace your abs like I was going to punch you in the stomach.
- *And:* Flex your butt like I was going to kick you in the butt.
- *Then:* Bring your belt buckle to the ceiling.
- *And:* Keep your pockets level the whole time.

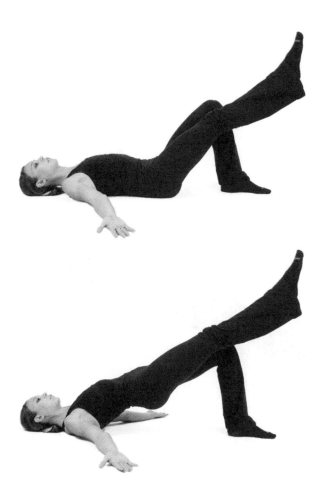

4: SIDE PLANK

Ready
- No equipment is required for this exercise.

Set
- Starting from one elbow and knee, move your feet back until your feet, hips, and shoulders all make a straight line on one side.
- Lengthen your spine, get tall, and replicate what perfect posture would look like standing up.
- Brace your abs hard, like you're doing a mini-crunch.
- Pull your ribs down and tuck your butt under.

Go
- Bring your hips up into a straight line from your head to your feet.

Josh Says
- *To start:* Brace your abs like I was going to punch you in the stomach.
- *And:* Flex your butt like I was going to kick you in the butt.
- *Then:* Bring your pants pocket up to the ceiling.

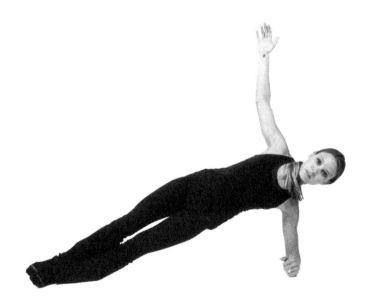

JOSH

CHAPTER 29

SHOPPING PLAN

First Sunday or Monday of the month

Protein	CHICKEN, FISH, BEEF, BISON, TURKEY
Nuts	ALMONDS, CASHEWS
Oils	FISH OIL, FLAX OIL, OLIVE OIL, AVOCADO OIL, COCONUT OIL
Pseudo-Grains	QUINOA, BROWN RICE, RICE, WILD RICE
Frozen Vegetables	ALL FROZEN VEGETABLES ARE AWESOME
Fresh Fruits, Vegetables, and Tubers	ALL FRUITS, VEGETABLES, AND TUBERS ARE AWESOME. DON'T FORGET AVOCADO FOR HEALTHY FAT.
Sauces	*MAKE YOUR HEALTHY FOOD TASTE GOOD! USE TOMATO SAUCE, SALSA, HOT SAUCE, PESTO SAUCE, AND SO ON.*
Spices	*PLEASE, MAKE YOUR HEALTHY FOOD TASTE GOOD! USE CAJUN SPICE, ITALIAN BLEND, PEPPER, SALT, CUMIN, RED PEPPER, OREGANO, BASIL, CILANTRO.*

Every Sunday or Monday

Protein	CHICKEN, FISH, BEEF, BISON, TURKEY
Nuts	ALMONDS, CASHEWS
Pseudo-Grains	QUINOA, BROWN RICE, RICE, WILD RICE
Fresh Fruits, Vegetables, and Tubers	ALL FRUITS, VEGETABLES, AND TUBERS ARE AWESOME. DON'T FORGET AVOCADO FOR HEALTHY FAT.
Sauces	*MAKE YOUR HEALTHY FOOD TASTE GOOD! USE TOMATO SAUCE, SALSA, HOT SAUCE, PESTO SAUCE, AND SO ON.*

Every Wednesday or Friday

Protein	CHICKEN, FISH, BEEF, BISON, TURKEY
Fresh Fruits, Vegetables, and Tubers	ALL FRUITS, VEGETABLES, AND TUBERS ARE AWESOME. DON'T FORGET AVOCADO FOR HEALTHY FAT.

WHAT TO GET, BY DEPARTMENT

MEAT SECTION OF THE MARKET

BUTCHER/FISH MARKET SECTION
SEAFOOD
POULTRY
BEEF
PORK
GAME

PRODUCE SECTION

PRODUCE SECTION
AVOCADO
ROMAINE/KALE/SPINACH
BROCCOLI/BRUSSELS SPROUTS/ASPARAGUS
BANANA/APPLE/ORANGE/BLUEBERRY/STRAWBERRY
ONIONS/TOMATOES/CILANTRO/BASIL/BELL PEPPERS/JALAPEÑO PEPPERS/GARLIC

FROZEN SECTION

FROZEN SECTION
FROZEN VEGETABLES
FROZEN FRUIT
SPROUTED-GRAIN BREAD
FROZEN ONIONS/PEPPERS

SHOPPING LIST

PROTEIN	FAT	VEGETABLES	CARBOHYDRATES
☐ BEEF	☐ ALMOND BUTTER	☐ ARUGULA	☐ APPLES
☐ BISON	☐ ALMONDS	☐ ASPARAGUS	☐ BANANAS
☐ CASEIN PROTEIN POWDER	☐ AVOCADO	☐ BEETS	☐ BLACKBERRIES
☐ CHICKEN	☐ AVOCADO OIL	☐ BELL PEPPERS	☐ BLUEBERRIES
☐ COTTAGE CHEESE	☐ BRAZIL NUTS	☐ BROCCOLI	☐ BROWN RICE
☐ EDAMAME	☐ CASHEW BUTTER	☐ BRUSSELS SPROUTS	☐ BROWN RICE PASTA
☐ EGG PROTEIN POWDER	☐ CASHEWS	☐ CABBAGE	☐ CHERRIES
☐ EGG WHITE	☐ CHIA SEEDS	☐ CARROTS	☐ CHICKPEAS
☐ EXTRA FIRM TOFU	☐ COCONUT BUTTER	☐ CELERY	☐ DATES
☐ FISH	☐ COCONUT OIL	☐ CUCUMBER	☐ GRAPEFRUIT
☐ GREEK YOGURT	☐ EGG YOLK	☐ GARLIC	☐ MELON
☐ HEMP PROTEIN POWDER	☐ FISH OIL SUPPLEMENT	☐ GREEN BEANS	☐ NECTARINES
☐ LAMB	☐ FLAX OIL SUPPLEMENT	☐ GREEN LEAF LETTUCE	☐ ORANGES
☐ NATTO	☐ FLAX SEEDS	☐ KALE	☐ PEACHES
☐ PEA PROTEIN POWDER	☐ GHEE	☐ ONIONS	☐ PEARS
☐ PORK	☐ KRILL OIL SUPPLEMENT	☐ PEAS	☐ PINEAPPLE
☐ ROE	☐ MACADAMIA NUTS	☐ RED LEAF LETTUCE	☐ PLAIN YOGURT
☐ SHELLFISH	☐ OLIVE OIL	☐ ROMAINE	☐ QUINOA
☐ SUPER FIRM TOFU	☐ OLIVES	☐ SPAGHETTI SQUASH	☐ RASPBERRIES
☐ TEMPEH	☐ PECANS	☐ SPINACH	☐ SPROUTED GRAIN BREAD
☐ TURKEY	☐ SUNFLOWER SEEDS	☐ SQUASH	☐ STRAWBERRIES
☐ WHEY PROTEIN POWDER	☐ WALNUTS	☐ TOMATO	☐ SWEET POTATOES
☐ WILD GAME			☐ YAMS

1. Plan your meals from left to right.
2. This list is not exhaustive—you *don't* need to restrict yourself to items on this list. This is to get you thinking about all of the great things you *can* have.
3. Don't forget your spices, sauces, and seasonings!
4. Some of the carbohydrates are as much as 25% protein, and that's awesome, but you're still going to treat these like a carbohydrate—a high-protein carbohydrate.
5. Some of the fats are as much as 33% protein, and that's awesome, but you're still going to treat them as a fat—a high-protein fat.
6. None of the foods on this table are magical. Foods that aren't on this list aren't evil.

JOSH

CHAPTER 30

THE ONLY GAME WORTH PLAYING

There's only one game worth playing: *How do we make it possible to eat the food we know we need to eat, in real life?*

The game is not what's the right food.

And it also isn't what's the right workout.

Almost always, the question I get is, "What do you think about XYZ food?" Although well intentioned—that's the wrong question. Nothing is always bad or always good. *We're playing a longer game than that.*

One piece of chocolate cake will no more derail your results than one meal of chicken with guacamole and steamed broccoli would make them. It's a 'most of the time' thing.

Look, what to eat we can handle in five seconds—

We use proteins like fish, beef, poultry, or pork.

We choose fats that are healthy, like avocado, nuts, olive oil, or flax oil.

Our carbohydrate choices are foods that are obviously healthy, like vegetables, fruit, brown rice, or quinoa.

We use fewer carbohydrates.

Once that's out of the way we can move on to what matters—creating the habits that help this kind of eating work.

As a blogger who reports on celebrity workouts and diets, I can tell you there are plenty more celebrities with awesome bodies because they have great nutrition habits than because they have great workouts.

Sure, lots of them do have great workouts—those are who I write about most often. But if I'm being honest, many have mediocre workouts and great food habits.

And the food habits always win.

We started this book saying, *Workouts are required but not sufficient for getting the body you want.*

So…do the workouts.

Here's the shocking truth about what your workout should do: *It should make you stronger.*

We don't care how sore you are or aren't the day after. We don't care if you're dripping buckets of sweat, or none at all. We don't care if it feels really hard, or completely easy.

What we do care about: *At the end of the month, you're lifting more weight or doing a harder bodyweight progression, or that you're doing more sets and more reps.*

And we care that when this rep range comes around again in six months, your starting weight or bodyweight progression is more than your starting weight or bodyweight progression was when you did it the last time.

Just get a little stronger, over time. Let the food do the rest.

Put *all* of your mental energy into staying on top of your food habits. Do that, and you'll win every time.

INDEX

action, emotion vs., 26
adrenaline, 104
advanced fat-loss food programs, 71–6
age, bodyfat and, 82–3
airborne lunges instructions, 252
airborne lunges, one-kettlebell instructions, 253
Allen, Woody, 90
Alpo Diet, 96
alternating periodization, 115–16
Anderson, Vince, 99
archer pushups instructions, 278
Asinof, Eliot, 23
Atkins diet, 19
attitude, 28–9
Avery, Kenny, 23
Augustine, Saint, 12
authority, training philosophy and, 9

"bad" vs. "good" food choices, 25–6
Bagrosky, Taryn, 62
Bailey, Covert, 94
Ballantyne, Craig, 99, 116
band assistance for pullups, 259
band resisted pushups instructions, 279
barbell deadlifts, 124, 196–7, 237–41
    instructions, 241
Basic Carb-Cycling Template, 73
basic human movements, 21–2, 113–14
basics, training philosophy and, 9–12
basketball, conditioning for, 24
Bass, Clarence, 5
Beck Diet Solution, The, 40
bent-over row instructions, 297
Berardi, John, 55, 59
Big 21 program, 9

bilateral deficit, 108
Blauer, Tony, 2
Body for Life diet, 17
body image, self-talk and, 40–1
bodyfat percentage, leanness
    age and, 82–3
    food quality and, 17–20, 33, 56–7, 74, 80, 106
    overall trend in, 55
    protein and, 53
    tracking, 63, 78–82
    women and, 82–5
bodyweight exercises
    bodyweight lunge & split-squat progression (original), 128
    bodyweight pushup progression (original), 128
    bodyweight squat instructions, 247
    fat loss and, 105–6
    original progression, 128
    resources for, 236
    time constraints and, 197–9
Boyle, Mike, 108
Bring It program
    basics of, 201–4, 219
    intensity in, 112
    nutrition in, 202–4
    Pull Your Weight program and, 201, 206
    refeeds and, 75
    rest during, 183
    workouts schedule for, 204–18, 220–32
bus-bench mentality, 3–5
By the Numbers strategy, 32–3, 42

caliper measurements, 79, 81–3
calories
    ideal intake of, 57–8

INDEX

maintenance, 53, 58, 74
minimum, 58
quantity of, 31, 33–4, 36, 38, 55, 57–8, 202
Campbell, Joseph, 11
carbohydrates
    carbohydrate cycling and, 71–4, 99, 203–4
    feeling full and, 37–9
    metabolism and, 60
    prioritization of, 51
    quality, 31, 33–4, 36–7, 55, 57, 202–3
    ratios of, 19
cascading, 9, 13
celebrities, 84
chin-ups instructions, 263–8
circumference measurements, 78, 80–1, 106
coaching cues, 237
competition, mindset for, 3–4
Compliance Grid, 59
Conrad, Chip, 8
cookbooks, diet, 56–7
cooking
    ahead of time, 29
    Bring It! program and, 204–5
    cooking games and, 44
    habit of, 31, 34, 36, 43, 51, 55
    priority of, 197–8
Conrad, Chip, 8, 113
Coonradt, Charles, 109
core work, direct, 190–1
corrective exercise, 193, 195–6, 236
Corrective Exercise Specialist (CES) system, National Academy of Sport Medicine's, 193
cortisol, 104
Cosgrove, Alwyn, 9, 116, 191, 197, 236
"could phase" of goal setting, 96
counting calories, 17
Cressy, Eric, 194
CrossFit, Fran work out of, 204

Darwin, Charles, 89
deadlifts
    barbell, 196–7, 237–40
    barbell alternative, 237
    kettlebells for, 108–9
    lifting to failure and, 187
    Romanian, 196–7, 239
    single-leg, 108–9
    single-leg assisted deadlifts instructions, 243
    single-leg, opposite-hand deadlifts instructions, 244
    single-leg, two-kettlebell deadlifts instructions, 245
    strength phase workouts and, 150
    trap-bar, 196–7, 241
deadlines, motivation and, 203
decisions, mission and, 90, 92

deductive logic, training philosophy and, 9–10
dehydration, 31–2
DeLorme, Thomas, 12
"density window," 201
Denver Kettlebell Bootcamp, 107
deprivation, ix, 10–12
DEXA scan, 80–1, 83
diaphragmatic breathing, 360-degree, 194
difficulty, workout, 21
discipline, developing, 41
doorway pull-up bars, 194, 258
double progressions, 185–90
downward dog, 192, 290
Durnin and Womersley method, 79
dysmorphia, 82

easy-to-hard monthly cycle, 186–7
easy workouts, long-term effectiveness of, 1, 111–12
eating program, effective, 57
"eighty-percent full" habit, 31, 38–9, 42, 55
either/or issues, 94
electronic impedance scales, 81
emotions, 11–12, 26–8
endurance goals, 41
endurance phase workouts
    basics of, 115–19, 140–1
    outline of, 139
    military presses and, 139
    pull-ups and, 139
    rest during, 183
    schedule for, 141–7
Enter the Kettlebell, 187, 236
epics, 89–90
Epictetus, 4
epistemology, training philosophy and, 7–14
external cues, 235

fads, conditioning, 11
failure, lifting to, 187–8
fast food, healthy, 54
fat
    feeling full and, 37–9, 53–4
    healthy, 31, 33–4, 36–7, 51, 53–5, 57, 203–4
    metabolism and, 60
    muscle vs., 77–8
    prioritization of, 51
    ratios of, 19
    vegetarian diet and, 54
Ferriss, Tim, 110
Fighter Workouts for Fat Loss, 186
"fit" vs. "fat" talk, 27
fitness industry, problems with, 93–8
food, central to fat loss, 17–19, 111–12
food games, 43–4

food journals
    coaching session with, 65–7
    effective, 25
    fullness and, 19, 37–8
    habit of keeping, 31–40, 42–4, 43, 51, 55, 202–3
    ideal calorie intake and, 58
    measuring progress and, 78–9, 81
    mindfulness and, 38–40
    online, 32–4, 37–8, 40, 54, 63–4, 66, 74
    priority of, 197–8
    protein intake and, 54
    refeeds and, 74
    re-planning and, 62–3
    scoring of, 63–5
    skills recorded in, 29–30
food preparation, skill of, 29–30, 198. *See also* cooking.
food pushers, 62
football, conditioning for, 24
forearm plank instructions, 301
forth-telling, 88
Fosbury, Dick, 12
Frankl, Viktor, 89
free days, 27, 47, 59–61, 73–4, 203
free meals, 59–61
front squats, kettlebell, 150 kettlebell front squats and, 150
full-down, knees-up pushup instructions, 273
fullness
    80% full habit and, 31, 38–9, 42, 55
    fat and, 37–9, 53–4
    food ratios and, 19, 37–9
    Fullness Leads to Fat Loss Strategy, 37–8, 42
Functional Movement Screen (FMS), 193
fundamentals, training philosophy and, 9–12

Gensel, Greg, 12
Get Off My Back (GOMB), 109–10
Gilgamesh, 89–90
givens, personal, 90–1
Gnoll Credo, 93
goals, goal-setting, 87–92, 94–8
goblet squats instructions, 292
gratitude, habit of, 31, 39–40, 43, 202
Greeley, Sean, 91
grids, for meal planning, 43, 59–60
gurus, fat-loss, 114

habits, diet as set of, x, 29
half-way down pushups instructions, 274
hex dumbbell handles, 194
Hierarchy of Fat Loss, 197–8
high-carb days, 72–3
High-Intensity Interval Training (HIIT), 191–2
Highland Games, 3–4, 94
hip bridge/side plank progression, 127

hip bridge instructions, 307, 309
Holmes, Sherlock, 12, 114
hormesis, 110
hydrostatic weighing, 81, 83

identity, transforming, 26–7
injury, pain from 192–4
integrity, 23
intensity, 1–2, 112, 201–2
internal cues, 235
interval training
    High Intensity Interval Training (HIIT) and, 191–2
    time constraints and, 197
intuition, training philosophy and, 9, 12

John Powell Discus Camp, xiii–xiv
judgment, 26

Kavadlo, Al, 236
ketogenic diet, 19
Kettlebell Fast Tens program, 186
kettlebells
    airborne lunges, one-kettlebell instructions, 253
    bent-over row instructions, 297
    deadlifts with, 108–9
    Denver Kettlebell Bootcamp, 107
    fat loss and, 105
    handles for pushups, 194
    interval training and, 191–2
    kettlebell front squats and, 150
    military press alternatives, 194, 290
    one-kettlebell military press instructions, 288
    one-kettlebell squat instructions, 293
    one-kettlebell swings instructions, 284
    pistol squat, one-kettlebell instructions, 255
    progressions, 129. *See also particular progressions under this entry.*
    push presses, one-kettlebell, instructions, 287
    rep range and, 185–6
    resources for, 236
    Russian military and, 140, 144
    safety with, 283
    shoulders, kettlebell military presses and, 194
    single-leg, two-kettlebell deadlifts instructions, 245
    split-squat, rear-foot-elevated, two-kettlebell instructions, 251
    squat progression, 126–7, 291–4
    thruster instructions, 300
    time constraints and, 197–8
    tripod row instructions, 297
    two-kettlebell military press instructions, 289
    two-kettlebell squat instructions, 293
    two-kettlebell squat progression, 292–5
    two-kettlebell swing progression, 125, 282–5

INDEX

two-kettlebell swings instructions, 285
women's military press progressions and, 107–8
working with two, 107–8, 289. *See also* two-kettlebell workouts.
Koch, Bill, 12
knee pushups instructions, 271

Landmark Education Self Expression Leadership Program, 25–6
leanness, muscle and, 77–8
Ledbetter, Steve, 87
long-term fat loss, basic program for, 115–19
low-carb days, 72–3
low fat diets, 19
lunges
    airborne lunges instructions, 252
    airborne lunges, one-kettlebell instructions, 253
    prisoner lunge instructions, 296
    bodyweight lunge & split-squat progression (original), 128
    lunge & split-squat progression, 125, 246–56
    walking lunges instructions, 249

MacDonald, Lyle, 75
macronutrient calculators, 72
macronutrient ratios, 17–20, 37, 56, 63
macronutrient timing, 71
maintenance calories, 53, 58, 74
maintenance habits, fat loss, 41–4
Marcel, Gabriel, 94
Mass Made Simple program, 9, 14, 22, 24
Maughan, Ralph, 9, 11, 23, 109–10
meal planning, 29–30, 31, 34–6, 43, 51, 55, 58–70, 197–8, 202–3
medium-difficulty workouts, effectiveness of, 1, 111–12
mental health counseling, 41
metabolic/endurance/strength phase workouts
    basics of, 115, 157–9
    outline of, outline of, 158
    schedule for, 159–75
    volume phase of, 176–83
metabolic phase workouts, 115–19
    outline of, 131
    pull-ups and, 132
    rest during, 183
    schedule for, 131–7
metabolism, 53–4, 60–1, 74–5
military presses
    alternatives to, 194, 290
    endurance phase workouts and, 142
    one-kettlebell, instructions, 288
    progression of, 107–8, 124
    two-kettlebell, instructions, 289
    women's progression for, 107–8

Mindfulness strategy, 38–9, 42
mindset, reaching goals and, 87–92
minimum calories, 58
mission, personal, 90–2, 94–5
mithridatism, 112
Montaigne, Michel de, 10–11
motivation, deadlines and, 203
movement choice continuum, 188
multi-adaptation phases, fat loss and, 119–20. *See also* periodization, undulating.
muscle
    fat vs., 77–8
    leanness and, 77–8
    ratio to food, 18
    rebuilding during refeeds, 74
    strength and, 53
    tone and, 77–8
muscle soreness, 192
muscle stretching, 192
"must phase" of goal setting, 96–8
mysteries, problems vs., 94–5
My Life Is My Message assignment, 91

"Nabi," 88
Naked Warrior, 236
negativity, 40–1
Never Let Go, 9
New Rules of Lifting for Abs, The, 191, 236
night time eating, 19
Nightingale, Earl, 23, 87–8
non-progression exercises, 295–301
Norton, Layne, 75
Notmeyer, Dick, 9, 14
nutrition, in Bring It! program, 202–4. *See also many other topics connected with nutrition, e.g.*, calories.
program, effective, 57

obesity rates, 57
obstacle, overcoming with structure, 35
One Change program, 202–3
one-kettlebell exercises
    airborne lunges, one-kettlebell instructions, 253
    one-kettlebell military press instructions, 288
    one-kettlebell military press instructions, 288
    one-kettlebell squat instructions, 293
    one-kettlebell swings instructions, 284
    pistol squat, one-kettlebell instructions, 255
    push presses, one-kettlebell, instructions, 287
online food journals, 32–4, 37–8, 40, 54, 63–4, 66, 74
online macronutrient calculators, 72
opposite-arm, opposite-leg raise instructions, 308

pain, dealing with, 192–4
pain avoidance, goals and, 96–7

Paleo diet, 109
park-bench mentality, 3–5
passion, 89
Paul, Jamie, 49
"Paydirt," 109
Pearson, Aaron, 46
Peele, Leigh, 75
periodization
    alternating, 115–16
    dietary, 74–5
    fat-loss, 115–19
    undulating, 115–16, 119. *See also* metabolic/endurance/strength phase workouts.
Phillips, Bill, 35
Photoshopped images, 84
pistol squat, box-assisted, instructions, 253
pistol squat instructions, 254
pistol squat, one-kettlebell instructions, 255
planks
    forearm plank instructions, 301
    front plank progression, 301–5
    hip bridge/side plank progression, 127
    plank progression, 127
    pushup plank instructions, 271
    shoulder-tap plank instructions, 305
    side plank instructions, 310
    side-plank progression, 306–10
    side-plank progression, 306–310
    single-leg plank instructions, 304
    tall plank instructions, 303
Planning and Preparing strategy, 34–5, 42
planning games, 43
plans, adaptation of, 58–9, 62–3
plant-based diets, 54–5
"plateauing," 28
Platinum Coaching Club Workouts, 186
pleasure, goals and, 96–7
Plummer, Thomas, 89
portion sizes, 17, 58
portioning, ahead of time, 29–30
posture work, 194
Power to the People, 187
preparation
    food pushers and, 62
    importance of, ix–x. *See also* food preparation.
    willpower versus, 61–2
prepositions, examining, 88, 94–5
prisoner lunge instructions, 296
problems, mysteries vs. 94–5
progress, gauging, 77–85
progressions
    barbell deadlift progression, 124, 237–241
    basics of, 121
    bodyweight lunge & split-squat progression (original), 128
    bodyweight pushup progression (original), 128
    deadlift progression, single leg, 242–5
    double, 185–90
    front plank progression, 301–5
    hip bridge/side plank progression, 127
    kettlebell progressions, 129. *See also under this entry.*
    kettlebell squat progression, 126–7, 291–4
    lunge & split-squat progression, 125, 246–56
    military press progression, 107–8, 124
    plank progression, 127
    pull-up progression, 122, 257–69
    push-up progression, 122, 270–80
    rationale for, 104
    side-plank progression, 306–310
    single-leg deadlift progression, 123
    two-kettlebell squat progression, 292–5
    two-kettlebell swing progression, 125, 282–5
protein
    adequate for fat loss, 51–3
    bodyfat percentage and, 17
    carbohydrate cycling and, 72
    effective nutrition program and, 57
    feeling full and, 37–9
    habit of daily consumption of, 31, 33–4, 36, 42, 55, 202–3
    prioritization of, 51
    ratios of, 19
    vegetarian diet and, 54
pull-ups
    band assistance for, 258
    door frame bars for, 257
    endurance phase workouts and, 140
    metabolic phase workouts and, 132
    partial, 151
    progression, 122, 257–69
    pull up hang instructions, 260–1
    pull-up instructions for, 268–9. *See also* chin-ups instructions
    strength and, 118, 150–1
Pull Your Weight program, 41
    Bring It! program and, 201, 206, 219
    core training in, 191
    during refeed, 75
"push, pull, squat, hip hinge," 189–90, 193
push presses, one-kettlebell, instructions, 287
pushup boards, 194, 281
pushup handles, 194, 281
pushup plank instructions, 271
pushups
    alternatives to, 194, 281
    bodyweight progression (original), 128
    instructions for, 271–81

INDEX

pain during, 193–4
progression, 122, 270–80
pushup boards, 194, 281
pushup plank instructions,
pushup-to-downward dogs and, 194
strength phase workouts and, 150

Quadrant Two, 24
quality, food
"free" meals and, 60
grade of, 63
leanness and, 17–20, 33, 56–7, 74, 80, 106
refeeds and, 74
quantity, food
tracking, 63
weight and, 17–20, 31, 33–4, 36, 38, 55–8, 77, 79–80, 106, 108, 202

RAMP: The 21st Century Warmup, 236
Rasmussen, Craig, 236
ratios, macronutrient, 17–20, 37, 56, 63
ratios, muscle-to-food, 18
Read, Andrew, 89
"real science," training philosophy and, 9, 12–13
"reasonable" diets, 22–4
"reasonable" workouts, 21–2
reassessment, 28
recipes, collection of, 56
re-feeds, 58, 60, 71–2, 74–6
regression, 9–12
Reifkind, Mark, 114
relationship to food, 40–1
renegade row instructions, 300
re-planning, 58–9, 62–3
reps
double progressions of, 185–90
range of, 185
varying, 113–14
responsibility, taking, 26–7
rest, 183, 201–2
results, measurement of, 78–81
Return of the Kettlebell, 236
rewards, food as, 11
Relaxed Carb Cycling Template, 73
Robbins, Anthony, 96
Rohn, Jim, 27, 35
Romanian, 196–7, 239
instructions, 240
rounds, circuits and, 202
rules, diet as set of, x
Russian military, kettleball system of, 140, 144

"safety zone," Coonradt's, 109–10

scale weight
food quantity and, 17–20, 31, 33–4, 36, 38, 55–8, 77, 79–80, 106, 108, 202
tracking, 63, 78
scheduling meals, 29
Schmidt, Paige Gaynor, 47
Schuler, Lou, 191, 236
self-image, 82
self-talk, body image and, 40–1
sense experience, training philosophy and, 9–11
sequences, eleven habits, 3
sets, cycles of, 186–7
Shiner, Sharon, 45
"should phase" of goal setting, 96
shopping, food, 29–31, 34, 36, 43, 51, 55, 198, 202–3, 311–313
shopping games, 43–4
shoulder-tap plank instructions, 305
shoulders, kettlebell military presses and, 194
side-plank progression, 306–10
side plank instructions, 310
Silvester, L. Jay, 12
Simple and Sinister, 236
single-leg assisted deadlifts instructions, 243
single-leg deadlifts, 108–9
single-leg hip bridge instructions, 309
single-leg, opposite-hand deadlifts instructions, 244
single-leg plank instructions, 304
single-leg pushups instructions, 276
single-leg, two-kettlebell deadlifts instructions, 245
"six small meals a day," 19
skills, diet and nutrition, x, 29–30. *See also* habits, eleven.
"skinny fat," 51–2, 78
sleep, adequate, 32
slow eating, habit of, 31, 39, 42, 55,
speech, actions aligned with, 26
spiderman pushups instructions, 277
split-squat instructions, 248
split-squat progression (original), bodyweight lunge &, 128
split-squat, rear-foot-elevated instructions, 249
split-squat, rear-foot-elevated, two-kettlebell instructions, 251
squats
bodyweight lunge & split-squat progression (original), 128
goblet squats instructions, 292
kettlebell front squats and, 150
kettlebell squat progression, 126–7, 291–4
lunge & split-squat progression, 125, 246–56
one-kettlebell squat instructions, 293
pistol squat instructions, 254
pistol squat, box-assisted, instructions, 253
pistol squat, one-kettlebell instructions, 255
"push, pull, squat, hip hinge," 189–90, 193
split-squat instructions, 248

split-squat, rear-foot-elevated instructions, 249
split-squat, rear-foot-elevated, two-kettlebell instructions, 251
two-kettlebell squat instructions, 293
two-kettlebell squat progression, 292–5
Staley, Charles, 14, 202
Stanton, J., 93
stick deadlift drill instructions, 238
stick hip-hinge drill, 196–7
story, personal, 90
strategies, effectiveness of, 28, 63–4
strength goals, 41
strength, muscle maintenance and, 53
strength phase workouts
- basics of, 115–19, 150–1
- deadlifts and, 150
- kettlebell front squats and, 150
- outline of, 149
- pull-ups and, 150–1
- push-ups and, 150
- rest during, 183
- schedule for, 151–6

strength standards for fat loss, 104–5
strength training, prioritization of, 51
stress, 102
structures, overcoming obstacles with, 35
"stubborn fat," 20
substitution, food, 44
System Six Easy Fat Loss, 186

tactical pull-ups instructions, 269
Taleb, Nassim, 13
talking about oneself, 26–7
tall plank instructions, 303
target density circuits, 201–2, 204–11
Thibadeau, Christian, 187–8
Thomas, Ash, 236
thoracic spine mobility, 194
thruster instructions, 300
time constraints, 197–8
timing
- macronutrient, 71
- meal, 19, 56

Todd, Terry, 113
tone, muscle, 77–8
"tough" diets, 22
"tough" workouts, 21
tracking food, 39–40
Trainer Certification, 24-Hour, 25
trap-bar deadlifts, 196–7, 241
- instructions, 241

tripod row instructions, 297
Tsatsouline, Pavel, 107, 114, 186–7, 236

two-kettlebell exercises
- single-leg, two-kettlebell deadlifts instructions, 245
- split-squat, rear-foot-elevated, two-kettlebell instructions, 251
- two-kettlebell military press instructions, 289
- two-kettlebell squat instructions, 293
- two-kettlebell squat progression, 292–5
- two-kettlebell swing progression, 125, 282–5
- two-kettlebell swings instructions, 285

undulating periodization, 115–16, 119. *See also* metabolic/endurance/strength phase workouts.

values, choice of, 9
vegetarian diets, 54–5
volume phase workouts, 115, 176–83

walking lunges instructions, 249
warmups, 189–90, 197
Warp Speed Fat Loss Program, 9
water, healthy intake of, 31–2
Waters, Valerie, 203
Watkins, Arthur, 12
weighted vest pushups instructions, 280
White, T.H., 23, 91–2
why, asking, 89, 91
willpower, preparation versus, 61–2
Win One Meat at a Time strategy, 35–7, 42
Winfield, Percy Henry, 23
Winkleman, Nick, 236
Wolf, Robb, 8–9, 13, 22
women, bodyfat percentage and, 82–5
Wooden, John, 9
wrist pain, during pushups, 193–4
Wulf, Gabrielle, 236
Wunsch, Mike, 236

yoga wedges, 194, 281

Zone Diet, The, 19